**HEALTH MAINTENANCE
ORGANIZATIONS:
DIMENSIONS OF PERFORMANCE**

HEALTH, MEDICINE, AND SOCIETY:
A WILEY-INTERSCIENCE SERIES
DAVID MECHANIC, Editor

Evaluating Treatment Environments: A Social Ecological Approach
  by **Rudolf H. Moos**

Human Subjects in Medical Experimentation: A Sociological Study of the Conduct and Regulation of Clinical Research
  by **Bradford H. Gray**

Child Health and the Community
  by **Robert J. Haggerty, Klaus J. Roghmann,** and **Ivan B. Pless**

Health Insurance Plans: Promise and Performance
  by **Robert W. Hetherington, Carl E. Hopkins,** and **Milton I. Roemer**

The End of Medicine
  by **Rick J. Carlson**

Humanizing Health Care
  by **Jan Howard** and **Anselm Strauss,** Volume Editors

The Growth of Bureaucratic Medicine: An Inquiry into the Dynamics of Patient Behavior and the Organization of Medical Care
  by **David Mechanic**

The Post-Physician Era: Medicine in the Twenty-First Century
  by **Jerrold S. Maxmen**

A Right to Health: The Problem of Access to Primary Medical Care
  by **Charles E. Lewis, Rashi Fein,** and **David Mechanic**

Gift of Life: The Social and Psychological Impact of Organ Transplantation
  by **Roberta G. Simmons, Susan D. Klein,** and **Richard L. Simmons**

Mentally Ill in Community-Based Sheltered Care: A Study of Community Care and Social Integration
  by **Steven P. Segal** and **Uri Aviram**

The Alien Doctors: Foreign Medical Graduates in American Hospitals
  by **Rosemary Stevens, Louis Wolf Goodman,** and **Stephen S. Mick**

Essays in Medical Sociology: Journeys into the Field
  by **Renée C. Fox**

Health Maintenance Organizations: Dimensions of Performance
  by **Harold S. Luft**

Health Maintenance Organizations: Dimensions of Performance

Harold S. Luft

Health Policy Program
University of California, San Francisco

A WILEY-INTERSCIENCE PUBLICATION

JOHN WILEY & SONS   New York · Chichester · Brisbane · Toronto

Library of Congress Cataloging in Publication Data:

Luft, Harold.
    Health maintenance organizations, dimensions of
performance.

    (Health, medicine, and society)
    "A Wiley-Interscience publication."
    Includes bibliographical references and index.
    1. Health maintenance organizations—United States.
I. Title. [DNLM: 1. Health maintenance organizations
—United States.   W275 AA1 L86h]
RA413.5.U5L83   362.1'0425   80-22420
ISBN 0-471-01695-0

Printed in the United States of America

10 9 8 7 6 5 4 3 2

TO LORRY

Preface

The primary issue in current policy discussions about the American medical care system is how to achieve control over accelerating expenditures. Many people see health maintenance organizations, HMOs, as a viable means to contain costs. The current system of fee-for-service payment of providers and extensive third-party insurance coverage insulates both providers and consumers from concern about the rising costs of medical care. In the HMO system providers have a fixed budget and are responsible for delivering appropriate services to an enrolled population. This represents a major departure from other existing health-care delivery systems.

The HMO concept has an inherent logic that makes it appealing for controlling costs. Eliminating fee-for-service payment removes the incentive for providers to deliver services of questionable necessity. More important, dealing with a fixed budget from which it must provide all services for a given population forces the HMO to make trade-offs between alternative ways of offering care. For instance, under conventional health insurance a physician frequently hospitalizes a patient in order to perform certain diagnostic tests that could be done on an ambulatory basis. Although hospitalization consumes far more resources, the patient's insurance covers these costs, but not the costs for outpatient tests. Within an HMO, however, the organization must provide the tests regardless of where they are performed, and it has an economic incentive to use the most efficient methods.

The HMO concept also is attractive to those who are concerned that questions of equity and accessibility will be pushed aside in an effort to contain costs. Increased cost sharing is believed to have a greater deterrent effect on the poor than on the rich, and gaps in current insurance coverage are thought to prevent some people from obtaining necessary care. HMOs cover essentially all services, both inpatient and outpatient, and in particular, preventive services. Since financial barriers to receiving care are removed within the HMO setting, there is a potential for containing costs as well as for increasing access.

The logic of the HMO concept is not the only thing that makes it appealing. There have been numerous reports of HMOs serving large populations with half the number of hospital beds and patient days as are used by age-sex matched populations with conventional insurance and fee-for-service payments to providers. This combination of logic and evidence has led to the development of an HMO strategy by the federal government, to the passage of legislation promoting HMO development, and to a continuing interest in encouraging HMO development as an alternative to more direct regulation over the medical care system.

Regrettably, HMO policy is based on discussions that contain more rhetoric than evidence. Having the information on hand allows policy-makers to base their decisions on a solid empirical framework. This book was written to help make informed choices. It provides a comprehensive review and analysis of what we know about HMO performance. It goes beyond what HMOs do, to examine those aspects of HMOs that explain their differential performance. Unfortunately, even a rapidly increasing body of research fails to answer all questions about HMO performance, so a final task of the book is to state what we do not yet know.

This book is the result of six years of research on the question of HMO performance. Work begain in 1974 when Alice Rivlin and Michael Timpane of the Brookings Institution requested a background paper on "what we know and need to know about HMOs." In due course, an extensive but conventional literature review was completed. While preparing the piece, I was impressed by two things. First, while the answers to many questions would require extensive research, it appeared that certain questions could be answered, or at least investigated, by some relatively simple analysis of data available in published articles. Second, the review had uncovered a substantial number of studies on some particular issues. Earlier reviews of HMO performance could summarize and integrate the data from the handful of studies available. Such summarization is difficult, if not impossible, when there are over fifty studies on one issue. This problem simultaneously created the opportunity for a methodological innovation: the reanalysis and juxtaposition of previously published material in order to identify patterns of performance.

Such an innovation was necessary because policy-makers ask about HMO performance in general, but research studies usually examine only selected aspects of performance in one or two HMOs. The review for Brookings convinced me that HMOs differ greatly, even when similarly organized. Therefore, generalizing from any one study, no matter how carefully executed, seemed comparable to discussing differences between the sexes based on observation of one couple. The belief that performance could vary widely from one HMO to another has an important corollary: a selective review of the evidence would be inadequate. When the goal is an understanding of how the generic HMO performs, all available evidence must be reviewed. If the findings are consistent, then we may be reassured in our interpretations. If results are not consistent, then it will be necessary to identify organizational characteristics that explain the differences. In several situations this approach seems to have succeeded, such as in explaining different patterns of ambulatory usage (Chapter 6) and preventive services (Chapter 9).

The underlying methodology of this book differs from that of most studies. Unlike the classic scientific situation, no crucial experiments provide a choice between two alternative hypotheses. Instead there are bits of evidence on various issues. The data must be collected and examined, and the consistency of findings must be determined. Under these conditions it is possible to find evidence that rejects simple hypotheses and leads to more subtle but more reliable explanations. Thus the research is truly exploratory, and while it may resolve some issues, it is designed to raise others. In order to provide a basis for further research, this book includes extensive references and, wherever possible, reproduces critical data.

While I have been led by the data, I have not accepted them at face value. Some studies have such poor designs that their figures merely muddy the waters. Most studies are of reasonable quality, but sometimes the nature of an issue leads to certain biases. For example, the fact that people can choose to join or disenroll from an HMO has both obvious and subtle effects on the measurement of consumer satisfaction. Since those who strongly dislike a plan can leave, measures of dissatisfaction will be underestimated. On the other hand, subtle aspects of the enrollment process may result in more vocalization of dissatisfaction. (A detailed discussion of these issues is included in Chapter 3.) Similar dynamics exist in the evaluation of quality of care. We find that some measures are inherently biased in favor of prepaid groups, and other measures are biased against them. (See Chapter 10.) Recognizing a potential bias does not eliminate it, but recognition allows a more appropriate interpretation of the data to emerge.

This book is multifaceted and contains messages at several levels. On the surface, it addresses various dimensions of HMO performance, such as cost, utilization, quality, satisfaction, and equity. Furthermore, while it seeks to outline what is known, it also decribes what is uncertain, thus laying a foundation for further studies. But the book has another purpose: to demonstrate that much can be learned by a methodical reanalysis of existing data. Moreover, this reanalysis can be accomplished with relatively simple and accessible analytical tools. In most instances, the crucial results are obtained with simple tables and graphs and through the application of common sense.

The process of doing the research was akin to that of detective work. I started with the common perception that HMOs provide medical care at lower cost. I proceeded to examine the evidence to support or refute this assumption, and then attempted to track down explanations for cost differences in terms of utilization patterns, efficiency, prevention, quality, and satisfaction. Having followed the trail as far as possible, I then examined a question of equity: can HMOs effectively serve the poor? It was also necessary to retreat from the notion of the generic HMO and consider the myriad organizational and environmental factors that influence HMO performance (Chapter 14). This long, sometimes tedious process uncovered an abundance of information about HMOs. It also revealed important areas about which very little is known.

The search was both intriguing and rewarding. Just as readers are spared the researcher's frustrations with misshelved books, balky computers, and uninterpretable data, they also miss the pleasure of seeing the results fall into place. In the next few pages I will highlight some of those more qualitative aspects of the book, emphasizing the flavor of each chapter.

My first mission was to identify an HMO. It became apparent that the term "health maintenance organization" was created as a political device to provide a new label for existing prepaid group practices and for the foundations for medical care that were attractive to independent fee-for-service practitioners. When Congress enacted legislation to foster HMOs, it too had to provide a definition. The requirements of the original legislation were sufficiently stringent that few existing plans applied. Even the current less restrictive requirements are unattractive for some well-established organizations. Because of these limitations, Chapter 1 offers a five-part definition of a generic HMO. This definition is designed to include most organizations commonly recognized as HMOs. The definition is based on the crucial economic and organizational aspects of HMOs and allows a wide diversity of organizational forms. It excludes organizations such as student health clinics and the Veterans Administration, which have some aspects of prepayment or group practice but are not generally considered HMOs.

There is wide variation within the two major categories of HMOs, prepaid group practices (PGPs) and individual practice associations (IPAs). To provide the reader with a sense of this diversity, brief descriptions of several HMOs are included in Chapter 1. These range from the Kaiser plans, with over 3.5 million enrollees, to the early Medical Care Group of Washington University, with only a few thousand enrollees.

Chapter 2 sets the stage for the analysis that follows. First, it outlines the various dimensions of performance that need to be considered in an evaluation of HMOs. Although the primary reason for policy interest in HMOs is their potential for constraining costs and utilization, other aspects require equal emphasis. For example, cost savings that are accompanied by a substantial reduction in quality would be unacceptable to policy-makers, as would a delivery system that pleased everyone but the doctors. Because HMOs exist within a larger medical care system, two additional dimensions were added. One examines the impact of HMOs on policies designed to promote equity. The other dimension is the influence of HMOs on the outside world through research, teaching, and, most important, a competitive impact on conventional providers and insurers.

The second part of Chapter 2 outlines some expectations concerning HMO performance that might be drawn from a consideration of economic incentives. If the organizations were less complex and the institutional settings less important, this chapter might set out a formal, theoretical framework. Under the circumstances, however, such an abstract exercise would have little relationship to reality. The expectations in Chapter 2, on the other hand, rely on common sense, theory, and an understanding of the HMO market. The discussion of these expectations is designed to guide the subsequent data analysis. As will become clear, there is a vast quantity of empirical evidence, and without some guidelines we would become lost in a morass of senseless correlations, associations, and random numbers.

Chapter 3 is the last detour before consideration of the empirical results. This discussion of the role of self-selection provides an important caveat that applies to everything that follows. Self-selection of HMO enrollees is guaranteed by the voluntary enrollment requirement. While politically necessary and ethically desirable, self-selection may influence every measure of performance, including cost, quality, and satisfaction. Selection can also occur among physicians, and here too it can affect performance. The difficulty is that we do not yet know the magnitude of selection effects and their impact on other measures. Our ignorance is not total, however. The selection effect appears to be greater in some areas than in others. Moreover, recognizing that selection may bias our results will help us interpret some data. Knowing the direction of the bias means that while some results are less solid than they appear, others are all the more firm, because the bias works against the observed outcomes.

An interesting story lies behind my development of the self-selection data. The first draft of this book was completed after nearly two years of writing. Because new data had been developed during that period, it was necessary to review this material and incorporate new findings into the manuscript. This included several new sources of data concerning self-selection. The interpretation of these figures led me to a reevaluation of the role of self-selection. Although the new version of Chapter 3 is not a complete about-face, it is at least a 120-degree change. That experience was chastening and served as a warning to avoid overinterpreting findings based on scanty evidence. No other change of comparable impact occurred in the rewriting.

The crucial HMO question is then addressed: are expenditures lower for HMO enrollees? Chapter 4 reviews the evidence, which indicates that HMO enrollees do indeed pay less. It is unfortunate that only six available studies present data on both premium and out-of-pocket costs, and only one examines the difference between community and experience-rated costs. Yet the results are consistent and are clearly supported by the utilization patterns described in the following chapters.

Hospital utilization differences appear to be the major factors in accounting for the lower costs for HMO enrollees. Fortunately, over fifty comparisons of hospitalization rates for people in HMOs and conventional plans are available for study in Chapter 5. Differences appear in almost every study; what is less apparent is their cause. Much of the chapter is devoted to an analysis of various explanations, such as shorter lengths of stay and fewer admissions. Although lower admission rates are the obvious answer, it is difficult to explain why they are lower. None of the simple explanations, such as disproportionately less surgery or discretionary hospitalizations, are satisfactory. Thus we must look at issues such as ambulatory care, prevention, and quality.

Chapter 6 reviews the evidence concerning ambulatory care utilization. Again there is a large number of studies, so we can begin to analyze patterns of ambulatory use. For example, IPA enrollees consistently make more visits per year than their counterparts with conventional coverage, and PGP enrollees are about evenly divided. In fact, PGP enrollees tend to have fewer visits than people with comprehensive third-party coverage for ambulatory services. This finding begins to separate two features of HMOs: (1) more comprehensive coverage for the enrollee; and (2) an incentive for the provider to do less.

It is often argued that HMOs have an incentive to be more cost conscious than the fee-for-service or cost-reimbursed provider. Claims are also frequently made for economies of scale in group practice. Chapter 7 examines the question of the relative efficiency of HMOs in producing medical services: does it cost an HMO less to produce a day in the hospital or a physician visit? In contrast to the preceding two chapters, the evidence here, especially concerning hospital costs, is exceedingly sparse. In this area new data were collected and analyzed because of the gaps existing in the literature. Since few consistent patterns appear, it is difficult to make the case for greater efficiency in HMOs. Moreover, the problems of biased data are particularly important in comparing hospital costs. The findings with respect to ambulatory services are only somewhat more firmly based, but again, there are few substantial differences in HMO performance. It is easier to write about research that finds significant differences, but we must also carefully review those areas in which the null hypothesis cannot be rejected; we can then move on to more fruitful areas.

Chapter 8 addresses HMO cost and utilization performance from a different perspective, that of trends over time. Are the differences in cost and utilization widening or narrowing? Or, from a policy perspective, have HMOs found the answer to slowing the inflation rate of medical care costs? Again, the data are sparse, and time-series from various sources have been compared. The results are not unambiguous. The chapter leaves some unanswered questions, such as why hospitalization rates have been falling in the last decade for *both* Blue Cross and Kaiser enrollees.

The name health maintenance organization suggests that the lower hospitalization rates might stem from more preventive care. If true, then the apparent cost savings would be real, and the arguments in favor of HMOs vastly stronger. Testing the hypothesis is difficult, because preventive care is not easily defined or measured. I chose to focus on those medical care services often considered preventive, such as checkups, immunizations, prenatal care, and screenings. (Primary preventive factors, such as exercise and diet, have more to do with lifestyle than medicine.) Fortunately, a number of comparative studies include data on these types of preventive services. Initially, the results were contradictory. Some studies showed more preventive services for HMO enrollees, while others showed the opposite. A simple cross-classification by type of coverage available to the *comparison* group provided the key. As in the case of ambulatory visits in general, HMO enrollees' greater consumption of preventive services seems to be a reflection of better coverage for such services. While explaining the different utilization patterns, this did not fully resolve the question of how effective these preventive services are. A review of the medical literature, however, indicated few situations in which such services were truly effective in reducing subsequent illness and costs. Moreover, the newer HMOs were experiencing low hospitalization rates upon opening their doors. Clearly, prevention could not explain those findings.

This led to an examination in Chapter 10 of quality of care. Three broad types of measures are considered in the literature on quality: structure, process, and outcome. One cannot take the published findings at face value, because some measures are inherently biased with respect to HMOs. For instance, multispecialty group practices score well on criteria that emphasize specialists. Groups offer more organizational continuity but less continuity with a specific physician. Also people who join HMOs may be slower in seeking care. These potential biases and the critical nature of quality assessments lead to an exceptionally cautious approach to the data. It appears safe to say, however, that HMOs provide care of at least comparable quality to that of conventional providers.

Consumer satisfaction is another outcome measure, but the framework for its evaluation is even less well established than that of quality of care. The analysis developed in Chapter 11 suggests two markedly different approaches. The first and most common approach is to use direct questions about satisfaction with specific aspects of plan performance or with the plan in general. In some instances these perception-based responses could be validated with objective measures, for example, by comparing satisfaction with waiting time to actual waiting time. The difficulty with these separate measures of satisfaction is that there is no way to compare them. HMOs tend to score higher on two dimensions and worse on others, but how does one compare satisfaction with financial coverage to feelings about the doctor-patient relationship? The second approach provides a simple, although crude response: watch what people do. Thus the second part of Chapter 11 examines out-of-plan use and enrollment and disenrollment behavior as indicators of overall satisfaction.

The focus on HMO performance is usually on the alleged impact on enrollees. Yet HMOs cannot develop and grow without some reasonable level of physician support. Chapter 12 addresses this issue in terms of physician satisfaction. As with consumer satisfaction, one can ask how people feel, compare that with reality, and examine behavior. And, as with consumers, any evaluation of physician satisfaction must take into account the realities of self-selection.

Chapter 13, which explores the ability of HMOs to serve the poor, is included for two reasons. First, much of the public debate about medical care is focused on programs for the poor and the elderly. Second, the fraud and abuse of the California prepaid health plan (PHP) program in the early 1970s cast doubt on the ability of HMOs to serve the poor. The PHP experience made the data for this chapter more difficult to evaluate, because most studies were done in a highly political atmosphere, and they usually involved advocates for one side or the other. In fact, HMO experiences with the poor could generally be placed in one of two categories: (1) demonstration projects with special incentives for both the HMO and the poor; and (2) standard settings in which no special incentives were present. As was the case in previous chapters, it became apparent that the evaluation of HMO performance often depended on the conventional medical-care sector. If the poor possess no viable alternatives, even the worst PHP would be an improvement.

The preceding chapters were based on a crucial simplifying assumption: that one could examine the performance of HMOs in general. That proved to be a reasonable assumption in many instances, and important patterns of performance were identified. Much remained unexplained, however, and upon closer examination it became apparent that HMOs, like people, have important individual characteristics. Various organizational factors, such as sponsorship, profit orientation, managerial skills, modes of physician payment, hospital control, and access to specialists might all have an impact on performance. Similarly, external factors, such as legal and regulatory constraints, sociodemographic characteristics of the population, and the local medical care market, also influence HMOs. Such influence is not unidirectional. HMOs often have an impact on the surrounding medical-care system through teaching and research and also through competitive pressures on conventional insurers and providers. Chapter 14 addresses these issues. Although evidence is scanty, this area is beginning to attract attention in research circles.

This book is a detailed, empirical analysis of issues that have significant policy implications. A brief summary of the crucial findings, while highly desirable, would ignore the uncertainties, caveats, and cautions that are part and parcel of the analysis. Chapter 15 offers a compromise. It provides a summary of the findings that is qualified by an indication of my own certainty about the results. Some are based on solid and highly consistent evidence. Other findings are tentative, and one good piece of counterevidence could shift my interpretation. The reader may reach different interpretations and attach different levels of certainty. In fact, the extensive tables and references throughout the book are designed to encourage readers to undertake new studies. Chapter 15 also harkens back to the original challenge from Brookings; in addition to outlining what we know, it describes what we do not yet know about HMOs. It can thus serve as an agenda for future research.

HAROLD S. LUFT

San Francisco, California
February 1981

Acknowledgments

A project of this magnitude would have been impossible without financial, collegial, and emotional support from many sources. The initial work on this project was supported by the Brookings Institution, with funds from the Edna McConnell Clark Foundation. Subsequent research has been supported by grant number 10-P-90335/9-01 from the Social Security Administration and the Health Care Financing Administration. The "Selection and Competitive Effects of HMOs" grant from the Health Care Financing Administration contributed substantially to the revisions of Chapters 3 and 14. Dr. Philip Lee, Director of the Health Services Policy Analysis Center, Health Policy Program, University of California, San Francisco, provided resources supported by grant HS 02975-02 from the National Center for Health Services Research for final revisions and editing. Dr. John Bunker, Director of the Health Services Research Program, Stanford University, also contributed through direct salary and other support.

Valuable research assistance was provided by Sandra Colville, Steven Crane, Jinnet Fowles, Polly Keller, Steven Penico, Zeil Rosenberg, and Harold Ting. Nancy Brown of the University of California, San Francisco Health Policy Program edited the entire manuscript and shepherded it through the final stages of production. Judy Todd, Health Policy Program librarian, helped track down sources and performed the painstaking task of reference checking. During the early years of the project at Stanford, Natalie Fisher provided excellent secretarial support through seemingly interminable drafts. Les Gates, at the Health Policy Program, carried on that tradition.

Many people provide the critical reviews necessary in this type of project. I am grateful for the comments and suggestions of the individuals who read various parts of the draft: Sylvester Berki, Mark Blumberg, Rachel Boaz, Robert Brook, John Bunker, Paul Densen, Joseph Dorsey, Diana Dutton, Alain Enthoven, Rashi Fein, Jinnet Fowles, James Fries, Douglas Gentry, Merwyn Greenlick, John Hershey, Halsted Holman, Helene Lipton, Susan Maerki, Keith Marton, David Mechanic, Paul Newacheck, Gerald Perkoff, Ernest Saward, Steven Schroeder, Anne Scitovsky,

Stephen Shortell, Paul Temple, Joan Trauner, Ralph Ullman, Frederick Wenzel, and Carol Winograd. In several instances analysis was made possible with valuable unpublished data provided by Donald Freeborn, Douglas Gentry, Shirley Harris, David Martin, John Newman, and Beverly Payne.

Some chapters in this book are revisions of work published elsewhere, and I am grateful for permission from the publishers to use these materials. Portions of Chapters 4, 5, and 6 appeared in a paper entitled, "How Do Health Maintenance Organizations Achieve Their 'Savings'?: Rhetoric and Evidence," *New England Journal of Medicine,* **298:** (June 15, 1978): 1336−1343. Chapter 8 is based on a paper entitled "Trends in Medical Care Costs: Do HMOs Lower the Rate of Growth?" *Medical Care* **18:** (January 1980): 1−16. Chapter 9 is adapted from a paper entitled "Why Do HMOs Seem to Provide More Health Maintenance Services?" *Milbank Memorial Fund Quarterly/Health and Society,* **56:** (Spring 1978): 140−168. An earlier version of a part of chapter 14 appeared in *Socioeconomic Issues of Health 1980,* edited by Douglas E. Hough and Glen I. Misek (Chicago: American Medical Association, 1980).

H.S.L.

Contents

**HEALTH MAINTENANCE
ORGANIZATIONS:
DIMENSIONS OF PERFORMANCE**

ONE

Definition and Scope of the HMO Concept

The term "health maintenance organization" (HMO) has a variety of interpretations. In part, this is by design. It was coined in the early 1970s as part of a strategy to win Nixon administration support and Congressional approval for prepaid health care as an alternative to the predominant fee-for-service (FFS) system with third-party reimbursement (Ellwood et al., 1971). A new name was needed because the term "prepaid" often was used specifically to refer to prepaid group practices, such as Kaiser-Permanente Health Plan, Health Insurance Plan of Greater New York (HIP), and Group Health Association (GHA) in Washington, D.C. Such prepaid groups were anathema to the medical care establishment. Also they represented only one of many possible types of prepaid plans. The new term was designed to improve the political viability of HMOs and to enhance understanding of the concept.

The HMO terminology had the distinct advantage of emphasizing the positive: "health maintenance" in contrast to the neutral "medical care" or negative "sickness care." The importance of such a semantic shift cannot be underestimated when one proposes a "comprehensive health policy for the 70s," as did President Nixon in 1971 (U.S. Office of the White House Press Secretary, 1971). However, because of its origins in political rhetoric, the term is necessarily imprecise. Some people use the term to refer to one specific category of HMOs, particularly to prepaid group practice. The federal government has provided a stringent set of guidelines to define those HMOs eligible for subsidies. This adds another dimension to the arena of HMO definitions. I use HMO in the generic sense to refer to any one of the many alternatives to traditional FFS practice that meet a small set of key criteria.

The first section of this chapter will provide some working definitions of HMOs and outline the major HMO categories. The second section will offer examples of the diverse HMOs contained within these definitions. A third section will describe briefly different types of HMOs and discuss their organizational characteristics.

DEFINITION OF A HEALTH MAINTENANCE ORGANIZATION

The key feature of Ellwood's health maintenance strategy is a contract between the enrollee and the HMO whereby for a fixed annual fee the HMO agrees to provide comprehensive health care services. The intent of the original strategy was to change some of the financial incentives within the medical care system. Under the usual FFS practice the provider's income is directly related to the number of services rendered. With a fixed payment per enrollee, the HMO's net income is inversely related to the number of services provided, and there is a financial incentive to reduce the number of unnecessary procedures. It is contended that the HMO also has a financial incentive to provide appropriate preventive services in order to avoid larger expenditures in the future. Thus the HMO theoretically emphasizes health maintenance, rather than simply sickness care.

The key features of the HMO concept are outlined below (Wetherille and Nordby, 1974).

1. The HMO assumes a contractual responsibility to provide or assure the delivery of a stated range of health services. This includes at least ambulatory care and inpatient hospital services.
2. The HMO serves a population defined by enrollment in the plan.
3. Subscriber enrollment is voluntary.
4. The consumer pays a fixed annual or monthly payment that is independent of the use of services. (This does not exclude the possibility for some minor charges related to utilization.)
5. The HMO assumes at least part of the financial risk or gain in the provision of services.

The role of each of these features in separating HMOs from other types of providers will be discussed in turn. In the process of this discussion it will become clear that the non-HMO sector is not a homogeneous group of physicians who provide medical care on a solo FFS basis.

The wide range of provider types in both HMO and non-HMO sectors makes comparisons between the two particularly complex. For the purposes of this volume, the term HMO will be used to refer to organizations that substantially meet the above five criteria. The HMO category of providers, of course, can be further broken down into subcategories, such as prepaid group practices (PGPs) and individual practice associations (IPAs), that will be discussed separately. The term "non-HMO" will be used to refer to providers outside of this category. The dominant type of non-HMO is the FFS provider; however, there are important types of non-HMO providers that do not operate on an FFS basis.

The first criterion defining HMOs is the *contractual responsibility* of the HMO to provide or assure medical care services; it implies that the member has the legal right to expect necessary treatment from the HMO. This may be contrasted to the situation in FFS practice, which is much like that in the normal marketplace—the provider has the right to decide whether to accept the patient and is under no obligation, other than an ethical one, to provide treatment. Some health insurance plans, such as Blue Cross and Blue Shield, provide service benefits. These plans have an obligation to pay for covered services; however, the enrollee is responsible for finding the service provider. In some areas it is difficult to find a provider even though one has insurance. In contrast to this catch-as-catch-can situation, most HMOs set geographic limits to insure that enrollees live within a reasonable distance. They also provide the equivalent of service benefits for members when they are travelling outside of the immediate area. Some non-HMO medical care providers also are obligated to make services available. For instance, the Department of Defense provides medical care for members of the armed forces, and the Veterans Administration operates an extensive network of facilities for veterans. Certain public clinics also have an obligation to provide care to whoever requires it.

The existence of a *defined enrollment* means that an HMO can know, at any point in time, for whom it is obligated to provide services, and it can estimate the demand for its services. This is critical for planning purposes. Enrollment is to be distinguished from registration, in which the provider merely has a record of people eligible to use its services. For example, Neighborhood Health Centers and clinics register clients and often determine eligibility on geographic grounds. Under such a system, when a client leaves the area or elects to use another provider, there is no incentive to withdraw the registration. HMOs, however, require periodic payments, which provide a clear incentive for members to disenroll when they change providers. The typical FFS provider usually does not have a registration list, but medical records are kept for each patient. Such records do not inform providers how many of their patients use them as a primary source of care, only how many patients they see per unit of time. The records can identify active files, but it is impossible to tell if an inactive file belongs to someone who has moved away, died, or has not required a physician's services (Densen, 1973).

The third criterion defining HMOs is that *enrollment be voluntary;* this requires that potential enrollees have a choice among alternative health care providers. Voluntary enrollment implies that the HMO is competing against other providers for members and thus has an incentive to meet their demands for services. If such choices were not available and the HMO were in a monopoly position, it is possible that services would deteriorate, or prices would increase.

The extent of voluntary enrollment or choice in the non-HMO sector varies substantially. Military personnel often have no choice, unless they exercise the option of paying for independent services out-of-pocket.

Traditional FFS providers emphasize freedom of choice, but that choice is limited by the availability of providers and their willingness to accept the potential patient. Many inner city and rural residents have insurance to pay for services (for example, Medicare and Medicaid) but cannot find providers; thus they may have no effective alternatives to public clinics.

Most private health insurance is obtained through employee group coverage (U.S. National Center for Health Statistics "Hospital and Surgical Insurance Coverage" August 1977). Voluntary enrollment implies that if members of an employee group are to be offered an opportunity to enroll in an HMO, they also must be offered one or more insurance alternatives. On the other hand, many companies and unions offer a single insurance plan with no alternatives. New federal regulations require that if federally certified HMOs are available in the area, employees must be offered an opportunity to join at least one of them. However, there are few such HMOs in existence.

The *fixed annual or monthly payment* to the HMO, which is made independently of the utilization of services, is a key feature of the definition. The HMO does not gain substantial revenue by providing more services. If it can provide less than the expected number of services, its net revenue after expenses will increase. Small copayments related to utilization may be required, but these usually are a small fraction of the cost of the service and are designed primarily to reduce the monthly premium or discourage frivolous utilization.

It is important to note the predominant role of third parties, such as insurance companies, in certain segments of the medical care sector. In 1975 only 8 percent of all hospital costs were paid for out-of-pocket by consumers; the remaining 92 percent were covered by third parties. Private health insurers paid 36 percent of the third party bill, and most of the remainder was paid for by the government (Mueller and Gibson, 1976a). Thus, while most hospitals are paid on an FFS basis, very few consumers pay for hospital services on an FFS basis.* Instead they pay fixed amounts for insurance or taxes. The same is true for people with complete insurance coverage who use physicians who charge by FFS.

The type of payment scheme used has important implications for the economic incentives present. A consumer paying FFS has a greater incentive to question whether a potential service is worth the fee, while if it is prepaid through a fixed premium, there is no financial barrier to seeking the service. A provider who is paid FFS has a financial incentive to maximize services, while one who is paid on a salary or other fixed basis has no incentive to increase the number of services. Examples of all four possible combinations exist: (1) The consumer pays FFS and the provider is paid FFS in the traditional ambulatory care setting. (2) The consumer has

*Many hospitals are reimbursed for costs incurred, rather than for charges. The crucial point for this discussion, however, is that they are paid more for doing more.

complete insurance coverage and has essentially prepaid for hospital and many surgical services, while the provider (the hospital or surgeon) is paid on an FFS basis. (3) Neither the consumer nor the provider is involved in an FFS transaction. This is best exemplified by some HMOs. Other provider types, such as Neighborhood Health Centers, the Veterans Administration, and industrial physicians, are paid on flat salary with no FFS payments by the consumer. (As will be noted below, some HMOs combine fixed payments to the organization with FFS payments to physicians within the HMO.) (4) The last combination, that of FFS payments by the consumer and fixed payments to the provider, is uncommon, but it does exist. For instance, hospital outpatient departments and clinics usually charge FFS, but the revenues may be absorbed by the hospital, while the staff is paid by salary. Similarly, National Health Service Corps physicians are paid a salary by the federal government, and their fees revert to the Treasury Department.

The fifth criterion of an HMO is that it assumes at least part of the *financial risk* or gain in the provision of services. This implies that the HMO, which provides or assures the delivery of services, also has a financial incentive to reduce their excessive use. If the provider is paid FFS this is obviously not the case; in fact the financial incentives are in the other direction—toward greater utilization. When there is no FFS incentive for the provider, and the consumer has complete insurance coverage, the former will be indifferent to costs. For example, if a patient requires minor surgery that can be performed either in the hospital or on an ambulatory basis, the surgeon's income is the same in both cases, and the insurance will pay for either the office care or the substantially higher hospital costs. Neither the patient nor the surgeon will have a financial incentive to reduce the total resource costs by having the procedure done in the office. If it is even slightly more convenient to operate in the hospital, that is probably where it will be done. The immediate loser in this case is the insurance company. In the long run, however, the consumer will pay higher premiums. The problem is that the surgeon does not share the financial risk involved in the provision of services; that risk is borne entirely by the insurer, and the company cannot provide appropriate incentives for the surgeon. This problem is typified in the Veterans Administration and in public hospitals, in which the staff is salaried and independent of the revenues and expenditures of the institution.

These five criteria define what I have termed a "generic HMO," or an organization that meets the minimum set of HMO characteristics. Within this minimum set there is great latitude for variation among organizations. Two important organizational characteristics that are explicitly excluded from the definition of an HMO should be noted: (1) no restrictions are made on the methods by which physicians are paid; and (2) the physicians may provide services in the context of a single group, or they may be dispersed over a large number of offices. These two dimensions help define two major types of HMOs: prepaid group practices (PGPs) and individual practice associations (IPAs).* Although there are a number of important exceptions, most IPAs are composed of physicians in private offices who are paid on an FFS basis by the HMO, and most PGPs pay their physicians on a salary or capitation basis.† The distinctions between PGPs and IPAs are sufficiently important that, when possible, they will be considered separately in both theoretical and empirical discussions.

Within PGPs and IPAs a number of characteristics may be important in determining how the organization performs. Such characteristics include (1) the method of paying key decision-makers, (2) the extent of risk sharing, (3) whether physicians are full or part-time, (4) the profit or nonprofit orientation of the HMO, (5) whether the HMO controls its hospital, and (6) the competitive market environment faced by the HMO. These and other characteristics will be considered separately under the heading of organizational characteristics, because it is expected that the impact of each of these factors on HMO performance is of secondary importance relative to that of the definitional characteristics. Also, given the small number of HMOs in existence and the much smaller number with available data, it is impossible to provide substantial evidence concerning the effects of these organizational characteristics.

The five-point definition of HMOs offered at the beginning of this section purposely leaves many of these organizational characteristics unspecified so that the policy discussion will not be limited to a narrow subset of potential health-care providers. This creates problems when policy implications are drawn about all HMOs from data that are limited to PGPs or to only one or two specific PGPs. The analysis of HMO performance in this book is often conditional to specific types of HMOs.

Before concluding this section on definitions, it is important to note that federal legislation provides a more stringent and exact definition of a health maintenance organization (U.S. Department of Health, Education and Welfare, 1974). This definition sets lists of services to be offered, such as basic inpatient and outpatient care, mental health services, alcoholism treatment, home care, dental services, and the like. Many HMOs do not offer the full range of such mandated services. Using a five-point definition similar to our own generic definition, Wetherille and Quale found that only 24 percent of HMOs met the minimum benefit package required by the 1973 HMO Act (1973). The regulations set limits on additional charges

---

*IPAs are sometimes known as foundations for medical care, or FMCs. There are two basic types of FMCs, those that only do claims review for an outside insurance company and those that offer a prepaid health plan of their own, as well as doing claims review. (See Egdahl, 1973). Only the second type, or comprehensive FMC, can be included in the HMO definition, and this is the type that will be discussed here as an IPA.

†Under a capitation scheme a physician is paid a certain sum per month to provide care for every subscriber on his or her list.

related to utilization; enrollment mechanisms and the extent of risk sharing also are specified. The 1976 Amendments to the HMO Act (P.L. 94–460) eased many of the restrictions, but some well-established HMOs, such as Group Health Cooperative of Puget Sound (GHCPS), have chosen not to seek federal qualification. The federal government's definition is too restrictive for the purposes of our discussion; if alternative policies are to be evaluated, a sufficient number of options must be available.

THE DIVERSITY OF HMOs

The five-point definition of an HMO allows a wide range of diversity because of characteristics explicitly excluded from the definition, such as the method of physician payment. Further diversity results from the fact that there is great variation in the degree to which the five points are met. This section will outline some of the variations among HMOs.

Guarantee of Services

The comprehensiveness and guarantee of service provision vary substantially among HMOs. Some HMOs only guarantee to provide ambulatory services directly, and they arrange for standard health insurance coverage of hospital care. For instance, when an HMO does not have arrangements with specific hospitals, as is often the case with IPAs, it may be difficult to guarantee the availability of inpatient services. Other organizations, such as the Health Insurance Plan of Greater New York (HIP), have not been at risk for hospital services; instead, their enrollees must carry companion health insurance coverage to pay for hospital care. (Because of this limitation, HIP is actually a quasi-HMO, but since it is the second largest organization in the country, with 760,000 enrollees, and has produced a wealth of data, it will be included in our discussion.) Although an HMO may offer the full range of services, the actual provision of such services may be constrained by organizational factors, such as long waiting lines and limited hours of availability, which tend to ration demand. (See, for example, the criticisms of California prepaid health plans in U.S. Senate Committee on Government Operations, 1975).

Enrolled Population

The defined populations served by HMOs vary widely. Operating HMOs range in size from 3000 to over 1,000,000 enrollees (U.S. Office of HMOs, 1978). In some cases enrollees are homogeneous populations ranging from university faculty and staff, on one hand, to Medicaid recipients, on the other hand. In other cases the population is very heterogeneous. The geographic base of the enrollment may be highly concentrated in a single city, such as Columbia, Maryland or Marshfield, Wisconsin, or it may be widely dispersed throughout an entire metropolitan area, such as the Kaiser plans and HIP, or a large rural region, such as the San Joaquin Foundation for Medical Care. Although the population at any time is known because of the capitation method of payment, it may range from being stable over time to being very unstable with extremely high turnover rates. For instance, the turnover rate for middle-aged Kaiser enrollees is about 3.5 percent a year, while in some plans the turnover rate has been about 75 percent a year (Cutler et al., 1973, pp. 198, 204; Breslow, 1975, p. 62). Also, the fact that an HMO treats a defined population on a prepaid basis does not preclude it from also treating individual patients on an FFS basis. In some cases this FFS component is a miniscule fraction of the total—about 1.4 percent for Kaiser in 1970 (Somers, 1971)—while in other cases the HMO operation is a sideline for a primarily FFS practice, as in the Marshfield Clinic, in which 85 percent of the income is from FFS (Broida et al., 1975).

The voluntary enrollment of subscribers in HMOs often does not fit the economist's model of perfect competition. For example, usually only one or two alternatives are offered. Rather than offering vouchers to members for use at any local plan, most employers allow enrollees to choose from one or two plans. On the other hand, most employers in Minneapolis offer a choice of six plans (Christianson and McClure, 1978). Legal alternatives may not be viable. In some states Medicaid reimbursement levels are so low that private practitioners refuse to accept Medicaid patients, and thus the government's offer to pay for services is somewhat hollow. For instance, a survey of California physicians indicated that 42 percent would probably or definitely refuse to treat new Medicaid patients (California Medical Association, 1977).

The fixed payment per enrollee is also subject to considerable variation. Copayments may be used to varying degrees by HMOs.* For example, California state employees were enrolled in HMOs that had coinsurance rates of 0, 20, and 25 percent, and deductibles of $0 and $2 per visit or $25 per illness (Dozier et al., 1973). In addition, the benefit packages of some plans do not offer certain items. The California state employees example mentioned above demonstrates the wide variation in coverage offered by different HMOs to the same group of people. Variation also exists among plans offered by a given HMO to different groups. The Southern California Kaiser Foundation Health Plan reported at least five different basic

---

*Several types of copayments may be involved. Coinsurance requires the enrollee to be responsible for a certain fraction of the costs of specific services. Deductibles require that the enrollee pay the first X dollars of the costs of specific services. Coinsurance and deductibles may be combined so that, as an example, the enrollee may pay the first $25 and 20 percent of all costs beyond the first $25.

benefit packages in 1971, with monthly premiums ranging from \$7.82 to \$16.60 per subscriber. Office visits ranged from no charge to \$2 per visit (a small copayment), maternity care costs were \$150 or \$350 (a substantial deductible); and inpatient services beyond a fixed number of days were half the prevailing rate (a 50 percent coinsurance rate). Federally certified HMOs now must offer a rather comprehensive basic benefit package. In addition, groups can purchase any combination of a whole range of special coverages for such things as eyeglasses, drugs, and mental health care (Somers, 1971).

It should be recognized that at times the implicit benefit package is much more extensive than that officially offered by the HMO. For instance, when Medicare or Medicaid recipients enroll in an HMO, they sometimes are allowed to retain their eligibility for FFS reimbursement, and thus their access to "free" medical care from outside sources.

The extent of risk and surplus sharing within the HMO is also subject to great variation. There are three major functional parts to an HMO that may even be legally distinct organizations: (1) the "plan" that contracts with enrollees, (2) the physician group that provides medical services, and (3) the hospital that provides inpatient services. The HMO definition merely requires that at least part of the overall financial risk be borne by one or more of the three groups and not be shifted entirely to an external third party through reinsurance.* Obviously, there are many different ways of allocating risk among the three parts of the HMO. Clearly, different incentives exist for physicians who bear a fraction of financial risk for medical or hospital expenses. In some cases physicians bear essentially all the risk and reap all the rewards, even though the mechanism may be indirect. (This is the case with the Ross-Loos Medical Group in Los Angeles, which is owned by the physician partners.) In other cases physicians receive a flat salary or capitation with little direct financial incentive. Even in the latter arrangement the physicians probably have a long-run interest in the success of the plan.

All of this variability is possible, considering the five defining criteria for an HMO; there is also the long list of special organizational characteristics, which will be discussed in Chapter 14. However, every HMO has unique features, and it is impossible to determine the extent to which the performance of a specific HMO is due to its general characteristics or to its special features.

---

*Reinsurance allows an organization that already serves an insurance function, as does an HMO through its financial obligations to provide services for a fixed premium, to purchase insurance from another company to protect itself against excessive losses. There are many ways in which this can be done, but one of the simplest is to negotiate a policy whereby all medical expenses that are X percent above those budgeted for by the HMO will be paid by the reinsurer. (See Burke and Strumpf, 1973).

EXAMPLES OF SPECIFIC HMOs

The HMO definitions and the overview of potential diversity in organizational characteristics provide a framework for our discussion. In order to bring these organizations into clear focus, this section describes seven distinct HMOs, giving the reader a view of the actual structure of specific organizations, and assisting in the interpretation of the data from these organizations. HMOs are constantly evolving, so a description of an organization may soon become outdated. In general the descriptions here refer to organizational structures in the early 1970s, the period of most of the quantitative studies used in subsequent chapters. (Up-to-date enrollment data on most HMOs are available in a census of HMOs published annually by the U.S. Office of HMOs, Department of Health, Education, and Welfare, now the Department of Health and Human Services.)

The Kaiser-Permanente Medical Care Program

The Kaiser-Permanente Medical Care Program (KPMCP) is the largest HMO in the country, with over 3.5 million enrollees in six regions. There are about 1.5 million enrollees in Northern California; 1.5 million in Southern California; 220,000 in Oregon; 110,000 in Hawaii; 120,000 in Ohio; and 100,000 in Colorado. Operations in the latter two regions began in 1969 (U.S. Office of HMOs, 1978). Its roots lie in the 1930s and 1940s when a prepaid practice was developed as a means for providing medical care to Kaiser Industries construction and shipyard workers. After World War II this industrial population diminished, and the plan was opened to the community. Since the late 1940s the plan's structure has evolved slowly, and to some extent it now reflects that history rather than the current environment.

The KPMCP is a complex organization that allows a substantial degree of autonomy for the six regions. During the period in question each region had four separate entities: The Kaiser Foundation Health Plan, Inc.; the Kaiser Foundation Hospitals, Inc.; the Permanente Medical Group; and the Permanente Services, Inc. (Recently, Permanente Services, Inc. has been disbanded and its functions absorbed by other Kaiser entities. The exact functions of the several units vary from region to region. (See Prussin, 1974; Somers, 1971.) The Kaiser Foundation Health Plan (KFHP) is a nonprofit administrative and contracting organization that does not provide medical care services. Its primary functions are: (1) entering into medical and hospital service agreements with groups and individuals, thereby enrolling members; (2) maintaining membership records; (3) collecting membership dues; (4) contracting with the regional Permanente Medical Group to provide medical and other health-care services; and (5) contracting with the Kaiser Foundation Hospitals to provide facilities and hospital services for plan members. The KFHP is governed by a self-perpetuating board of directors that includes members of the KPMCP staff, Kaiser Industries personnel, and prominent community leaders who are not necessarily enrolled in the plan.

The Permanente Medical Group (PMG) in each area is independent and takes full responsibility for all professional health care services as well as for associated paramedical services. This includes responsibility for services in physicians' offices and the hospitals and for home care. When necessary the PMG arranges for and purchases the services of outside specialists and facilities.

Kaiser Foundation Hospitals, Inc. (KFH) is a nonprofit corporation that owns and operates over twenty-five hospitals in five of the six regions. (Kaiser Colorado uses community hospitals in its service area for the provision of hospital services.) It is responsible not only for inpatient hospital facilities but also for outpatient office facilities attached to the hospitals. In some regions it also manages freestanding ambulatory care centers. Overall responsibility for KFH is vested in its board of directors, which is the same as that of the KFHP, but broad authority is delegated to regional manager, who supervises the administrators of each facility.

Permanente Services, Inc. (PSI) is a separate, for-profit service corporation in each region. The entire stock is owned by the KFHP and the KFH of the region. PSI provides business and administrative services, such as central purchasing, accounting, internal audit, payroll, and data processing. In addition, because of tax regulations, PSI operates retail pharmacies and optical shops at the freestanding ambulatory centers, and in some regions it manages the freestanding centers. PSI operates on a break-even basis, deriving its revenues from service charges to the various KPMCP entities.

The KPMCP central office coordinates legal policies and governmental affairs for all regions. The central staff provides assistance in rate setting, personnel management, and benefit package development. Each region is responsible for maintaining quality of care, for determining benefits and rates, and ultimately for achieving financial success. Primary decision-making authority is vested in the medical director of the regional PMG and the regional manager, who has responsibility for the health plan and hospitals in that region.

Prepaid dues and other revenue from plan members are pooled by the health plan, and about 2.5 percent of this is applied to the administrative costs of the KFHP. The remainder is used to pay the medical groups and Kaiser Foundation Hospitals for contractual health-care services, and for certain services provided by KFHP. Each year the KFHP negotiates a budget with the medical groups and the hospitals. Contract payments to the medical group are composed of a fixed per capita payment based on the actual membership during the year and a contingent or incentive payment. The incentive payment is established at the beginning of the year and is a part of the total planned compensation for physicians, of which this portion is placed at risk. The actual amount of the incentive payment is determined at the end of the year and is based upon actual results. The incentive payment is divided among physicians in the group and varies by year and region. In general, it represents about one-quarter of each physician's compensation. The PMG is responsible for outpatient services, outside specialists' fees, laboratory and X-ray departments in and out of hospitals, physical therapy, and various service expenses on an allocated cost basis.

KFH also establishes budgets based on its net financial requirements. These take into consideration revenue from nonplan sources and two systematic earnings factors, one based on 4 percent of the historical cost of all facilities and the other based on a planned amount. Both are used for capital generation. KFH pays for various service expenses on an allocated basis.

Regional differences occur in the delivery of services as well as in administrative structure. For example, the two California plans are approximately equal in size, yet they operate differently. Southern California has fewer but larger hospitals, with numerous outpatient medical offices spread throughout its region. Northern California has fewer outpatient medical offices, most of which are in or adjacent to the Kaiser Foundation Hospitals. Southern California does most of its laboratory work in a few central facilities, and Northern California began centralizing its laboratory services in 1977. Southern California does almost all of its own open heart surgery in a single hospital, while Northern California contracts with Stanford University and other medical centers to do its open heart operations.

Group Health Association, Inc.

The Group Health Association, Inc. (GHA) is a nonprofit membership corporation based in Washington, D.C., with about 110,000 enrollees. (See Prussin, 1974; Riedel et al., 1975; U.S. Office of HMOs, 1978.) About 75 percent of its members are federal employees covered under the Federal Employees Health Benefits Plan; an additional 12 percent are transit workers. In contrast, while federal employees are also the largest single enrollee group in Kaiser Northern California, they comprise only 11 percent of the enrollees (Somers, 1971). Ambulatory care is provided at four outpatient centers in the District of Columbia and in suburban Maryland and Virginia. Inpatient care is provided at local community hospitals, although most admissions are made at major teaching hospitals. Blue Cross of Washington, D.C., is the fiscal agent for processing and paying hospital claims, and GHA pays Blue Cross about 4 percent above claims for these services. GHA, however, is at risk for these hospital costs.

The GHA governing body is composed of nine subscribers who are elected by the membership. This board of trustees appoints an executive director and, with the approval of the medical group, a medical program administrator, who is responsible for supervision of the medical aspects of the program.

Medical services are provided by full-time employed physicians who are primarily in the specialties of pediatrics, internal medicine, and obstetrics-gynecology. Since 1977 GHA physicians have been members of an independent union that bargains with the board of trustees. Disagreements over salaries and physician independence led to a strike in April 1978 (Peck, 1978). Physicians who are not full-time members of the group, principally those in surgery and highly specialized areas, are paid on a per capita, fee-for-time, or retainer basis. All nonpremium income, such as FFS revenue, is retained by the health plan in order to reduce costs or increase benefits.

Group Health Cooperative of Puget Sound

The Group Health Cooperative of Puget Sound (GHCPS) is a nonprofit, consumer-owned corporation that provides medical services to approximately 250,000 enrollees in the Seattle, Washington area. (See Prussin, 1974; Handschin, 1971.) The GHCPS was founded as a consumer cooperative in 1947 and strongly retains an orientation toward consumer control. Only about 30 percent of its enrollees are actually cooperative members who provide capital investment dues of $200 per family, $175 of which is refundable upon termination of membership. Most of the remaining enrollees are in employee groups, and their capital costs are included in the monthly dues structure. The cooperative membership directly elects a governing board, and all board actions are subject to review and ratification or rejection at annual membership meetings. Consumer members take an active part in working committees that serve the board.

The GHCPS owns and operates a 301-bed hospital and nine neighborhood medical centers throughout the three counties served by the cooperative. Well over 90 percent of hospital care is provided in the GHCPS hospital. The board of trustees of the cooperative acts as the hospital board and appoints the hospital administrator.

Although medical staff are technically employees, they essentially operate as a partnership and contract with the board to provide all medical services covering the full range of specialties. The medical staff and the board bargain each year to determine the capitation rate per enrollee. A key factor in this bargaining is the expected rate of growth, because negotiations include the staffing ratio of physicians to enrollment as well as the mix of specialties. Salary schedules and fringe benefits also are subject to negotiation, based on capitation and staffing rates, taking into consideration general market competition. Salary schedules recognize differences among specialties as well as lifetime earning patterns developed by the physicians. Income from FFS practice (about 5 to 6 percent of total income), exceptionally rapid enrollment growth, and special cost savings from such efforts as the use of physician assistants, are split evenly between the plan and the medical group. There are no direct financial incentives for the physicians to reduce hospital expenses.

The health plan is directly responsible for paying out-of-area and emergency claims. It also pays for outside specialists and referral services. Most allied health personnel, such as nurses, laboratory technicians, and X-ray technicians, bargain with the health plan through their unions.

Health Insurance Plan of Greater New York

The Health Insurance Plan of Greater New York (HIP), founded in 1947, is the second largest group practice plan in the country, with about 750,000 subscribers and their dependents. (See Prussin, 1974; Health Insurance Plan of Greater New York, 1970.) HIP is actually a quasi-HMO, because it is not at risk for hospital care, although this is changing. Members are required to have a basic hospitalization plan, such as Blue Cross, that pays for their hospital claims.

Members sign up with one of the approximately forty medical groups associated with HIP. The groups contract with HIP to provide all physician and ancillary services to plan members. The groups own or lease their facilities and provide for all necessary ancillary personnel. (HIP leases facilities to the groups at rates substantially below the market rate.) HIP pays the groups a basic capitation rate plus capitation incentives for various purposes. These incentives are designed to increase pediatric utilization, concentrate hospital admissions in a single hospital, provide extensive office hours, reduce the dropout rate, encourage Pap smears, provide full-time physicians, and increase office visit utilization. For a typical group in 1970, these incentive payments would add $16.07 per person per year to the basic capitation rate of $45.13 (Health Insurance Plan of Greater New York, 1970, p. 27). The medical groups are allowed to provide FFS care for non-HIP enrollees in the group center; however, HIP is attempting to convert its groups to full-time HIP practice. Each group selects its own formula for net income distribution.

The Health Plan is governed by a thirty-member unpaid board of directors composed of community leaders, no more than three of whom may be physicians practicing in the plan. A Medical Control Board is appointed by the board of directors to set professional standards. It is composed of medical group physicians as well as outstanding physicians from the medical community. A Joint Committee for Improved Medical Care made up of five physicians, two appointed by HIP and three by the groups, evaluates the quality of medical care of all groups, institutes continuing education programs for physicians, and receives and acts upon consumer complaints. Although members are not directly represented on the board of directors, new HIP contracts with the medical groups call for the establishment of a consumer council in order to provide a formal mechanism for feedback to the specific group.

HIP provides a number of special services to the groups, such as health education, nutrition counseling, social services, and a central emergency answering service; and it shares with participating medical groups the costs of a central clinical laboratory and of specialty referral services. Out-of-area emergency services are paid for by HIP.

Greater Marshfield Community Health Plan

The Greater Marshfield Community Health Plan (GMCHP) began operation in 1971 in Marshfield, Wisconsin. (See Lewis, 1973; Broida et al., 1975; Broida, 1975.) The plan is sponsored jointly by the Marshfield Clinic, St. Joseph's Hospital, Blue Cross, and Blue Shield, At the time of the plan's inception, the Marshfield Clinic was a multispecialty FFS group of 102 physicians that served as a major referral center and provided primary care for most of the Marshfield area population. All active physicians on St. Joseph's Hospital staff were members of the clinic, except for three who practiced in the town of Colby, twenty miles away. The population within a fifteen-mile radius of Marshfield is about 35,000, and it accounts for about 20 percent of the clinic's total income (Lewis, 1973). Since 1954 clinic physicians have used a salary scheme based on equal distribution, with surpluses distributed as bonuses.

In the late 1960s clinic physicians began to consider the possibilities of providing care at reasonable cost to everyone in a specific geographic area. Their plan was developed as an alternative to existing types of HMOs. At the same time, Blue Cross of Wisconsin was concerned about the potential impact of some of the more radical national health insurance proposals and decided to participate in an experimental prepaid group practice in order to gain experience and demonstrate their capabilities. Along with St. Joseph's Hospital, the two groups combined to design a comprehensive plan with periodic open enrollment for everyone within the defined geographic area on either a group or individual basis. This was to be accomplished by holding two thirty-day open enrollment periods annually, at which time any resident under the age of sixty-five could join the program. There were to be no preexisting illness clauses, no co-pays or deductibles. The program was to be community-rated, and funding was sought to assist those on limited incomes.

Enrollees have free choice of physicians within the clinic and also the option of using the Colby Clinic, which is reimbursed by GMCHP on an FFS basis. Similar arrangements exist with three other practitioners who are located some distance from Marshfield. About a third of the Marshfield area population belongs to GMCHP, and they represent about 15 percent of all clinic patients. The clinic maintains a policy of not making the enrollee's source of payment known to the physician, and it appears that in about 80 percent of the cases the physician does not know the patient's payment status (Broida and Lerner, 1975).

The original set of financial arrangements divided the total premium into capitation payments to the Marshfield Clinic, St. Joseph's Hospital, Blue Cross, and out-of-area and referral services. The clinic and St. Joseph's were guaranteed their audited costs plus 4 percent. If the plan could not cover those costs, they would be made up in later years. Surpluses were to be shared at the rate of 25 percent each for the clinic and hospital and 50 percent for Blue Cross and Blue Shield. The arrangements have gone through a number of changes since then, as the GMCHP ran substantial losses in the initial years. The 1975 agreement gives the clinic a capitation as payment in full for all services rendered; St. Joseph's, along with two affiliated hospitals, is paid an inpatient per diem plus 90 percent of outpatient charges as full payment, and Wisconsin Blue Cross and Surgical Blue Shield of Milwaukee receive a capitation for all administrative services and hospital and physician services rendered outside the GMCHP. Surpluses, if any, are distributed as before (Broida, 1975).

The Medical Care Group of Washington University

The Medical Care Group of Washington University, St. Louis (MCG) was established in 1969 as an experimental plan to develop controlled studies of the costs of medical care under FFS and prepaid practice with comparable groups of people. (See Perkoff, 1971; Perkoff, Kahn, ,and Mackie, 1974; Perkoff, Kahn, and Haas, 1976). The experiment was supported by the Metropolitan Life Insurance company and the W. K. Kellogg Foundation. As originally constituted, the MCG was not really an HMO, because it was not at financial risk; however, its experimental design and data availability make it of substantial interest. In fact, in the plan's design potentially favorable effects of risk-sharing arrangements were deliberately avoided.

The MCG plan offered comprehensive family care by four internists, four pediatricians, and one obstetrician, who provided primary ambulatory, hospital, emergency, and home services. These nine physicians worked part-time for the MCG on a salary basis and provided 2.2 full-time physician equivalents. The MCG ambulatory care offices were located in the Washington University Medical Center, and inpatient admissions were made to the medical center. Specialists on the Washington University School of Medicine faculty provided consultations, surgery, laboratory, X-ray, and other procedures and services. The MCG paid for these services on an FFS basis, but the revenues went to the departments; the consultants themselves were salaried. The MCG physicians and patients had complete access to hospital beds in the medical center, just as is the case with community physicians and their patients. The MCG physician retained responsibility for inpatient care.

The experimental nature of the program is clearly indicated in the enrollment patterns. Members were enrolled from three companies in the metropolitan St. Louis area. Each company originally offered its employees a health insurance package underwritten by the Metropolitan Life Insurance Company. A limited number of places in the MCG were offered to each employee group, and enrollees were randomly selected from those who volunteered to become members. Those who were not selected retained their standard coverage and served as a control group. Those who were selected to become MCG members lost their insurance coverage for services offered by the MCG. Hospital insurance was the same for both groups.

San Joaquin Foundation for Medical Care

The San Joaquin Foundation for medical care (FMC) was established in 1954 as the first IPA type plan in the nation. (See Egdahl, 1973; Morozumi, 1971; Steinwald, 1971, Harrington, 1971; Sasuly and Hopkins, 1967). The San Joaquin Foundation was developed by the county medical society when the local Longshoremen's and Warehousemen's Union proposed to invite Kaiser-Permanente to establish a clinic for union members. Faced with this threat, local physicians established the foundation in order to provide comprehensive physicians' services for a fixed capitation rate. At the same time, the physicians maintained their dedication to the principles of FFS practice and free choice of physician. The foundation now provides services for about 180,000 persons, 60 percent of the area population. This includes 95,000 people in 80 commercial plans sponsored by eleven insurance companies, 36,000 Medicare beneficiaries, 4000 federal employees, and about 50,000 Medicaid eligibles.

Participation in the foundation is open to all physicians who are members of the county medical society; about 96 percent of the practicing physicians are members. The physicians retain their usual mode of practice, but they bill the foundation for their services, rather than billing the patient. The FMC performs several interrelated functions. It designs a set of minimum standards in terms of the types of services that must be covered by sponsoring health insurance packages. These minimum benefits are designed to cover on an outpatient basis many services that are traditionally covered only on an inpatient basis, including diagnostic X-ray, laboratory services, and outpatient surgery.

The expansion of coverage, as well as the guarantee to provide services for members, necessitates a means of control over expenses. This control is carried out in three ways: a fee schedule, peer review of claims, and risk sharing. Physician participants agree to abide by a standard fee schedule that is based on the California Relative Value Studies of usual and customary fees. All physician-generated claims are reviewed according to established peer review criteria. These are used as guidelines by the clerical staff. Claims that fall outside the guidelines and those in which the patient profile is unusual are referred for peer review. About 15 to 20 percent of all claims are forwarded for review by a physician who may then approve payment or refer it to the full peer review committee for further consideration. Only 1 to 2 percent of all claims are sent to this panel.

Another incentive for the control of expenses is the risk sharing that the

FMC undertakes with some of its groups. This has been the case with its coverage of about 50,000 persons under Medicaid in a four-county area. In the first year (1968) the FMC was responsible for the cost of all physician services, which were billed at usual and customary fees. At year's end the FMC returned $200,000 in savings to the state based on total payments of about $5 million. The second year resulted in a net loss, which was absorbed by participating physicians on a pro-rata basis. Beginning on August 1, 1974, the FMC assumed the risk for hospital and nursing-home costs under its Medicaid contract. This contract was canceled by the foundation in January 1975 because the premiums for hospital costs were inadequate. Although the foundation is at risk for physicians' services and shares in the savings attributable to reduced hospitalization for other enrollees, it is not at risk for hospital inpatient costs beyond projected levels.

SUMMARY

While it is desirable to keep one's definitions simple, the discussion in this chapter has been necessarily complex, reflecting the complexity of the HMO issue. A narrow HMO definition would be relatively easy to provide, but it would be sterile and could offer little to the policy discussion. Our broad definition includes the key features that are essential in distinguishing HMOs from traditional health-care providers. These features are: (1) the contractual responsibility to provide or assure the delivery of medical care; (2) a population defined by enrollment in the plan; (3) voluntary enrollment of subscribers; (4) a fixed premium independent of the use of services; and (5) the assumption by the HMO of part of the financial risk or gain.

This definition allows great diversity both in terms of what is and is not part of the definition. For each of the five points there is a substantial variation in the degree to which any particular HMO meets the ideal. Furthermore, the definition is purposely silent about a number of characteristics. For instance, HMO physicians may practice in a group setting, or they may be widely dispersed in individual offices. Similarly, the physicians may be paid on the basis of anything from a straight salary to pure FFS. These two characteristics—group versus solo and salary versus FFS—are often fighting issues in discussions about HMOs. Yet there is room for them all within the generic HMO model. A number of other characteristics are of interest, but they are not crucial to the definition and thus are considered to be fine-tuning characteristics. Among these are whether or not physicians are full-time, the profit orientation of the HMO, whether it controls its own hospital, and the extent of consumer participation.

The last section of this chapter breathes life into the dry process of setting out a definition by describing seven different HMOs and quasi-

HMOs. These organizations were chosen because of their differences and because many of them will be referred to in later chapters. They range from the Kaiser-Permanente program, with 3.5 million members in five states, to the Medical Care Group of Washington University, with a total of 500 families. Some, such as Kaiser, GHA, GHCPS, and HIP, were developed solely as HMOs, while others, such as GMCHP and the San Joaquin FMC, developed from an existing FFS system. The organizations have widely varying degrees of centralization and consumer input, and their relationships with physicians offer great contrast. The next chapter examines the theoretical implications and empirically measurable differences that may be attributable to these varying characteristics.

TWO

Dimensions of Performance: Claims, Expectations, and Initial Conjectures

As is the case with any innovation, HMOs have advocates and detractors. The claims made for and against them cover the spectrum from near panacea to a major threat to liberty in the United States. The following statements illustrate the contrast.

Of the various health-care systems currently available to the American people, Health Maintenance Organizations (HMO's) most nearly meet the objective of providing access to high-quality comprehensive medical and health-care services at the most reasonable cost possible. (MacLeod and Prussin, 1973, p. 439)*

The corporate contract practice of medicine controlled by laymen is the gravest threat now to the practice of private medicine.

The Health Maintenance Organization concept is the most recent and salable name used for per capita prepayment group practice schemes, which is corporate contract practice through politics . . .

There is only one key to countering this threat to liberty in the United States—*understanding*. (Dorrity, 1972, p. 265)

HMOs are neither as good nor as bad as such claims would suggest. To put later empirical discussions into perspective, this chapter outlines how HMO performance can be expected to differ from that of the conventional system. The first section delineates the major dimensions of performance that should be examined. The second section discusses the nature of theoretical expectations and how they are used to focus our examination of the data. The third section outlines expectations concerning HMO performance along each dimension and points out that these expectations are better developed in some areas than in others. A final section offers a brief summary.

*Reprinted by permission from the *New England Journal of Medicine,* **288**:9 (March 1, 1973): 439.

DIMENSIONS OF HMO PERFORMANCE

When confronting alternative social policies, one is rarely faced with a choice between two strategies, one of which is clearly better than the other in every dimension. Of course, this can happen if one examines only a single dimension, but life is rarely so uncomplicated. This section outlines some key dimensions of HMO performance that should be investigated prior to any attempt to evaluate HMO achievement in comparison to the alternatives. There are five key factors of interest: cost, quality, consumer satisfaction, distributional equity, and externalities. Individual policy analysts and policy-makers vary in the manner in which they weigh the relative importance of the various dimensions. My purpose here is to identify the relevant issues, raise the important questions, and provide the data. This information should aid those who must decide which factors are most critical in order to determine an appropriate balance.

Costs

Perhaps the first consideration of a government policy-maker is the cost of the HMO versus that of alternative providers. The cost question has at least five aspects that should be distinguished. These are (1) total costs, (2) out-of-pocket costs, (3) number and mix of services rendered, (4) cost per unit of service, and (5) long-term cost trends. Each of these will be discussed in the context of national expenditures on health care.

Total Costs. The total costs of a medical care delivery system are obviously key issues in national health policy. For the year ending December 1980 health care expenditures were projected at $245 billion or 9.5 percent of the gross national product (Freeland, Calat, and Schendler, 1980). Of this total, about $216 billion is attributable to personal health-care expenditures; this excludes expenses for public health programs, research, and medical facilities construction.

Table 2-1 presents the aggregate and per capita expenditures for personal health care in fiscal year 1977.* These data may be viewed from various perspectives, and a discussion of the different viewpoints on total cost will help to explain the cost controversy.

The true economic costs of the resources involved in providing personal health services is best approximated by the total figures, $150 billion in the aggregate or $680.41 per capita. However, government expenditures came to only 39 percent or $266.73 per capita, and in an era of balanced budgets and tax revolts this may be the figure of primary interest to politicians. Government payments are not allocated in the same fashion as total

---

*Although total health care costs are increasing rapidly, the distribution of these costs by type of expenditure and source of payment is relatively constant.

Table 2-1 Aggregate and Per Capita Expenditures for Personal Health Care, by Type of Expenditure and Source of Payment, Fiscal Year Ending September 1977[a]

Type of Expenditure[b]	Total	Direct Payments	Third Party Payments				
			Total	Private Health Insurance	Government Federal	Government State and Local	Philanthropy and Industry
			Aggregate Amount (in Millions)				
Total	$150,157	$ 48,509	$101,650	$ 39,299	$ 41,253	$ 17,610	$ 3,487
Hospital care	65,626	3,866	61,761	24,021	25,715	10,484	1,540
Physicians' services	32,184	12,502	19,682	11,817	5,807	2,016	42
Dentists' services	10,020	7,965	2,055	1,554	311	190	—
Drugs and drug sundries	12,516	10,401	2,115	973	613	529	—
Prepayment and administration	7,572	5,233	2,339	—	1,430	313	596
All other health services[c]	22,238	8,542	13,698	934	7,377	4,078	1,309

22

Per Capita Amount

	$680.41	$219.81	$460.62	$178.08	$186.93	$79.79	$15.80
Total							
Hospital care	297.38	17.52	279.86	108.85	116.52	47.51	6.98
Physicians' services	145.83	56.64	89.19	53.55	26.32	9.13	0.19
Dentists' services	45.40	36.10	9.31	7.04	1.40	0.86	—
Drugs and drug sundries	56.72	47.13	9.59	4.41	2.78	2.40	—
Prepayment and administration	34.31	23.71	10.60	—	6.48	1.42	2.70
All other health services	100.77	38.71	62.07	4.23	33.43	18.47	5.93

SOURCE: Robert M. Gibson and Charles R. Fisher, "National Health Expenditures, Fiscal Year 1977," *Social Security Bulletin*, 41:7 (July 1978), Tables 2 and 3.

[a] Preliminary estimates.

[b] Prepayment and administration expenses are usually not included in total health care expenditures but are included in total health expenditures.

[c] Includes "other professional services," with $3,212 million total expenditures; "eyeglasses and appliances," $2,086 million; "nursing home care," $12,618 million; and "other health services," $4,322 million.

expenditures. Although hospital care accounts for 43.7 percent of the total, it accounts for 62.3 percent of federal and 59.5 percent of state and local government expenditures. On the other hand, dental services and drugs, which account for 15.0 percent of all expenditures, require only 1.5 percent of the federal and 3.0 percent of state and local health budgets. Thus it is not surprising that the interest of government policy-makers is focused primarily on the costs of inpatient services.

Consumer interest is focused on two columns of the table, direct payments and payments through private health insurers. Direct payments are just that, consumer out-of-pocket expenditures for medical care. Only a small proportion of these direct payments goes for hospital services; most out-of-pocket expenditures are for physicians, dentists, and drugs—the items for which health insurance coverage is the least extensive. Health insurance is purchased directly by the consumer, and it is often paid for indirectly by employers through payroll deductions or fringe benefits. When health insurance is included as a fringe benefit, there are substantial tax advantages. Theoretically, those benefits could be converted into cash payments that would allow workers to purchase care directly or through the health plan of their choice (Feldstein and Allison, 1972). The average health insurance benefits of $178.08 per person are obtained at a price of $23.71 in expenses for prepayment and administration. In fact, this last figure is not truly an out-of-pocket cost, but rather is the net cost of insurance, or the difference between premiums and benefits, that is eventually borne by the consumer.

If tables such as these were developed for people who use HMOs and the conventional system, which of these costs would be relevant to the comparison of the two methods of financing services? Ideally, one would examine the total cost figures in each group to assure that there are no hidden subsidies, such as government or private grants, which artificially lower the costs in one program or the other. Similarly, one should not ignore administrative costs, which total about 13 percent for conventional health insurance and about 7 percent for independent plans, most of which are HMOs (Carroll, 1978, p. 14). This is the ideal; in practice, the best available estimates are usually based on premium costs, plus out-of-pocket expenses for people in each group. As will be seen below, more detailed analyses of the mix of expenditures for various services can provide clues about the way different programs operate.

Out-of-Pocket Costs. It should be apparent from this discussion that for a given expenditure level, out-of-pocket costs and insurance payments are inversely related. The more the consumer has to pay at the time a service is purchased, the greater the financial deterrent to purchasing the care. Although physicians control much of the decision-making in medical care and many treatment choices are made on the basis of clinical necessity, there is overwhelming evidence that as out-of-pocket costs increase, overall medical care consumption falls. (See Newhouse and Phelps, 1975; Scitovsky and Snyder, 1972; Coffey and Hornbrook, 1977). How one interprets this relationship is a matter for debate. It could mean that when people must pay for medical care out-of-pocket, they are deprived of treatment that they should receive but cannot afford. Or it could mean that when people pay out-of-pocket they receive exactly the amount of care that they think is necessary, and the extra care consumed as the price (net of insurance) falls is unnecessary and not worthwhile. To a substantial degree, the debate stems from differences in ethical or philosophical position, rather than from economic or medical facts. (See Newhouse, Phelps, and Schwartz, 1974). The important point is that out-of-pocket expenditures are an important dimension of cost that must be considered.

Number and Mix of Services Rendered. Total and out-of-pocket costs focus on who pays the bill, rather than on what is being purchased. These figures may be misleading if used alone, because expenditures can be reduced in several ways, each of which has different implications. To calculate total cost, multiply each service times its cost and accumulate these costs for each service rendered. Total cost can be reduced in three ways: (1) a reduction in the total number of services rendered; (2) a reduction in the costs of individual services; and (3) a reduction in the number of expensive services only partially offset by an increase in less expensive services, so that while the total number of services may even increase, their total cost decreases.

Again, measuring changes in the number of services is one thing; evaluating the changes is another. For example, across-the-board reductions in all services would seem desirable to someone who believes the medical system does too much of everything. It is more likely that certain types of services are less necessary than others. For example, some observers would be more concerned if HMOs reduced the hospitalization rate for heart attacks than if they reduced the rate for hernia operations. The third way to reduce costs, changing the mix of services, is also subject to discussion. In this case the organization does not reduce what appear to be unnecessary services; instead it substitutes less expensive but supposedly equally efficacious services for more expensive ones. Thus patients may be treated over time with medication and ambulatory care, rather than with surgery. Whether such a substitution is efficacious is rarely empirically tested, and thus the continuing controversy.

Cost per Unit of Service. Improvements in the cost per unit of service approximate the economist's concept of technical efficiency, or movement toward the least-cost method of producing a given service. Such improvements are, in theory, to be desired by everyone, because they imply a reduction in the waste of resources that produce no benefit. Unfortunately, the existence of slack, or the inefficient use of inputs, usually benefits someone, either on the production or the consumption end. This is not measured in the usual calculations. For instance, using more than the minimum number of people in an office staff may provide relief from pressure and thus produce happier workers. Such workers may or may not be more helpful in dealing with patients. Is a patient's experience in a doctor's office affected by an unresponsive or unpleasant receptionist? If it is, then the cost savings obtained by reducing "excess staff" is, in part, a reduction in quality, and the two services are not the same.

Long-Term Changes in Cost.   Although much concern about health-care expenditures is due to their sheer size, as reflected in Table 2-1, the growth rate of expenditures is of even more concern. Health-care expenditures are growing at a rate that is 30 percent higher than the GNP growth rate. Thus the fifth area of concern about costs is whether a specific program can reduce the rate of growth in costs. It may be worthwhile to invest in a more expensive alternative that promises to reduce substantially the rate of growth in health-care costs. For example, the large capital investment required to develop HMOs might be worthwhile if it allows the organizations to reduce the rate of growth in costs.

Qualilty

Most economic analysis generally assumes that there is a trade-off between quality and cost (or quantity). This assumes that pure waste in the production of services is rare and that improvements in quality require more effort, which implies more cost, or a reduction in other things, such as the quantity of services. One major exception to this trade-off is when an innovation in the production process allows an improvement in quality or quantity. Usually, such innovations are equally accessible to all producers. However, in some cases they are applicable only to certain types of organizations, such as large groups of physicians.

The current state-of-the-art in quality assessment of medical care is inadequate to measure the quality-quantity trade-off. (See Brook, 1973a; Huntley and Howell, 1974; Donabedian, 1978). Any thorough evaluation of HMOs probably will require the development of new tools for measuring quality. This important issue will be discussed later, but it must be remembered that some measures of quality are inherently biased in favor of certain methods of providing health care. For instance, two commonly used groups of quality measures focus on (1) the "structure" or setting in which care is provided and (2) the "process" of care. The structure approach generally concerns itself with such factors as board certification of physicians and the adequacy of facilities. The process approach is based on the appropriateness and completeness of information obtained through clinical history, physical examination, and diagnostic tests; justification of diagnosis and therapy; technical competence in the performance of various procedures; evidence of preventive management; and coordination and continuity of care. Only rarely are measures of outcomes of care available (Donabedian, 1966, 1968). To the extent that structure and process measures are based on accepted traditional practice standards, they will be biased against innovative uses of personnel, such as utilizing allied health professionals who have less training than physicians, and changes in the practice of medicine that provide fewer rather than more services.

Consumer Satisfaction

Consumer satisfaction is clearly related to quality of care and is in fact an outcome measure. The weight given to satisfaction in the evaluation of HMO performance varies widely. Some people argue that patient satisfaction would be the key variable in evaluation. Others argue that most people have little knowledge about medical services; thus their evaluations are of little value. But most people who go to "quacks" are satisfied with the services they receive. In many instances, this is not out of ignorance, but because standard medical providers cannot or will not provide the services they desire (Cobb, 1954; Parker and Tupling, 1977).

Measures of consumer satisfaction can be broken down into various components of care and the delivery of services. It is true that most consumers do not have much expertise in judging the technical quality of care that is provided. However, consumers' evaluations of such things as courtesy and their ability to gain information about their condition and treatment are usually valid. Another key set of consumer-measured variables concerns the ease of access to care. The typical consumer faces a variety of nonmonetary barriers to getting care in any system—the length of time necessary to wait for an appointment, the difficulty in contacting a physician, travel time to the provider's office, and waiting time in the office. All are relevant factors that affect consumer satisfaction. An entirely different approach to evaluating satisfaction looks not at what people say but at what they do, in terms of out-of-plan usage and disenrollment.

Physician Satisfaction

Measures of performance concerning costs, quality, and satisfaction have been considered from the consumer's perspective. In one sense they are all factors to be included in a consumer's utility function. Most economic analyses would not go on to evaluate the producer's utility, but in the case of medical care, with the dominant role of the physician, such an evaluation is necessary. For instance, a medical care system that is optimal from the consumer's perspective might be infeasible because of a physician boycott. Usually, such issues are included in theoretical analyses through the cost variable. In the above example, the price demanded by physicians for their participation could be infinite, or at least beyond any reasonable range. In a more empirically based discussion, it is worthwhile to consider explicitly those factors that influence physician satisfaction and thus affect potential implementation of the HMO concept.

Distributional Equity

Many people are concerned about equity—whether various subgroups in society receive a "fair share." Arguments about equity often focus on proposals concerning the redistribution of income and wealth to benefit the poor. Similar arguments arise about whether the poor get their share of health services. Of course, how one measures fair share is subject to much debate. Should it imply equality in services per capita, services per health problem, or something else? Equity questions also arise with respect to geographic distribution of services; for instance, even if people in rural areas are not poor, they may be medically underserved because there are few providers close by.

A number of issues must be evaluated when examining distributional equity in the context of designing a national health-care strategy. For instance, in addition to questions of whether benefits accrue to the people for whom they are intended, one must ask who bears the cost of the program. Are these costs financed through out-of-pocket payments, premiums, or taxes? Furthermore, equity issues may be raised concerning not only who is allowed into a program, but who is allowed to opt out of a program, and if such decisions are to be voluntary. Other issues include supplementation of benefits and the possible income effects for providers. (For a consideration of this type of analysis with respect to national health insurance, see Berki, 1971.) The question of who stands to gain and to lose is of particular interest for predicting whether a plan will be implemented successfully (Luft, 1976a).

Externalities

The above measures of performance address issues internal to the organization and its members, the costs and quality of care, consumer satisfaction, and distributional equity. The last measure of performance deals with the effects of the organization on others—its externalities. These take many forms. The introduction of a new type of medical care delivery system in competition with the existing system may result in substantial changes in the latter's behavior. For instance, the mere threat that Kaiser might establish a clinic in San Joaquin County led to the development of the San Joaquin Foundation for Medical Care. Similarly, competition from HMOs may lead conventional providers and insurers to become more cost conscious. Other externalities could occur through the effects of HMOs on medical research and on the training of medical practitioners.

Thus the evaluation of alternative methods of health care delivery should be multidimensional and include a broad definition of costs, quality, consumer satisfaction, distributional equity, and externalities. Some of these can only be measured imperfectly for lack of an appropriate methodology (e.g., quality) or a crystal ball (e.g., long-term trends in costs and competition), while others have difficulties of their own. The remainder of this book will be oriented toward recognition of the importance of these multiple measures of performance.

USING THEORY TO GUIDE THE ANALYSIS

The reader should understand the general framework within which theoretical implications are drawn. The expected performance differences need not occur all of the time. They may take a while to appear; when they do they may be of little importance, and they may not appear at all. These caveats are not based on any particular problems in terms of HMOs, but instead are based on standard methods for theoretical predictions. Thus when an economist predicts that the demand for services will rise as the price falls, or when a sociologist predicts that bureaucratic controls will be resisted by professionals, the predicted outcome is meant to be a *tendency* in behavior, *other things being held constant.*

The notion of tendency can be interpreted in several ways. For instance, in the example of the price reduction, it means that more rather than fewer people will want to purchase a service, or that they are likely to demand more rather than fewer units of service. It does not mean that everyone will demand more units. Furthermore, tendency may be interpreted in a probabilistic sense that allows for normal random variation. Suppose that consumer decisions involve an element of pure chance, totally unrelated to price. From day to day the consumer's demand for services will fluctuate randomly around some mean value. If the price is lowered, this mean will tend to shift upward, even though on a given day the observed demand of a particular consumer or even a group of consumers may be lower because of random variation. If the theoretical predictions are correct, and nothing else has changed, observation of a large number of consumers over time should show an increase in their average demand.

Time is important in the notion of tendency, because behavior rarely changes instantaneously for at least three reasons. First, many decisions normally are made infrequently, so a change in a variable such as price cannot have an effect until the consumer makes another purchasing decision. Second, not everyone learns about price changes. Information transfer is imperfect. Thus some people make decisions based on what used to be the case but is no longer true. Eventually, more and more people will learn about the new prices. Third, many people are creatures of habit, and even if they know about the new price, they may still make the old choices for a while. (Some people, of course, never will change their behavior in response to the price change under discussion; it may be too small for it to matter to them, or it may be irrelevant. Decreasing the price of chocolate sundaes will increase the number purchased for most people, but even free sundaes will not induce consumption among people allergic to chocolate.)

Even after this tendency has time to work itself out completely and behavior is at a new equilibrium, the observable change may be small. This is usually an empirical rather than a theoretical issue. At best, one may offer theoretical predictions concerning the relative size of a behavior change. For instance, one would predict, for obvious reasons, that the demand for appendectomies will be less sensitive to price than the demand for cosmetic surgery. However, the responses of both to a given price change may be so small as to be of negligible importance.

The second key factor in these predictions is that *other things are held constant*. If other things change at the same time as the variable of interest, then they too may have an effect on behavior. That effect may be in the opposite direction, and it may be dominant. Thus if the price of a service is reduced but simultaneously the waiting time to receive it is increased, the net change in demand will be the result of the increased demand attributable to the price reduction and the decreased demand attributable to the time increase. Without empirical estimates of these two effects, it is impossible to predict the net change in demand. Moreover, with the exception of a few carefully designed and controlled experiments, other things are not held constant.

With all these caveats, why should one even consider theoretical predictions? Of what use are they? Perhaps the most important role for such predictions is to focus our attention on certain key variables and thus help to make sense out of an almost endless set of data. Furthermore, predictions can be used to test hypotheses. Even if several changes occur at once, their predicted effects may be in the same direction, and if the expected results are found, they will tend to support the hypotheses. More importantly, if the predicted results are not found or if they are in the opposite direction, we should have less faith in the hypothesis or at least suspect that the magnitude of the predicted effects are small.

WHAT DIFFERENCES IN PERFORMANCE WOULD BE EXPECTED?

Given the characteristics of HMOs outlined in Chapter 1, how would performance be expected to differ from that of the traditional forms of medical practice? Most of the predictions in this section are drawn from the application of economic theory, primarily because a knowledge of the detailed characteristics of particular HMOs is necessary in order to examine their noneconomic behavior. (See Pauly, 1970, and Reinhardt, 1973, for excellent theoretical discussions of the economic incentives in health care.) Whenever possible, I have drawn upon the insights of other disciplines. This section outlines the manner in which the five characteristics that define a generic HMO might be expected to influence HMO performance. The impacts of group versus solo practice and salary versus FFS payment of physicians are also considered.

Expectations Concerning Costs

The major expectation about HMO behavior, both theoretically and in terms of policy importance, is that HMOs will tend to reduce the overall cost of providing medical care. This prediction is derived from an examination of the incentives with respect to both the number and mix of services and the cost per unit of service. In traditional FFS practice the health care provider's income is positively related to the number of services provided and the net revenue per service. Thus there is an incentive to provide more services, much like any business. When observed in the medical care sector, this seemingly standard type of transaction is the source of much concern for two reasons: disbelief in consumer sovereignty and the presence of insurance. Some researchers argue that patients are exceptionally ignorant consumers, and with the high degree of risk associated with medical care, they must rely upon their physicians to be both agents and providers. (See Arrow, 1963, and Feldstein, 1974.) The extent of consumer ignorance in medical care is largely unknown, and it is possible that with effective educational programs, it may be no greater than that in relation to other goods and services. It is true, however, that most patients do not know much about the technical aspects of care or alternatives to specific treatments. Furthermore, when one's life or the life of a family member is or is thought to be at stake, it is unlikely that even someone who is usually a model of economic rationality would continue to be so.

Problems of the consumer's lack of information and the emotional situations that often surround the provision of medical care are compounded by the widespread use of insurance, which substantially reduces the effective price of care (Pauly, 1968). Thus in many instances in which the consumer acts as if cost is no object, it is the insurance company that bears the direct expense. Therefore, even without the consumer ignorance issue, the presence of health insurance will tend to reduce the consumer's sensitivity to price and total cost in much the same way that auto collison insurance reduces cost sensitivity.

The low net price of insured care and the financial incentives of the provider combine to convince some observers that there is a bias toward providing too many services in the FFS system with extensive insurance coverage. (See Eisenberg and Rosoff, 1978.) Other people argue that alternatives such as HMOs, provide too few services (Schwartz, 1978). Obviously, it is difficult to define how much medical care is too much. It is clear that the conventional financial incentives lead to more medical care than would be the case if patients paid the full cost, rather than the price net of insurance. While a patient may realize that "excess utilization" will lead to higher premiums in the future, the effect of his or her own decision will seem negligible.

One argument can be made against this definition of "too much." A consumer may be willing to pay a substantial amount in extra premium cost in order to guarantee low out-of-pocket costs when decisions about medical care must be made. Thus, after the fact, there will be no regrets about not having had "the best care possible" because of financial constraints. In other words, the consumer expects that utility functions or preferences will be distorted or painful to examine at some future decision point when the care is necessary, and thus buys an option for a low price in the future. (For a discussion of "option demand" in other contexts, see Weisbrod, 1964.) One may also question the extent to which financial incentives influence providers, especially when one considers the role of professional ethics.

The fixed monthly payment to an HMO implies that the marginal or extra revenue for additional services is zero, while there will be additional costs for each extra service rendered (Monsma, 1970). Thus it is relatively easy to predict that HMOs will tend to reduce the utilization of medical care services relative to FFS practice. A key link in this prediction is the requirement that the HMO bear at least some of the financial risk or gain. It also assumes that consumer demand for services is comparable—that the net price to the consumer is the same so that a major factor, demand, is held constant, and the prediction is based solely on the provider's incentives. However, consumers often have different effective coverage, especially for ambulatory care, under the two types of plans. If they face no costs for HMO visits and they pay substantial fees under the alternatives, their utilization might well be higher in the HMO. (This is an important example of two predictions that work in opposite directions).

It is possible to make some predictions about the ways in which HMOs will attempt to reduce health-care costs in terms of the number and mix of services rendered. First, while the average American has about 4.8 physician visits per year and a hospital admission every 7.1 years, the per capita yearly cost of physicians' services was only $146, relative to $297 for hospital care in 1977 (U.S. National Center for Health Statistics, 1978; Gibson and Fisher, 1978). Second, the average consumer tends to be more knowledgeable about problems requiring only ambulatory care than those requiring hospitalization, because the former tend to be less technically involved. Third, the consumer can directly initiate an ambulatory physician visit, while only a physician can admit a patient to a hospital. [These two factors imply physician control over hospitalization. The control is not absolute; consumers who think they know what treatment they need often will search until they find a physician who is willing to provide it. Similarly, many patients refuse surgery even after it is recommended by two physicians (McCarthy and Finkel, 1978).] Finally, the sheer number of

physician visits makes them much more difficult to monitor and control.*
All of these factors suggest that the major cost savings of HMOs will take
place through reductions in hospital utilization, rather than physicians'
visits. Note that our argument does not rest on the efficacy of specific types
of care; there are inefficacious procedures in both inpatient and ambulatory care settings.

Not only can it be predicted that HMOs will place a greater effort on
reducing hospital utilization, but there is also the expectation that when an
HMO has the choice between providing inpatient or outpatient care, it will
choose the less costly outpatient mode of delivery. This is a substitution of
one type of service for another. Thus the observed number of ambulatory
visits in an HMO may include some services that "normally" would have
been performed in the hospital. Because there is still a financial incentive
for an HMO to reduce unnecessary ambulatory visits, the observed number
of visits will represent the net effect of these two incentives. It should be
possible, however, to examine subsets of visits in order to test the two
predictions. For instance, one should be able to observe in HMOs a relative
shift away from admitting patients for routine workups and minor surgery
that could be done in the physician's office. One may also find a reduction
in the overall number of certain discretionary procedures, both inpatient
and outpatient.

It is substantially more difficult to develop clear predictions concerning
the technical efficiency, or cost per unit of service, in HMOs relative to
non-HMOs. In part, this is because both types of producers have an
incentive to reduce pure waste in the provision of services. More importantly, particular predictions are dependent on the special characteristics of
the HMOs and non-HMOs in question. For instance, most hospitals
operate on a not-for-profit basis and are often paid by cost reimbursement.
The cost reimbursement aspect of this arrangement suggests that there is
little incentive for a hospital to try to reduce costs, and the not-for-profit
aspect further reduces incentives for a hospital administration to be
efficient. (See Dowling, 1974, for a discussion of hospital incentives.)
However, the payment scheme for hospitals can be independent of HMOs;
in both HMO and non-HMO systems hospitals can be paid on a cost-
reimbursement, flat fee per day or per case, incentive contract, or other
scheme. Similarly, hospitals may be operated on a profit or not-for-profit
basis in either system. Thus predictions concerning the costs of hospital
services will depend on questions related to organizational factors. (A
detailed discussion of organizational factors is contained in Chapter 14.)

Questions of efficiency may also be raised about physicians' services. The
key issue here concerns the number of physicians who share in the costs

---

*For example, using the data presented above, preventing one physician visit would save
about $30.42, while preventing one hospital admission would save $2121.43, a greater than
seventyfold difference.

and benefits of specific items. For instance, consider the depth of the carpet in a physician's office or the presence of a full-time secretary. These benefits accrue directly to the physician. One would expect a physician to ask for more such benefits when their costs were to be shared with ninety-nine partners than if they were to be borne on an individual basis. Thus there is likely to be more inefficiency in large groups than in small groups, especially when costs are shared equally (Newhouse, 1973; Sloan, 1974). Sloan points out, however, that as the number of physicians in a group increases, they are more likely to hire full-time administrators to help control costs and to protect themselves from the collective costs of their individual incentives. Again, the question of group versus solo practice arises both in and out of HMOs.

One efficiency advantage can accrue to HMOs through their defined population and enrollment mechanisms. Because of these features, the HMO can plan more effectively for the health-care resources required to service its population. Thus it can purchase new facilities and hire new staff only as they are needed. Individual FFS providers have much less information. They may enter the market with few patients and work substantially below capacity for several years. Similarly, hospitals may compete for physicians by acquiring specialized equipment that may be underused. One would expect an HMO (or a well-functioning resource allocation agency) to set up a specialized service, such as an open heart unit, only when it could be fully employed, thus reducing slack in the system.*

The remaining cost questions concern out-of-pocket costs and long-term cost changes. Because the definition of an HMO requires that there be only minimal out-of-pocket charges, the first issue appears to be moot; however, that does not allow for utilization of services outside of the plan. Such utilization may be designed into the benefit package, such as when certain services are not covered, or it may occur because of patient dissatisfaction with the availability or quality of services. There also may be a certain expected level of out-of-plan use. Whether HMO enrollees have more or fewer out-of-pocket costs than a companion group depends on too many individual factors to allow us to predict the outcome on a theoretical basis.

Long-term changes in costs are the result of several factors. Obviously, the cost of producing a given medical service will partially depend on the costs of the materials and labor that go into the service. In turn, these will reflect the general level of prices in the economy and any special changes associated with medical care inputs. For instance, in the last decade the salaries of nurses and other health personnel have increased more rapidly than wages and salaries in general. The cost of production also depends on

---

*Slack has its advantages at times for most systems, especially in providing a cushion for emergencies. One would suspect that if an HMO did not have the option to purchase extra services in the FFS sector during an emergency, it would tend to operate with more slack than would otherwise be the case. As usual, the focus here is on "relatively" more or less slack.

the degree of technical efficiency or slack in production, and this may change over time within a given organization. Of course, the total costs of medical services over time will reflect changes in the number or mix of services.

It is difficult to make strong predictions concerning HMO performance with respect to long-term cost changes, because many variables are likely to fluctuate. But some predictions are possible. All medical providers tend to face the same increases in the costs of inputs; however, if an HMO is more efficiently managed, it may be better able to alter its mix of inputs in order to reduce the effects of increased costs. For example, efficient organizations may more rapidly introduce new, lower-cost allied health personnel to perform some tasks usually performed by more expensive personnel, such as physicians. Changes in technical efficiency are more difficult to predict, especially because there is a limit to the possible reduction of slack, so that efficient organizations will have more difficulty improving than will inefficient organizations. There is an expectation, however, that competition among providers usually will increase their collective efficiency over time. Thus one would predict less rapid cost increases over time for both HMOs and non-HMOs in areas where there is effective competition among provider types than in areas where no such competition exists. Competition within provider type does not seem to be effective. For example, many observers point to the competition among hospitals for physicians; this often results in overrapid adoption of new technology by too many hospitals, so that there is idle capacity and greater waste. (See Lee, 1971; Lee, 1972.) Given the cost incentives faced by HMOs, one could predict that they would constrain purchases of new technology so that idle capacity would be minimized. Such a prediction depends, of course, on the HMO having control over the purchase of new equipment; this may be the case only if it controls or has substantial influence over the hospitals it uses.

Expectations Concerning Quality

As was discussed above, it is difficult to measure quality; however, it is possible to make some predictions concerning the potential quality of HMOs relative to non-HMOs. Because HMOs include some organizational structure, either through group practice or the peer-review mechanisms of the IPAs, they have the capability to enforce higher quality standards among their physicians than is the case among individual practitioners. There are several important qualifications to this prediction. First, it refers to capabilities and not whether an HMO actually exercises quality control. Second, such control probably is most effective in weeding out poor quality practitioners; it may even serve as a disincentive for the very best practitioners. Thus HMOs can reduce the size of the low end of the quality curve, but it is unclear whether the average quality level will be higher or lower than in non-HMOs. Third, the institution in solo practice of peer-review mechanisms, such as Professional Standards Review Organizations (PSROs), may have the effect of reducing poor quality in FFS practice, thus eliminating the HMOs' advantage.*

One frequently used quality measure is preventive care, and a great deal of discussion has centered around the HMO's supposed incentive to provide preventive health services. This argument implicitly rests on the assumption that the costs of preventive and therapeutic care, and the efficacy of the former, are such that it is less expensive to prevent illness than treat it. If this is the case, then the financial incentives are such that an HMO will emphasize preventive services, while an FFS physician will tend to emphasize therapeutic care (Pauly, 1970).

Of course, the argument cuts both ways; if the cost of prevention, say through mass screening for presymptomatic disease, exceeds the cost of treatment, the HMO will tend to offer less prevention, in contrast to the health maintenance rhetoric. In fact, if FFS physicians were driven by purely economic incentives, they might even provide ineffective preventive services as long as they were profitable (Warner, 1977). However, such incentives only operate on the margin; more important factors are involved, especially since the medical care system is not very competitive on economic factors. A physician's professional ethics and concern for the patients and also the desire to avoid a malpractice suit, are likely to be the dominant factors among incentives to provide preventive care under FFS practice. (After all, if complications do arise, it is likely that a patient will be referred to another physician, thus the revenue will be lost entirely.) Another important factor is that preventive care procedures are often rather dull and uninteresting for the physician who has been trained in medical school to track down and cure rare diseases. Even if the net income for preventive care were as high as for curative care, one might expect such physicians to prefer a case-mix that favored curative care.

Expectations Concerning Consumer Satisfaction

Consumer satisfaction with various health plans must be measured along several dimensions. In terms of satisfaction with cost, the lower expenses and in particular the lower out-of-pocket expenses for many HMO members, should be seen as creating a substantial advantage. However, because HMOs cannot use fees to ration care, it may be expected that other means will be used, such as delays in appointments and other types of queues. This may result in consumer dissatisfaction about the responsiveness of the HMO to demands for care. It should be expected that an HMO will be less responsive to such demands than FFS practitioners. In part, such consumer dissatisfaction may merely reflect the fact that most people

---

*Currently PSROs are limited to the review of institutional services and cannot review office practice; however, even such review may substantially improve quality if vigorously pursued. Just how vigorously the PSRO concept will be implemented remains in question.

want more for less. If they pay FFS, they complain about cost; while if they do not have price rationing, they complain about queues. Some scheme for rationing resources must be used, but the two have different implications. Price rationing may lead to inequity for the poor; while queues may make it difficult to distinguish among more or less necessary care, as seen by the patient.

A key factor that affects consumer satisfaction is voluntary enrollment in the HMO. This suggests that consumers think they will prefer the HMO; otherwise they would not join. If they become too dissatisfied, they will leave the HMO. Thus the organization has an incentive to maintain a reasonable level of satisfaction. Given that membership is voluntary, one would expect HMO enrollees to be fairly satisfied. But non-HMO members also have a choice among plans and, aside from the financial mechanism, they can select among all available FFS providers. Further analysis of the satisfaction question is intertwined with the self-selection issue and will be discussed in the next chapter.

Expectations Concerning Physician Satisfaction

The economic incentives of an HMO are likely to affect a physician's perception of medical practice in several ways. Complete coverage of all services allows a physician to assume that patients can afford prescribed tests and procedures. The fixed total budget, however, is the opposite of what most physicians experience. The typical situation is one in which the physician is rewarded financially for doing more. Hospital financial well-being also depends on high utilization. HMO physicians therefore might feel constrained in their practice options.

A number of implications for physician satisfaction depend upon the type of HMO in question. Physicians who are paid FFS by an IPA may see little difference in their day-to-day practice, with the exception of a more detailed claims review. Such a review by a physician-controlled organization, however, is likely to be preferred to reviews by insurers or the government. Salaried physicians in prepaid group practices may respond differently. There may be substantial dissatisfaction if salaries are thought to be too low, but lower salaries may be offset by more leisure and rotating coverage. The solo physician has almost complete autonomy and control over patient scheduling and the style of practice. This autonomy is lost in a group setting. A major factor in determining the satisfaction of physicians will be their expectations of practice and their ability to select a setting they find congenial.

Expectations Concerning Distributional Equity

Most predictions concerning the effects of HMOs on equity depend on specific plan characteristics and their alternatives. For instance, FFS payments can impose a substantial burden on the poor, but adequate insurance coverage can be provided to eliminate that problem. Certain types of HMOs, such as groups, may provide one-stop care that may be more effective for the poor, but FFS groups can do the same. On the other hand, groups may impose bureaucratic hurdles that are more difficult to overcome for the poor than for the middle class. If one is concerned about the poor underutilizing services because of lack of knowledge, then HMOs, with their incentives to reduce utilization, may cause equity problems. Although an HMO can provide a base for outreach programs to bring in the underutilizers, it is not clear that there would be an incentive to do so. FFS providers may not be as well organized, but they have a more obvious incentive to encourage the poor to increase utilization.

Expectations Concerning Externalities

The most important expectation concerning externalities is that competition between HMOs and non-HMOs within a region is likely to produce lower costs than would exist without such competition. The benefits of such lower costs would accrue to both HMO and non-HMO members. There are, however, certain perverse situations in which competition could lead to increased costs. For instance, an HMO might introduce new resources to an area and attract a substantial fraction of the population, thereby increasing excess capacity, costs, and perhaps unnecessary utilization in the non-HMO sector, at least in the short run.

An enrolled HMO population can provide an excellent data base for epidemiological research that is usually unavailable. Similarly, an HMO has responsibility for the full range of medical services and thus can provide an ideal base for medical education and training. The question is: do such research and training programs cost the HMO resources and provide benefits outside the HMO? Unless the HMO is paid separately it will probably underinvest (from a social viewpoint) in research and training. This is a general problem when externalities exist, and a producer can neither capture all the benefits nor be paid by others for the benefits they receive.

SUMMARY

This chapter was designed to establish a framework for the rational analysis of the vast body of data concerning HMOs and their performance. The first step was to outline the various dimensions of performance that are of interest to the policy-maker and to discuss how HMOs are predicted to perform on each. Perhaps the most important dimension in terms of policy is cost and its various components. HMOs are expected to result in a reduction in the total cost of medical care for their enrollees. This cost reduction can be expected to occur, in large part, through a reduction in the number and mix of services. It appears that the greatest cost savings would be forthcoming through a reduction in hospital services, although HMOs have an incentive to reduce all services. They may, however, substitute ambulatory care for more expensive inpatient care. Predictions concerning savings from increased efficiency are much less clear and depend on the specific characteristics of the organizations in question. The same qualifications hold for discussions of out-of-pocket costs and long-term cost trends.

Predictions concerning HMO performance on the other four dimensions are even less firm than those on cost. HMOs have a greater potential for monitoring and eliminating low-quality care, but they also may lose the best practitioners. Financial incentives concerning preventive care (another quality measure) depend on the relative costs of prevention and therapy. Consumers may be expected to be more satisfied with the financial aspects of most HMOs, but they also will be less satisfied with some aspects of the HMO's method of rationing services. Physicians may find the HMO's financial incentives either constraining or liberating. The prepaid group practice setting has an even greater potential influence on satisfaction, but this may be offset by the physician's choice of the style of practice. The impact of HMOs on distributional equity depends largely on the specific organization, but the HMO incentives may lead to underutilization by the poor. While HMOs may be well equipped to establish outreach services, it is unclear what incentives exist for them to do so. A similar set of problems exists for the potential of HMOs to serve as bases for research and training. The potential is there, but the incentives to follow through may not be present, as is usually the case with externalities. The incentive problem is less severe in terms of HMO competition with other providers, but there is the possibility that, in the short run at least, such competition would raise rather than lower total expenditures.

The available data are hardly adequate to support rigorous tests of these predictions. The data are drawn from a rather biased group of HMOs and represent a collection of incomplete case studies. Recognizing the limitations of the data leads us to be more cautious in our analysis; nonetheless, by combining the available evidence with our predictions, we should be able to increase substantially our understanding of HMO performance.

THREE

The Self-Selection Issue

People are not assigned randomly to HMOs and conventional insurance plans. In fact, the generic definition requires that an HMO voluntarily enroll its members from among populations who have at least a dual choice. This implies self-selection. If people who expect to increase their requirements for medical care join a plan with more comprehensive coverage, the data will reflect the net effects of their greater need and the special incentives of the plan. However, if people chose health plans based on some factor that would not be expected to affect their medical care utilization, such as hair color or astrological sign, then self-selection would not create a problem in interpreting utilization and cost data. Even in these trivial cases, the mere fact that people can self-select has substantial implications for the organization and for measures of consumer satisfaction.

Numerous studies have shown that observing different outcomes in two settings is not sufficient to identify the causes of the difference in performance (Campbell, 1969; Mahoney, 1978). The observer may introduce subtle biases into the interpretation of the data, or the subjects may behave differently because of the nature of the experiment, rather than because of the new treatment. (The latter often is called the Hawthorne effect.) Problems mount when people can select the treatment, whether surgery versus drug treatment or HMO versus FFS. It is commonplace in medical literature to discount claims that one treatment is better than another unless the evidence is derived from a randomized, controlled trial (Cochrane, 1972). To my knowledge, only two such true experiments have been undertaken with HMOs. One is the Medical Care Group of Washington University, which is described in Chapter 2. The other is part of the RAND Health Insurance Experiment, from which data are not yet available.

The empirical evidence in this book is drawn almost entirely from nonexperimental settings involving self-selected populations. Experimental evidence would allow us to determine the true effect that HMOs have on utilization, cost, and satisfaction. However, it is probably more useful to explore the behavior of HMOs and other providers in the natural setting that allows for selection, rather than in the artificial environment of an experiment. Given the present political environment, it is difficult to imagine a national health policy that would assign people to HMOs; the most that can be expected are policies that would increase the options and encourage people to select HMOs.

This chapter will present some of the theoretical issues associated with self-selection and then examine data from various settings to help put the question into perspective. A third section will examine some theoretical issues concerning disenrollment, or the option to select out of a plan.

REASONS FOR JOINING HMOs: THEORETICAL CONSIDERATIONS

Since all HMO enrollees have some choice of plans, it is reasonable to assume that the HMO option is more attractive to them than the alternatives. (Strictly speaking, this can be assumed to be true at the time they join, especially if they take some positive action to switch plans. Those people who remain in a traditional plan either prefer it, are indifferent, or do not want to make a decision.) Because there is generally substantial inertia in situations concerning choice of plan, it is likely that HMO enrollees see the plan as having a clear advantage and that the others perceive less of an advantage in favor of the HMO or positive disadvantages to it.* Four factors have been raised as having a potential influence on the choice of plans: (1) risk-vulnerability; (2) attitudes toward illness and medical care; (3) neuroticism or the "worried-well" hypothesis; and (4) lack of integration in the present system. As will become apparent, all four factors could be included under an expanded concept of risk-vulnerability. Because of the different theoretical bases of the various factors, we will consider them separately.

The risk-vulnerability hypothesis is closest to a purely economic analysis and has the clearest implications for the interpretation of utilization data. In brief, it argues that people who consider themselves to be at high risk in terms of expected illness and who feel financially vulnerable because of potentially high out-of-pocket costs are more likely to join prepaid plans. (See Bashshur and Metzner, 1967, 1970; Metzner, Bashshur, and Shannon, 1972; Moustafa, Hopkins, and Klein, 1971; Bice, 1975; Berki et al., 1977a, 1977b; Tessler and Mechanic, 1975b.) In more formal terms, it suggests that a factor in the choice of plan is the expected cost of medical care in a probabilistic sense. This expected cost is the product of the

---

*A good example of this inertia and the advantages of being the "first plan" are given in Burke (1973, p. 34). A group of West Coast longshoremen were covered exclusively by a PGP for three years. When given a dual choice option, only a few shifted. In fact, after ten years 93 percent were still PGP members. In contrast, warehousemen of the same union who had had dual choice from the beginning split about equally between the two options.

probability of requiring care times the cost of care. If the HMO premium is greater than that of the alternative plans, then the expected cost savings from joining the HMO would have to more than compensate for the premium difference, thus increasing even further the impact of self-selection on expected utilization.

Certain aspects of the risk-vulnerability hypothesis become especially important in the empirical analysis. In particular, the hypothesis is really based on two interactive factors. The first may be termed the "risk-perception hypothesis," which states that "the higher an individual's a priori subjective probability assigned to future events regarding medical care, the more likely the person is to enroll in a plan which, other things being equal, offers a more comprehensive, more accessible benefit package." The second is the "financial loss hypothesis," which states that "the larger the expected utility loss associated with a given expected financial loss, the more likely that individual is to enroll in a plan which, other things being equal, reduces the financial costs of utilization" (Berki et al., 1977, p. 98). The financial loss hypothesis builds upon the view that a given out-of-pocket cost is a greater burden for people with fewer financial resources or more commitments on their resources.

Within this framework, if the same financial risk exists under both plans, then there will be no financial incentive to join one rather than the other, regardless of differentials in expected illness. In most dual choice cases conventional insurance plans offer fairly complete coverage of inpatient services, but much less often do they offer comprehensive coverage of ambulatory services, particularly preventive or "well" care. Thus it is more likely that the risk-vulnerability effect will be greater for ambulatory than for inpatient care.

An important factor in the economic calculations implicit in the risk-vulnerability hypothesis is the premium cost to the enrollee. Although the true cost of a health plan is the premium plus expected out-of-pocket costs for the year, some people may focus primarily on the premium and discount future out-of-pocket costs. This may be because they believe themselves to be healthier than average, are excessively optimistic, or live day-to-day. To the extent that this is true, the allocation of costs between premium and out-of-pocket may be crucial. This issue is further complicated by the role of employer contributions. In many instances the employer pays a fixed amount toward whichever plan the employee chooses, and the employee pays whatever additional amount is required. This fixed contribution often covers just the least expensive premium. Thus, while the total premiums for two plans might differ by only 10 percent, say $80 versus $88, the net premium for the more expensive plan would be $8 per month. The additional $96 per year might seem much larger than a 10 percent difference. Based upon this logic and the previous discussion of the risk-vulnerability hypothesis, we might expect people who perceive themselves as healthy to be particularly sensitive to small premium differentials. In some cases, however, the employer pays the full premium regardless of cost differences, so employees have no incentive to weigh premium versus out-of-pocket costs. This situation often occurs when a labor union contract includes contributions to cover a specific plan's premium, which over time has shifted from being least to most expensive. For example, Kaiser Industries in San Francisco contributes more for employees who choose conventional coverage than for those who choose the Kaiser-Permanente plan.

Attitudes toward illness and medical care are, in theory, likely to affect utilization patterns. (See Andersen, 1968; Anderson, 1973; McKinlay, 1972.) Faith in physicians, perceived control over illness, and propensity to use medical services when ill should affect the decision of whether or not to seek care when an illness episode occurs. One would predict, therefore, that people with high ratings on such scales would tend to prefer HMOs, with their more comprehensive ambulatory coverage. It is less likely that such attitudes will have a major influence on the choice of plan with respect to more serious conditions requiring hospitalization. A second set of attitudes concerns the importance of immunizations, checkups, and preventive health care—services that often are not covered by the more traditional health insurance plans. These attitudes, if they are sufficiently important to influence self-selection, could make it difficult to use data concerning such preventive visits to compare quality in HMOs and non-HMOs. While most of these attitudes affect the consumer's perception of risk and vulnerability, attitudes favoring innovative over traditional forms of practice may also influence choice of plan.

The concept of the *worried well* was developed by Sidney Garfield to describe those people who seek medical care when they are not really sick (Garfield, 1970; Garfield et al., 1976). Such people often have medical complaints but not clinically important abnormalities, and in many cases the complaints stem from psychological causes. It may be expected that people who are neurotic or hypersensitive to symptoms would want more readily available care, and the comprehensive ambulatory coverage of HMOs would be attractive to them.

Lack of integration into the traditional medical care system has several aspects. First, people who are well integrated have a usual provider with whom they have established ties. They are unlikely to want to change systems and give up a known provider with whom they are satisfied (This will not be an issue when the choice is between conventional coverage and an IPA or similar arrangement that allows enrollees to retain their own physicians.) Second, people who do not have a usual provider may find it difficult to obtain care. If they shift to an HMO in which the availability of care is guaranteed, they may increase their utilization. This is especially likely with respect to ambulatory care.

Data from the 1974 Health Interview Survey indicate the major reasons for not having a regular source of care (Blumberg, 1978). Overall, 15.6

percent of the population reported no usual source. Over half of these, or 8.5 percent, said no doctor was needed; another 2.8 percent saw a variety of doctors. Within a third category 0.2 percent said it was too expensive; 1.2 percent were unable to find the right doctor; and 1.2 percent said the previous doctor was no longer available. This suggests that most people without a usual doctor are unlikely to seek much medical care.

Reasons for Joining HMOs and the Adverse Selection Issue

The adverse selection issue has always been a key element in the HMO debate. This refers to the concern that the comprehensive coverage of HMOs will attract sicker people. In essence, this is described in the risk-vulnerability hypothesis. A counterargument, primarily based on the lower utilization rates of HMO enrollees, is that for some reason HMOs attract healthier people. To the extent that any self-selection occurs, whether it is adverse or preferential, it is no longer valid to compare HMO enrollee utilization rates with those of people in conventional plans. (The implications of selection for policy-making are even more important, but that discussion will be postponed until Chapters 14 and 15).

As will be apparent in this review, the evidence concerning self-selection is mixed. In part, this seems to be because the various studies are drawn from different settings with highly divergent market situations. But even if this discussion is far from the last word on the self-selection issue, it should cause us to be particularly alert to its potential presence in other studies.

The risk-vulnerability hypothesis often is tested in several ways. At the crudest level, demographic factors such as age, sex, and marital status are examined. Some such studies indicate that people who join HMOs are likely to be young, married, and have young children (Bashshur and Metzner, 1967; Moustafa, Hopkins, and Klein, 1971, p. 40; Gaus, 1971, p. 10; Hetherington, Hopkins, and Roemer, 1975; Berki et al., 1977a; Richardson et al., 1976). Other studies indicate the reverse (Scitovsky, McCall, and Benham, 1978; Moriarty, Venkatesan, and Sicher, 1977). Still others indicate no significant differences in such variables among plans (Tessler and Mechanic, 1975; Roghmann et al., 1975; Yedidia, 1959; Gaus, Cooper, and Hirschman, 1976).

A second level of analysis compares perceived measures of health status. This can be done with direct questions concerning health status or with specific questions concerning chronic and acute illness. Some studies indicate no differences in the evaluation of health status (Anderson and Sheatsley, 1959; Tessler and Mechanic, 1975; Gaus, Cooper, and Hirschman, 1976; Berki et al., 1977a; Scitovsky, McCall, and Benham, 1978). Studies that focus on chronic and acute conditions indicate either no differences among plans (Gaus, Cooper, and Hirschman, 1976) or mixed results with more of certain types of illnesses reported by HMO members and no differences in other measures (Tessler and Mechanic, 1975; Dozier et al., 1973; Roghmann et al., 1975; Hetherington, Hopkins, and Roemer, 1975, p. 66). A third group of studies finds less illness among HMO enrollees (Richardson et al., 1976; Bice, 1975; Berki et al., 1978).

Attitudes toward illness and medical care have been much less frequently examined as factors in the self-selection question. Moreover, in the few studies that tried to examine attitudes toward care explicitly, few significant differences were found among enrollees in various plans (Tessler and Mechanic, 1975, p. 166; Scitovsky, McCall, and Benham, 1978). While the Tessler and Mechanic study indicates no significant differences in attitudes toward preventive services, a significantly higher percentage of PGP enrollee children were fully immunized at the time they enrolled. Berki et al. (1977a, 1977b, 1978) found that IPA enrollees expressed no greater health concern than those who stayed in Blue Cross-Blue Shield (BC-BS), while those joining a PGP had the highest level of health concern. Moreover, health concern was an important predictor of the use of preventive services. Roghmann et al. (1975, p. 526) indicate that a substantial percentage of those who joined three particular prepaid plans mentioned preventive care as one reason for their choice.

There is also limited evidence concerning the role of the worried well in self-selection. Hetherington, Hopkins, and Roemer (1975) use an index of hypersensitivity that registers somewhat higher for members of one of the two PGPs they examined. Unfortunately, the derivation of their index is unclear, and they provide no significance tests. Tessler and Mechanic (1975, p. 167) used a measure of neuroticism and found no differences among groups. Results from studies of two Kaiser plans indicate that between 12 and 19 percent of ambulatory visits were classified as worried well (Garfield et al., 1976; Jackson and Greenlick, 1974). Whether this is considered high depends on one's perspective. It is not clear if psychosomatic problems are clinically unimportant; they may, however, have a substantial impact on physician behavior and satisfaction, as will be discussed in Chapter 12.

Lack of integration was explicitly tested by Roghmann et al. (1975), using a number of measures. People who joined HMOs were found to have a significantly shorter length of residence in the area, were less likely to have a family physician as a regular source of care, and were more likely to have no usual source of care. Furthermore, they were more likely to rate as important such access variables as twenty-four-hour availability of care and comprehensiveness of services, as well as short appointments, short office waits, and convenient hours. Ullman (1978) reassessed Roghmann's data on geographic mobility and found them consistent with the hypothesis that newcomers to an area are more likely than long-term residents to join a PGP. Gaus (1971) presents data that show a greater propensity to enroll in the Columbia PGP among people who moved from outside the Baltimore-Washington area and thus could not remain under the care of their previous physicians.

Richardson et al. (1976) found little difference between enrollees in two plans in the number of years they lived in the area. Those who joined the PGP, however, were only half as likely to report a private physician as their usual source of care. Scitovsky, McCall, and Benham's study (1978) of Stanford enrollees in Kaiser and the Palo Alto Medical Clinic (PAMC) indicates that the longer one had worked for Stanford, the less likely one was to be a Kaiser member. In part, this reflects the fact that Kaiser had been an option for only four and a half years at the time of the study. Of those employees who joined Stanford before Kaiser became available, only 39 percent were in Kaiser, whereas among those who started work after Kaiser was available, about 66 percent were Kaiser enrollees. (These are not market shares; an unknown number of employees chose a third enrollment option.) This finding is supported by the fact that 40 percent of the PAMC enrollees rejected Kaiser because they did not want to change physicians. Berki et al. (1977a, 1978) found that having a private physician was the best single predictor of choice of plan. Not having a private physician was the best predictor of joining a PGP, while having one was the best predictor of joining an IPA. It should be noted, however, that this doctor-patient relationship may well be built on the presence of chronic conditions and consequent ambulatory care use (Berki et al., 1978, p. 694).

A synthesis of these factors concerning adverse selection is necessary, yet difficult. One problem is the fact that there is no single determinant of enrollment choice, so examining one variable at a time is bound to produce conflicting findings. Berki et al. (1978) and Scitovsky, McCall, and Benham (1978) provide excellent multivariate analyses of enrollment choice that examine the simultaneous influence of several factors. In general, the multivariate findings are similar to those of more simple, bivariate tests. Aside from the interacting roles of multiple variables, an important factor resulting in inconsistent findings across studies is the influence of the external circumstances surrounding the choice situation. One crucial external factor is the premium differential, which in turn is influenced by the employer contribution. Another factor is the nature and reputation of the alternative plans. Fortunately, there have been a number of studies concerning choice among plans by employees in specific firms in Rochester, New York (Berki et al., 1977a, 1977b, 1978; Roghmann, 1975; Roghmann, Sorensen, and Wells, 1977; Wersinger, 1975; Ullman, 1978). These studies include not only the typical proxy variables, such as sociodemographic factors, attitudes, and integration, but also direct measures of medical care utilization.

The Rochester area has a history of active health planning and community interest in the medical care delivery system. About 87 percent of the population under age sixty-five is covered by Blue Cross. This represents the greatest market penetration in the nation (Blue Cross-Blue Shield Fact Book, 1976). Moreover, with the exception of the General Motors plant, all firms have a single community-rated premium, a situation quite unlike that of most areas in which each firm obtains a premium based on the utilization experience of its own employees. Beginning in 1973, three new HMOs were offered as options to certain employee groups. The Monroe Plan, or Health Watch, was an IPA-type plan sponsored by the Medical Society of Monroe County. It included somewhat more than half the physicians in the area. The plan went out of existence in June 1976. Genesee Valley Group Health Association (GVGHA) is a centralized multispecialty group practice sponsored by Blue Cross and Blue Shield. Rochester Health Network (RHN), a decentralized group practice with numerous locations, is sponsored by a former Office of Economic Opportunity (OEO) Neighborhood Health Center. Enrollment decisions can be examined with surveys of specific employee groups and verified with review of their hospital utilization, because all of the HMOs use Blue Cross as their fiscal agent for hospital care.

Because the employer contribution and basic BC-BS package varies across firms, it is useful to examine homogeneous populations. Roghmann et al. (1975) report on a 1973 survey of photographic company employees who were not unionized and who received a moderate employer contribution. The monthly family premiums for 1973 were as follows: Basic Blue Cross, $34.49; GVGHA, $49.68; Monroe Plan, $60.10; and RHN, $56.54 (Roghmann, Sorensen, and Wells, 1977, p. 6). The coverage offered by the three HMOs was generally comparable and much more extensive than the basic Blue Cross plan (Berki et al., 1977a). This 1973 survey presents the classic situation of higher HMO premium for better coverage. Furthermore, the Rochester situation included a special factor: those potential enrollees whose physicians were members of the Monroe Plan could continue with their usual source of care and merely obtain more complete insurance coverage, although at a higher premium. Enrollment in the two PGPs generally required a change in physician.

The 1973 survey results provide some crucial direct data concerning risk-vulnerability and self-selection. Actual out-of-pocket expenses in the preceding year for HMO enrollees were somewhat higher than for those who stayed in Blue Cross. Disaggregating by type of HMO, the higher preenrollment expenses were more obvious for enrollees in the IPA than for those who joined the PGPs. Enrollees in GVGHA in fact had substantially lower out-of-pocket hospitalization expenses. Survey data on utilization support these expense differences. Monroe Plan enrollees had slightly higher hospitalization rates before enrollment than did the "nonjoiners," while GVGHA enrollees had substantially lower hospitalization rates. The situation was somewhat different for visits to physicians and other providers. Monroe Plan enrollees had substantially more visits (4.32 versus 3.05), and both sets of PGP enrollees had somewhat more visits than those who stayed in Blue Cross. Moreover, with the exception of the RHN plan, which attracted a substantially poorer group of people, the HMO enrollees were substantially less likely to have had no visits to physicians.

The above data suggest adverse selection for both hospital and ambulatory care by IPA enrollees, while the situation for GVGHA enrollees was mixed: they had a more favorable hospitalization record but were somewhat higher users of ambulatory care. Somewhat different findings can be drawn from a set of Rochester studies undertaken by Berki et al. (1977a, 1977b, 1978; Ashcraft et al., 1978). While their survey occurred a year later, the crucial difference is that its focus was on workers in the local General Motors plant, who had complete employer contributions for all plans. This eliminated premium differentials. For the preenrollment period, the findings with respect to hospitalization are similar: there were no differences between the Monroe Plan and BC-BS enrollees, but enrollees in the two PGPs (combined) had significantly fewer hospital episodes, days of care, and out-of-pocket costs. Monroe Plan enrollees again had higher utilization rates for ambulatory care and out-of-pocket costs. The PGP enrollees, however, were significantly lower users of ambulatory services, particularly for illness visits. They had about the same rate of preventive visits and had significantly lower out-of-pocket costs.

These different responses make sense in light of the different premium costs faced by the two employee groups. The General Motors employees faced no additional costs when joining any of the HMOs and could realize substantial savings. Thus it is not surprising that a large fraction of General Motors families opted for the IPA. While the PGPs offered somewhat better coverage, enrolling in them required a change in physician. In fact, the primary determinant of PGP enrollment, even when controlling for health status and prior utilization, was the lack of a usual private physician (Berki et al., 1978). It is not surprising that General Motors PGP enrollees were relatively lower utilizers of ambulatory services. For employees in the firm studied by Roghmann et al. (1975), joining any HMO entailed additional premium costs, with the Monroe Plan being the most expensive. With the exception of maternity and psychiatric coverage, the BC-BS inpatient coverage was fairly complete; the major difference was in ambulatory care. Thus it is not surprising that those people willing to pay the extra premiums were higher users of ambulatory care.

Both the Roghmann and Berki studies are based on samples and rely on recall. While recall of hospitalization is generally good—see U.S. National Center for Health Statistics, Series 2, Nos. 6 (1965), 8, (1965), and 69 (1977)—hospital use is relatively infrequent, and a small sample may be subject to substantial statistical variability. Roghmann, Sorensen, and Wells (1977) provide an extremely useful supplement to this discussion with their cohort data on hospital utilization. Because all three HMOs used Blue Cross as an intermediary, it is possible to examine utilization both during HMO enrollment and in 1972 when everyone had Blue Cross coverage. The data are also disaggregated into those who were General Motors employees and those who were not. (See Tables 3-1 to 3-3). The age-standardized rates for all services support the survey data (Table 3-1). Prior

Table 3-1   General Motors and Non-General Motors Utilization Rates Before and After Joining HMOs 1972-1974-1975 Final Cohort, Inpatient Days per 1000 Enrollee Years, Age Standardized Rates, All Services (Obstetrics, Nursery, Medical, Surgical, Psychiatric)

	1972 (Before)	1974 (first year)	1975 (second year)	Percentage Change	
				1974/ 1972	1975/ 1974
Blue Cross					
GM	931 ± 13	894 ± 13	812 ± 12	− 4	− 9
Non-GM	618 ± 1	633 ± 1	640 ± 1	+ 2	+ 1
Total	625 ± 1	638 ± 1	642 ± 1	+ 2	+ 1
PGP (GVGHA)					
GM	448 ± 19	396 ± 22	410 ± 18	−12	− 4
Non-GM	517 ± 10	413 ± 12	345 ± 9	−20	−16
Total	491 ± 9	414 ± 11	360 ± 8	−16	− 1
Medical Foundation					
GM	796 ± 9	594 ± 14	930 ± 12	−25	+57
Non-GM	727 ± 12	1268 ± 19	1123 ± 18	+74	−11
Total	760 ± 7	940 ± 12	979 ± 10	+23	+ 4
NHC (Network)					
GM	439 ± 40	634 ± 49	1010 ± 50	+44	+59
Non-GM	474 ± 19	719 ± 28	762 ± 24	+52	+ 6
Total	480 ± 17	694 ± 25	789 ± 21	+45	+14

SOURCE: Roghmann, Sorensen, and Wells, *A Cohort Analysis of the Impact of Three Health Maintenance Organizations on Inpatient Utilization*, Final Report for Contract No. HEW-100-77-0021, 1977.

to joining the two PGPs, General Motors enrollee hospitalization rates were less than half that of their fellow workers who kept their Blue Cross coverage (448 and 439 versus 931). General Motors workers who joined the IPA had substantially higher usage, 796 days per 1000, but below that of the stayers. (This may be a reflection of pure inertia, or of the mix of patients seen by those physicians who chose not to join the Monroe Plan.)

Among people who did not work for General Motors the pattern is also clear: those joining the IPA had substantially higher hospitalization rates in 1972; the PGP enrollees' 1972 hospital usage was much closer to that of the BC-BS "stayers" than was the case for General Motors employees. Utilization of inpatient obstetrics and psychiatric care (Table 3-2) shows an even more striking selection pattern, because it is for these services that the HMOs offered the greatest increment in coverage for those outside of General Motors. IPA enrollees increased utilization by 143 percent, and GVGHA enrollees increased usage by 62 percent. Other data from these files, although not segregated by employer, indicate that the fertility rate per 1000 women aged fifteen to forty-four among Blue Cross members was 30.9, while the rates in the three prepaid plans were 75.1, 81.5, and 148.8

Table 3-2   General Motors and Non-General Motors Utilization Rates Before and After Joining HMOs 1972-1974-1975 Final Cohort, Inpatient Days per 1000 Enrollee Years, Age Standardized Rates, Other Services (Obstetrics, Nursery, Psychiatric)

	1972 (Before)	1974 (first year)	1975 (second year)	Percentage Change 1974/ 1972	Percentage Change 1975/ 1974
Blue Cross					
GM	212 ± 6	219 ± 6	217 ± 6	+ 2	− 1
Non-GM	142 ± .7	153 ± .7	157 ± .7	+ 8	+ 3
Total	143 ± .7	153 ± .7	157 ± .7	+ 7	+ 3
PGP					
GM	142 ± 11	62 ± 9	24 ± 4	−56	− 61
Non-GM	132 ± 6	214 ± 9	121 ± 5	+62	− 44
Total	133 ± 5	184 ± 7	102 ± 4	+38	− 45
Medical Foundation					
GM	164 ± 5	164 ± 8	245 ± 6	0	+ 49
Non-GM	261 ± 7	634 ± 14	414 ± 11	+143	− 35
Total	195 ± 4	417 ± 9	311 ± 6	+114	− 25
NHC (Network)					
GM	155 ± 19	40 ± 19	673 ± 34	− 74	+158
Non-GM	79 ± 9	343 ± 20	159 ± 13	+333	− 54
Total	87 ± 8	302 ± 17	223 ± 12	+247	− 26

SOURCE: Roghmann, Sorensen, and Wells, *A Cohort Analysis of the Impact of Three Health Maintenance Organizations on Inpatient Utilization,* Final Report for Contract No. HEW-100-77-0021, 1977.

(Wersinger, 1975, p. 21). The potential for self-selection for maternity care is obvious, but the data in Table 3-3 suggest that PGP enrollees were also lower utilizers of medical surgical services.

Two additional settings provide corroborative evidence on self-selection. Broida et al. (1975) examined utilization of people in the Greater Marshfield area who in 1971 were offered HMO coverage through their usual source of care, the Marshfield Clinic. Thus, while the setting was one of a prepaid group practice (albeit embedded within a predominantly FFS group), the enrollment situation was like that of an IPA, in which patients could retain their physicians. The only change was an improvement in coverage. In the period prior to the prepayment option, hospital use for the subsequently prepaid group was essentially the same as that of the continuous FFS group. Ambulatory use of the prepaid group, however, was significantly higher, suggesting some adverse selection in response to more complete coverage at higher premium cost.

Richardson et al. (1976) surveyed utilization in the Seattle Model Cities area. These low income (but not Medicaid) people were offered the choice

Table 3-3 General Motors and Non-General Motors Utilization Rates Before and After Joining HMOs 1972-1974-1975 Final Cohort, Inpatient Days per 1000 Enrollee Years, Age Standardized Rates, Medical and Surgical Admissions Only

	1972 (Before)	1974 (first year)	1975 (second year)	Percentage Change	
				1974/ 1972	1975/ 1974
Blue Cross					
GM	716 ± 12	676 ± 11	594 ± 11	− 6	−12
Non-GM	475 ± 1	481 ± 1	483 ± 1	+ 1	0
Total	481 ± 1	483 ± 1	484 ± 1	+ 0	+ 0
PGP					
GM	306 ± 16	335 ± 21	386 ± 18	+10	+15
Non-GM	385 ± 16	199 ± 9	224 ± 7	−48	+13
Total	358 ± 8	230 ± 8	258 ± 7	−36	+12
Medical Foundation					
GM	632 ± 8	430 ± 12	684 ± 10	−32	+59
Non-GM	467 ± 9	634 ± 13	710 ± 13	+36	+12
Total	565 ± 6	523 ± 9	668 ± 8	− 7	+28
NHC					
GM	284 ± 35	595 ± 46	337 ± 37	+10	−43
Non-GM	395 ± 17	375 ± 20	604 ± 20	− 5	+61
Total	393 ± 15	392 ± 18	566 ± 18	− 0	+44

SOURCE: Roghmann, Sorensen, and Wells, *A Cohort Analysis of the Impact of Three Health Maintenance Organizations on Inpatient Utilization,* Final Report for Contract No. HEW-100-77-0021, 1977.

of enrolling in Group Health Cooperative (GH) or a conventional plan sponsored by King County Medical/Blue Cross (KCM-BC). Both plans offered nearly identical comprehensive coverage, and the entire premium cost was absorbed by the project. As reported above, the GH enrollees were substantially less likely to have a private physician before enrolling. The prior utilization experience of the two groups fits a now-familiar pattern: the GH enrollees had somewhat fewer ambulatory visits in the preceding month (0.37 versus 0.42) even though the proportions with at least one visit were identical (0.23) (Richardson et al., 1976, p. 234). Nine percent of the GH enrollees had been hospitalized in the preceding year, in contrast to 10 percent of the KCM-BC enrollees. A greater number of multiple hospitalizations among the KCM-BC enrollees exacerbated the difference in the number of discharges per 1000 enrollees, 104 for GH enrollees and 132 for KCM-BC.

In summary, this review suggests that self-selection can be an important factor influencing comparisons of utilization in HMOs and other plans. Predicting the type of selection that occurs, however, is much more difficult. Three major determinants are: (1) the premium differential faced by the potential enrollee; (2) whether alternative plans require the enrollee to switch physicians or to obtain services in a different geographic setting; and (3) the type of options available. All evidence points to the importance of the preexisting physician-patient relationship. People with strong ties are unwilling to break them and will prefer to retain their old coverage, unless an HMO is structured to change only the financial linkages rather than the personal ones. IPAs and FFS groups converting to PGPs follow this model. It seems to be the case that within an employed population strong physician-patient ties are associated with poorer health status. More precisely, employed people without a private physician as their usual source of care are usually healthier than average, or at least lower utilizers of medical care.

The more comprehensive coverage of HMOs is often associated with higher premiums. When this is the case, people must trade off the certainty of an increased payroll deduction against projected out-of-pocket costs for future medical care. This leads to adverse selection into HMOs by people who anticipate using services such as preventive or ambulatory visits and maternity care, which are not covered or are poorly covered by their conventional insurance. While using more of certain services, these people tend to be relatively low users of hospital care. This finding is reinforced if the HMO option is a PGP that entails switching physicians. IPA-type plans are particularly attractive, so long as their premium costs are not excessive; but if they continue to attract higher utilizers, low premiums cannot be sustained. If PGPs can offer enrollment with little extra premium cost, either because of lower utilization or employer contributions, then they are even more likely to attract a favorable enrollment mix; the physician switching factor remains, and the lack of a premium differential makes the plan even more attractive to people who anticipate little medical care use. This argument is based on the view that some people perceive themselves as being very healthy. For instance, in 1977 it was estimated that 13 percent of the U.S. population had not seen a physician in at least two years (U.S. National Center for Health Statistics, "Current Estimates from the Health Interview Survey: United States, 1977" 1978, p. 31). For such people health insurance is merely catastrophic coverage for illnesses or accidents that are not expected to occur. Since they probably have no strong ongoing relationship with a physician, the choice of plan is essentially unimportant, and the extra premium cost is the only major factor.

The self-selection issue is important, but it should not be overemphasized. As will be seen in the next section, disenrollment must also be considered. Moreover, even if an HMO attracts relatively healthy people, over time they will begin to utilize services, and many will develop ties to their new physicians. Thus the influence of selection is likely to be greatest among new enrollee groups and new HMOs. As the organization matures, the influence of each year's cohort of new enrollees becomes insignificant.

While comparisons among plans can control for many of the factors that affect the demand for care—age, sex, marital status, chronic illnesses, attitudes, and the like—there may still be some uncontrolled-for biases toward more or less utilization by particular types among HMO enrollees in specific circumstances. The effects of the potential biases on hypothesis testing are shown in Table 3-4. It is apparent that the bias both helps and hinders, depending upon the hypothesis and the empirical results. It is important to remember these effects when evaluating the cost and utilization data in Chapters 4 through 8.

SELF-SELECTION, SATISFACTION, AND DISENROLLMENT

Most concern with self-selection has traditionally focused on the decision to enroll in a plan and how that might affect utilization patterns. A less obvious but nonetheless important aspect of self-selection has to do with decisions to leave an organization. Albert Hirschman (1970) has presented

Table 3-4   The Effects of Potential Self-Selection Biases on Testing Hypotheses Concerning the Impact of HMOs on Utilization

If the Evidence Indicates That Utilization is:	Hypotheses to Be Tested	
	HMOs Increase Utilization	HMOs Decrease Utilization
Self-Selection of Higher Utilizers into HMOs (e.g., for maternity care or preventive services)		
Higher in HMOs	Bias *reduces confidence* in the support given the hypothesis by the data	Bias could explain the observed results: thus *more difficult* to reject the hypothesis
Lower in HMOs	Bias works against the observation so *more confidence* in rejecting the hypothesis	Bias *strengthens* confidence in the support given the hypothesis by the data
Self-Selection of Lower Utilizers into HMOs (e.g., people without strong physician ties into PGPs)		
Higher in HMOs	Bias *strengthens* confidence in support given the hypothesis by the data	Bias *strengthens* confidence in rejecting the hypothesis
Lower in HMOs	Bias could explain the results, thus *more difficult* to reject the hypothesis	Bias *reduces confidence* in support given the hypothesis by the data

some theoretical discussions that may have substantial implications for HMO performance, particularly for measures of consumer satisfaction. Hirschman argues that most economic analyses consider consumer preferences to be expressed by the overt behavior of "voting with their feet;" if consumers no longer like the services of one organization, they will leave it for another that serves them better. He points out that they do have another alternative, that is, staying within the organization, complaining, and working for improvement. Political scientists usually focus on the latter view of behavior. Hirschman terms the two types of behavior "exit" and "voice," respectively, and demonstrates that they are intimately related to one another.

The key to analysis of exit and voice is the recognition that markets for some goods and services are not atomistically competitive (that is, there are not always many producers and consumers) and that quality is an important variable. Furthermore, quality is not evaluated in the same way by all people. At any point in time there will be a mix of consumers, some of whom value the quality of the service highly and some of whom see quality as less important. Hirschman then expands upon this simple observation:

That appreciation of quality—of wine, cheese, or of education for one's children—differs widely among different groups of people is surely no great discovery. It implies, however, that a given deterioration in quality will inflict very different losses (that is, different equivalent price increases) on different customers; someone who had a very high consumer surplus before deterioration precisely because he is a connoisseur and would be willing to pay, say, twice the actual price of the article at its original quality, may drop out as a customer as soon as quality deteriorates, provided a nondeteriorated competing product is available, be it at a much higher price.

Here, then is the rationale for our observation: in the case of "connoisseur goods"—and, as the example of education indicates, this category is by no means limited to quality wines—the consumers who drop out when quality declines are not necessarily the marginal consumers who would drop out if price increased, but may be intramarginal consumers with considerable consumer surplus; or, put more simply, the consumer who is rather insensitive to price increases is often likely to be highly sensitive to quality declines.

At the same time, consumers with a high consumer surplus are, for that very reason, those who have most to lose through a deterioration of the product's quality. Therefore, they are the ones who are most likely to make a fuss in case of deterioration until such time as they do exit. (1970, p. 49).

Much of Hirschman's effort is devoted to an analysis of when people choose to exit rather than use voice when they become dissatisfied with quality. The decision as to which type of response to use depends on the perceived cost and efficacy of each alternative. If good alternative organizations offer a similar service, then, unless the costs of change are too high, exit will generally be preferred. If there are no acceptable alternatives, incentives to work for change within the organization increase. Similarly, the effectiveness of the voice strategy depends on the relative power of the individual. In an organization with relatively few buyers it is substantially easier for a consumer to exert influence than it is in an organization with many independent customers. This is true both because the cost of expressing dissatisfaction is less in a small group and because voice is often backed up by the threat of exit. The more the exit will hurt the organization, the more effective the threat. It is apparent that the presence of the exit option sharply reduces the likelihood that the voice option will be used, because exit is often easier for the consumer, and because exit rids the organization of those people who are pressuring it to change.

Hirschman also introduces the concept of "loyalty." Loyalty makes the customer less likely to leave the organization, and it also may lead the individual to become more influential, thus raising the perceived effectiveness of the voice option. Loyalty thus leads to a greater reliance on the voice option than would otherwise be the case. Many factors can lead to loyalty behavior, but it is important to distinguish between conscious and unconscious loyal behavior. In the former the consumer-member is aware of the deterioration in the organization but chooses to remain, at least for a while, in the hope that things will improve. In the latter the problems are not even recognized and thus cannot lead to either voice or exit. In some organizations it may be possible to increase the amount of unconscious loyalty through the imposition of severe initiation rites. In part, this is predicted by cognitive dissonance theory. A corollary to this prediction is that while expensive or severe initiation may delay voice through unconscious loyalty, it will also make the resort to voice more active, because membership is more valuable.

Hirschman's concepts of exit, voice, and loyalty have a number of important implications for the analysis of self-selection behavior in the medical care sector. Before these are examined, it is important to consider some characteristics of providers and consumers that are relevant to the application of his model. Medical care has an important quality component for most people, and it is likely that, as with most connoisseur goods, those people who especially value the quality of care may be willing to pay substantially more than the going price. (Note that the argument here rests not on the ability of consumers to judge the true quality of medical care, but merely to know what they like and feel strongly about. In this instance much of the perceived quality probably reflects physician-patient relations rather than technical expertise.) The costs of changing providers are often considerable as it is usually difficult to get information about the quality of care offered without actually becoming a patient. (See Arrow, 1963). It is, however, substantially easier to change providers within the FFS sector than it is to change from FFS to HMO or vice versa. The difficulties in changing provider types, rather than individual physicians, stem from the

limited options, periodic enrollment schemes, and probably most importantly, the ideologies and beliefs surrounding the two systems. Individual
FFS physicians are usually termed "private physicians," in contrast to
practitioners in PGPs, even though the PGP patient may have a personal
physician.

Combining Hirschman's theory and our understanding of medical care
providers and HMOs leads to a number of predictions. First, the voice
option is unlikely to be important among patients of dispersed FFS
providers for several reasons: exit to other FFS providers is easy; the
consumer is only one of many and cannot easily organize collective action;
and communicating dissatisfaction is often difficult, especially given the
status and power of the physician. The difficulties in comparing the quality
of various providers suggests that dissatisfied consumers continue changing physicians and do not use the voice option to improve the situation.
The physicians get no clear message from the exercise of the exit option,
because new patients generally replace the old. In fact, physicians tend to
write off such behavior as "doctor-shopping," as if it conveyed no information about their practices. Second, the voice option may be of substantial
importance for people who join HMOs for several reasons. The exit option
is costly (through out-of-pocket payments) until the next time that plans
can be changed during a periodic open enrollment period. Loyalty may be
encouraged through the severe initiation of choosing an unconventional
delivery system and choosing a new provider. Voice may be more effective
in HMOs because it can be focused at a single organization, and the threat
of exit may be more powerful if voice may result in the renegotiation of
group contracts. Freidson (1973) notes the difficulties in dealing with
patients who use their influence with negotiators. Kaiser representatives
also note that "dual choice provides a means for avoiding the member
dissatisfaction that inevitably surfaces when people are captives of a system,
particularly a system they do not like" (Phelan, Erickson, and Fleming,
1970, p. 800).

The predictions lead to two implications concerning HMOs and FFS
practice. Increased availability of the voice option may lead to greater
responsiveness to consumer preferences on the part of HMOs, whether or
not there are formal roles for consumers in the organization. If there is a
consumer board, however, that influence may be more direct and more
finely tuned; for example, with a lower cost of transmitting complaints,
consumers are more likely to use voice for relatively minor issues, rather
than waiting for a major "do or die" issue. Regardless of whether or not an
HMO is more responsive to consumer demands, the great difficulties
surrounding entry and exit are likely to lead to more vocalization of
complaints, rather than constant doctor shopping. Thus consumer satisfaction surveys may be biased toward showing more complaints among HMO
members. This potential bias must be taken into consideration when
making comparisons among various provider types.

SUMMARY

Our expectations concerning HMO performance represent tendencies of behavior that may or may not be empirically significant. Such expectations also assume that everything else is held constant. But the open enrollment characteristic of HMOs implies that everything else may not be a constant; in particular, people who self-select to enroll in HMOs may well be different from those who choose not to enroll. In theory, those people who feel they have a high risk of illness and are financially vulnerable, those with particular attitudes about medical care and preventive medicine, those who seek care out of neurotic needs, and those who are not well integrated into the traditional system may be more likely to join an HMO. All of these people are likely to have greater than usual demands for some types of medical care and less demand for others, and thus may bias the data concerning HMO costs and utilization.

The theoretical presence of a potential bias is enough to cause us to be careful when interpreting data. Moreover, this concern is bolstered by evidence that supports the risk-vulnerability hypothesis—a somewhat greater orientation toward prevention on the part of HMO enrollees and a somewhat lower level of integration into the medical care system prior to joining and different patterns of utilization prior to enrolling.

A second aspect of self-selection deals with decisions to leave an organization, rather than work for change within. An application of the theory concerning exit, voice, and loyalty suggests that while unsatisfied patients of solo FFS practitioners are likely to move on from one physician to the next, causing little change in the system, unsatisfied HMO enrollees are likely to be much more vocal about their dissatisfaction and also to try to change the organization.

FOUR

Overall Measures of Cost and Utilization: Total Expenditures, Out-of-Pocket Costs, and the Number and Mix of Services

The most common question raised about HMOs is, do they save money? While this seems to be a simple question, the answer is very complex, and it accounts for most of this book. To begin to answer the question, one first must examine the questions of costs from a global perspective. It is relatively easy to exhibit "cost savings" by shifting the responsibility of certain costs to other parties. Yet, from an overall perspective, this does not really lower costs and may even raise them because of additional administrative costs.

This chapter will focus on overall measures of the financial aspects of HMOs. The total cost of a medical-care system may be examined from two perspectives: that of society and that of the consumer. The social perspective is concerned with the total cost of care, including all premiums, copayments, and costs for out-of-plan use. (The social view also includes an evaluation of nonfinancial costs and externalities, but these additional issues will be discussed in later chapters.) The consumer as a citizen shares the social concern for total costs, but the consumer as an enrollee may be concerned only with out-of-pocket costs and that portion of the premium not covered by the employer. One level below that of total expenditures is the composition of expenditures, that is, the number and mix of services provided by HMOs and the conventional system. Even if total expenditures were the same, people might prefer a system that emphasizes ambulatory care over a system that emphasizes hospital care.

TOTAL HEALTH CARE EXPENDITURES

The first step in obtaining an overall picture of HMO performance with respect to costs is a comparison of the total annual expenditures for health care by people enrolled in different plans. When making this comparison it is important to combine the premium and out-of-pocket expenses to obtain the total costs to the individual. Such results are relatively difficult to obtain because they require household surveys to determine the cost of out-of-plan utilization. Table 4–1 presents comparative data on the total yearly costs of medical care under alternative plans.

A number of important caveats must be remembered when examining these data. First, it must be emphasized that we have a limited ability to generalize these results, because in five of the six cases the major HMO is a Kaiser-Permanente plan. In some instances data are available for other HMOs, including IPAs, but the California experience dominates. Second, these data are best interpreted as crude estimates of cost that do not adjust for differences in the populations that join the various plans—the self-selection issue. Studies two, three, five, and six involve comparisons of costs for people who chose from among all the plans mentioned, while the Hetherington, Hopkins, and Roemer study, number four, involved samples of members of the different plans, rather than applying an employer/employee base. Third, the Columbia University study involved geographically distinct members of blue-collar unions. These differences in the populations under study have implications both for the self-selection and population-mix issue and for the role of competition among plans.

These six studies all indicate lower total costs of medical care for PGP members. Yearly costs for BC-BS enrollees are from 16 to 88 percent higher than for enrollees in the lowest cost PGP under study, be it Kaiser or GH. Enrollees in the major medical-indemnity plans have an intermediate position, with costs that range from 5 to 48 percent above Kaiser enrollees. Data for another prepaid group practice, Ross-Loos, indicate enrollee expenditures about 15 percent above those of Kaiser in both the 1973 Dozier and Hetherington, Hopkins, and Roemer studies, and 6 percent above Kaiser enrollees in the 1964 Dozier study.* The Dozier studies also provide two estimates of enrollee medical care costs in IPAs. In 1962–63 these were close to the level of BC-BS enrollees, 27 percent above the Kaiser level; while in 1970–71 they were in a more intermediate position, 24 percent above Kaiser.

Some differences in the findings of the various studies are attributable to differences in what is included in the measure of total cost. For instance, the Hetherington, Hopkins and Roemer data include only out-of-pocket expenses for doctor and hospital bills, while the Wolfman and 1973 Dozier studies are much more comprehensive and include diagnostic tests, drugs, and eyeglasses. The Hetherington, Hopkins, and Roemer data can also be computed using two different premium measures (See Note *d* to Table 4-1.) But neither of these differences explains the much larger observed

---

*The increasingly higher costs for Ross-Loos enrollees may be a reflection of a long-term policy of no growth. From the early 1950s to the mid-1970s overall enrollment remained nearly constant at about 135,000. This may have led to an increasingly aged and less healthy population relative to comparison groups.

Table 4-1 Yearly Medical Care Expenses by Type of Health Insurance Plan

	Premium	Direct Costs	Total	Ratio of Total Cost to Minimum Total Cost
Blue-collar union members, expenditures/person, 1958[a]				
Blue Cross-Blue Shield—New Jersey	$ 38	$ 51	$ 89	1.25
Major Medical—several midwestern cities	5-38	44	79-82	1.11-1.15
Kasier-Northern California	39	32	71	1.00
United Auto Workers' members, Oakland, California, dual-choice option, expenditures/person, 1959[b]				
Blue Cross-Blue Shield	$ 58	$ 63	$121	1.27
Kaiser-Northern California	57	38	95	1.00
California state employees, multiple-choice option, expenditures per typical person in a typical family, 1962-63[c]				
Cal-Western-Occidental (Indemnity Plan)	$ 57	$ 47	$104	1.12
Blue Cross-Blue Shield	71	50	121	1.30
Kasier-Northern and Southern California regions	71	22	93	1.00
Ross-Loos (PGP)	68	31	99	1.06
Foundations for Medical Care	77	41	118	1.27
Enrollees in six Southern California plans (not multiple choice), expenditures per person, 1967-68[d]				
Large commercial	$104	$ 79	$183	1.48
Small commercial	91	69	160	1.29
Hospital sponsored (Blue Cross)	127	108	235	1.90
Physician sponsored (Blue Shield)	157	74	231	1.86
Large group (Kaiser)	111	13	124	1.00
Small group (Ross-Loos)	92	50	142	1.15

California state employees, basic plan, multiple-choice option, expenditures per person, 1970-71[e]

Indemnity plans			
Blue Cross-Blue Shield—statewide	$176	$102	$74	1.03
Kaiser—Northern and Southern California	242	161	81	1.42
Ross-Loos and Family Health Plan (PGPs)	171	136	35	1.00
Foundations for Medical Care	199	139	60	1.16
	218	128	90	1.27

Low-income residents of Seattle Model Cities Area, dual-choice option, costs per person, 1971-74[f]

King County Medical/Blue Cross	$279	—	—	1.52
Group Health Cooperative of Puget Sound	184	—	—	1.00

[a] Columbia University, 1962a, p. 177. These data are adjusted for price differences in the three regions. The relative weights are New Jersey, 111; Midwest, 100; and California, 125.

[b] Wolfman, 1961, p. 1187. Out-of-pocket expenses include hospital and physician charges, prescribed drugs, laboratory and X-ray, household drugs, and other medical services, primarily eyeglasses. Data were given for families and converted to a per capita basis, using average family sizes of 3.8 for Kaiser and 3.4 for Blue Cross.

[c] Dozier et al., 1964, p. 77. These data refer to a typical family of one employee and three dependents and are developed from individual data for employees and covered dependents. Costs include physician services, in-hospital care, and prescription drugs, if the patient saw the physician within the questionnaire period. Excluded are dental care, eyeglasses, and nonprescription drugs. Costs associated with maternity care are also excluded.

[d] Hetherington, Hopkins, and Roemer, 1975, pp. 204, 233. Hetherington, Hopkins, and Roemer do not name the plans in their study, but their descriptive information provides sufficient data to identify four of the six. Two sets of data are presented concerning premium costs. Those shown in the table are derived from the out-of-pocket and total expense data shown on pages 204 and 223, respectively. Annual premium costs per family are given on page 64, and converting these to per person rates (using the family size data on page 66) yields the following premium estimates: $73, $71, $90, $108, $88, $70 for the six plans. While these are substantially lower than the other data, they are in the same pattern, and do not alter the overall rankings or relative expenses in each plan.

[e] Dozier et al., 1973, pp. 44, 99. The total costs, out-of-pocket, and premium costs are derived from the weighted average of premium cost per family (p. 99) and average family size (p. 44) for basic plan employees and their beneficiaries only.

[f] McCaffree et al., 1976, p. III-52. These are "experience-rated" costs and include claims paid under a coordination of benefits provision between the Prepaid Project and KCM-BC. KCM-BC administrative costs of about 9 percent are included as are GH administrative costs. Both plans offered very comprehensive benefit packages with no copayments. The cost figures, however, do not include any out-of-plan expenditures. About 10 percent of all visits reported by GH enrollees were to non-GH providers, and it is estimated that out-of-plan costs amount to about 5 percent of total GH costs. KCM-BC enrollees also used some out-of-plan services at free clinics or through Medicaid (McCaffree et al., 1976, p. III-61). If the figures in this table are age-sex adjusted, the differential is reduced by less than 2 percent.

difference in expenses for enrollees in the plans in the Hetherington, Hopkins, and Roemer study, with BC-BS enrollee expenditures being nearly 90 percent above those of Kaiser enrollees. It is possible that the sample design used by Hetherington, Hopkins, and Roemer accounts for a substantial part of the differential, because most of the BC-BS enrollees were not in a dual-choice situation. This problem in interpreting their data should be remembered in later analysis.

One additional set of data that is relevant to the question of total expenditures derives from the experience of Medicare beneficiaries (Corbin and Krute, 1975; Weil, 1976; Goss, 1975). Data are available for Medicare reimbursements to enrollees in seven PGPs across the country and for other Medicare beneficiaries residing in the same counties, but the data do not include direct, out-of-pocket expenditures. However, given the relatively complete coverage offered by Medicare, it is useful to examine the results as outlined in Table 4-2. (Similar findings are available for 1969.) With the exception of the two New York PGPs, Medicare reimbursements were lower for PGP enrollees than for the control groups. The average savings was 13 percent for all seven plans. The primary source of these savings was in lower reimbursements for inpatient services. This more than compensated for higher expenditures for physician and related services. It should be noted that none of the plans was at risk for all medical care costs. Instead, they received capitation payments to cover in-plan physicians' services only. In addition, the beneficiaries retained their usual Medicare coverage for out-of-plan services and hospitalization. Thus the observed "savings" are primarily reflective of different practice patterns by physicians in HMOs, rather than specific HMO incentives.

The substantially lower costs for Kaiser and GH enrollees are crucial findings for policy purposes. It must be remembered, however, that cost *differences* are not the same as cost *savings* because of the self-selection factor. The Seattle Model Cities Project data allow a rough estimate of the potential impact of self-selection. Table 4-3 presents the results of a crude adjustment of KCM-BC costs in Year I of the project to reflect differential utilization patterns of KCM-BC and Group Health enrollees prior to the study. The raw figures show nearly 50 percent higher costs for enrollees in KCM-BC, but after adjusting for higher preenrollment admission and outpatient utilization rates, the differential is narrowed to 25 percent. This suggests that half the apparent "savings" may be attributable to self-selection. (Moreover, as indicated in the note to Table 4-3, this estimate is probably conservative.) While this is a potentially important finding, before resorting to generalization, the reader should consider the discussion in Chapter 3 concerning the crucial role of enrollment options and context. The first-year experience of any cohort is likely to show a much larger self-selection effect than would be the case with comparisons of the total, predominantly long-term enrollments in various plans.

Theoretical considerations led to the prediction that HMOs would lower

Table 4-2 Medicare Reimbursements per Beneficiary in Prepaid Group Practices and Comparison Populations, 1970

	Medicare Reimbursement per Beneficiary			PGP Reimbursement as a Proportion of Control Reimbursement[b]		
	All[a] Services	Inpatient Hospital	Physicians	All[a] Services	Inpatient Hospital	Physicians
Union Family Medical Fund, New York City	$507	$313	$175	104%	95%	125%
Health Insurance Plan of Greater New York	431	254	161	102	91	126
Kaiser-Southern California	388	200	149	94	77	115
Kaiser-Northern California	331	186	123	82	72	102
Community Health Association-Detroit	312	189	110	78	66	113
Kaiser-Oregon	226	107	95	67	48	113
Group Health Cooperative of Puget Sound	196	90	95	66	47	110
Average	$342	$191	$130	87%	73%	116%

SOURCE. Corbin and Krute, March 1975, p. 7.

[a] Includes extended care facility, hospital outpatient, and home health services.

[b] Reimbursements for each control group are adjusted to the age-sex distribution of the matched PGP.

Table 4-3   Annual Medical Care Costs for Enrollees in the Seattle Model Cities Project Adjusted to Reflect Different Preenrollment Utilization Patterns

	Group Health	KCM-BC	KCM-BC÷ Group Health	KCM-BC÷ Expected KCM-BC
Hospitalization				
Preenrollment admission rate/1000	104	132	1.27	
Year I Hospital cost/person	$48.94	$103.17	2.11	
Year I Inpatient physician cost	6.44	26.31	4.09	
Year I Total inpatient cost	$55.38	$129.48	2.34	$101.95
Ambulatory care				
Preenrollment physician visits/month	0.372	0.415	1.12	
Year I Outpatient professional cost	$64.88	$64.50	.99	
Year I Outpatient prescription drugs	14.29	19.61	1.37	
Year I Emergency room	13.53	8.34	.62	
	$92.70	$92.45	1.00	82.54
Total costs				
Actual	$148.08	$221.93	1.499	
Adjusted for higher preenrollment utilization among KCM-BC enrollees	148.08	184.49	1.245	

SOURCE.   McCaffree et al., pp. III – 15; Richardson et al., 1976, pp. I – 136, I – 139.
NOTES.   The expected costs for KCM-BC enrollees are computed by dividing their actual Year I costs by the appropriate ratio of preenrollment utilization (e.g., $101.95 = $129.48/1.27). For hospitalization, this may be a rather conservative adjustment, because only admission rates are taken into consideration. The Year I admission rate for KCM-BC enrollees was 1.47 times that of GH enrollees, but the KCM-BC patient-day rate, which includes length of stay differentials, was 2.11 times that of GH (Diehr et al., 1976, pp. II – 108, II – 187). The current adjustment assumes that prior to the experiment the two groups of enrollees had identical lengths of stay and differed only in their admission rates. If the LOS for KCM-BC enrollees prior to enrollment was also 27 percent higher, their expected inpatient costs are only $80.42 = 129.48/1.61, and their total costs are only 10 percent above those of the Group Health enrollees.

the total costs of medical care. It is impossible to test this prediction rigorously with these data, because the populations are self-selected, and there is no way to determine precisely what fraction of the observed lower costs are due to the HMOs, rather than to their particular populations. Furthermore, while in each instance for which there are complete data, the Kaiser plans and GH had the lowest costs, results for the other HMOs were mixed. Ross-Loos, a prepaid group practice, had costs that were 15 to 16 percent higher than Kaiser, but they were still lower than any other plan except for the indemnity plans in the 1973 Dozier study. The IPAs fared considerably worse, with costs 24 to 30 percent above those of Kaiser enrollees. This places them at or near the top of the range.

OUT-OF-POCKET COSTS

The major reason for examining total costs is to obtain an estimate of the cost to society for providing medical care; when the focus shifts to the effects on consumers, out-of-pocket costs become a major concern. Thus one must not only consider the magnitude of medical care costs but also who pays for them. The primary reason for the analysis of cost distribution is one of consumer utility and welfare. This raises two questions: (1) what is the appropriate unit of observation? and (2) what costs are relevant, and do they all count equally?

In the data concerning the total costs of care, the individual was used as the unit of observation wherever possible. However, it must be recognized that the choice of the individual rather than of the family was not unambiguous. Health insurance policies rarely are designed with more than three steps (self, self plus dependent, self plus two or more dependents), so the per capita premium cost drops for large families. On the other hand, total costs for health care rise with family size. However, marginal costs for extra family members tend to be low, because larger families are composed mostly of children, who tend to require relatively inexpensive medical care. (See Cooper and Worthington, 1972.) Thus plans with a disproportionately high number of large families will have higher total costs per family and lower total costs per person than would otherwise be the case. When the interest is focused on well-being, it is probably reasonable to consider the family as the decision-making unit. This is particularly true in the case of health insurance, which often has family rates and is obtained through the place of employment of the primary worker. The choice of unit is still not unambiguous, because within any one year, larger families are statistically more likely to have someone with a major illness.* In some sense, what is desirable is a well-being measure that is independent of family size. Unfortunately, none exists, and we must use various measures, such as costs per family and costs as a percentage of family income.

The second question concerns what costs are relevant to the family's welfare. Should they be long-run or short-run costs? Most economic analyses show that almost all costs of employer-purchased health insurance

---

*Keeler, Relles, and Rolph (1977), however, indicate that when the family's out-of-pocket risk is considered after taking into account deductibles and copayments, there is little difference in the standard deviation of payments under either family or individual deductibles.

eventually are borne by labor. (See Mitchell and Phelps, 1976.) Thus, in the long run, the employee pays the full cost of health care—the total premium, plus direct costs, as shown in Table 4−1. However, it may be that employees are conscious only of the net premium cost to them, that is, the portion that the employer does *not* pay (Krizay and Wilson, 1974). Thus a second figure of interest is the out-of-pocket premium cost for the worker; this may be a uniform proportion of the total premium, or it may be what remains after the employer pays a fixed amount per worker. The measurement of direct costs also is subject to long-run and short-run considerations. In the long run, an average family can expect to pay in direct out-of-pocket costs the average amount paid by a large group of similar families, as shown in column 2 of Table 4−1. However, an important aspect of medical expenses is that they are not uniform and, in fact, can vary a great deal. Most people are willing to pay someone else to average out the variation in medical costs, hence the development of health insurance (Arrow, 1963). Thus it is reasonable to expect that if two plans involve the same average direct cost and one has a greater variance than the other, consumers will prefer the one with the lower variance. Table 4-4 presents some data concerning both premium costs borne by the family and the distribution of direct costs. The available data suggest that HMOs not only are associated with lower overall expenditures, but they sharply reduce both the average direct cost to the consumer and the variation in cost.

The unadjusted data concerning out-of-pocket expenditures per family in the Columbia University study indicate substantially lower expenditures for Kaiser members than for people in the Blue Cross or major medical plans. Adjusting these data for differences in the cost of medical care in the three regions widens the differential between Kaiser and the other plans. With either the adjusted or unadjusted data, the differential is statistically significant at better than the 5 percent level. Adjustment for family size widens the difference. Distribution of families by expenditure levels also indicates that Kaiser enrollees had a lower probability of large expenditures.

In the study of United Auto Workers, overall premiums for Blue Cross and Kaiser were relatively close, and the employer paid half the premium cost of each; so the net extra premium per Kaiser family was $10 per year.* The lower average total costs per Kaiser family more than make up for this difference. Of more interest is the distribution of expenditures; the

---

*The arguments concerning the shifting of the cost of employer-paid health insurance to the workers refers to the average cost. Employers are unlikely to hire workers differentially based on their prospective choice of health insurance plan. Thus, to the extent that the premium costs are shifted back equally, the Blue Cross enrollees are implicitly subsidizing the Kaiser enrollees. This is not the case when the employer pays a fixed amount per worker regardless of the choice of plan.

Table 4-4   Measures of Out-of-Pocket Costs for Premiums and Direct Charges by Type of Health Insurance Plan

Blue Collar Union Members and Their Families: Out-of-Pocket Expenditures per Family, 1958[a]

Distribution of Families by Expenditures Not Covered by Plan under Study	Blue Cross-Blue Shield New Jersey	General Electric Plan Major Medical	Kaiser—Northern California
Under $50	29%	30%	39%
$50-99	18	21	20
100-199	26	26	23
200-299	11	12	8
300-399	10	8	5
500 and over	5	3	4
Mean out-of-pocket expenditure	$161	$137	$126
Mean out-of-pocket expenditure per person	55	44	40

United Auto Workers and Their Families, 1959: Cost per Family[b]

	Blue Cross	Kaiser
Average Total Premium	$198	$217
Average Net Premium	99	109
Total out-of-pocket costs		
Average	$312	$255
Range	$93-1646	$84-774
Proportion of families in each category:		
$0-199	37%	40%
200-299	19	30
300-399	22	20
400-499	9	2
500+	13	7
Out-of-pocket cost as a percent of family income		
Average Percent	5.3	4.3
Range	1—38%	1-17%
Proportion of families in each category:		
1.0-2.4%	20%	28%
2.5-4.4%	29	35
4.5-6.4%	29	22
6.5-8.4%	9	6
8.5-10.4%	7	5
10.5% and over	6	3

continued

Table 4-4 (cont.)

California State Employees and Dependents, 1962-63 [c]

	Statewide Service Plans	Indemnity Plans	Prepaid Group Practices	Individual Practice Associations
Distribution of extra Charges for Out-of-Hospital Care for People Who Used Such Services, and mean cost per user, Jan-Mar 1963				
$0	0.0%	0.4%	0.1%	0.4%
1-9	36.1	42.2	88.8	45.7
10-24	37.7	33.2	6.7	36.3
25-49	16.4	17.4	1.2	11.8
50-99	6.5	5.2	1.3	4.5
100+	3.3	1.6	1.9	1.2
Mean Cost Per User	**$24.44**	**$19.09**	**$7.61**	**$16.56**
Distribution of extra Charges for In-hospital Care for People Who Used Such Services, and mean cost per user, July 1962-Mar 1963 (Except for Maternity Care)				
$0	11.8%	10.6%	63.0%	21.1%
1-24	19.2	12.3	20.6	32.7
25-49	16.5	11.7	4.3	21.1
50-99	18.0	28.2	2.6	11.5
100-299	22.7	27.3	4.8	3.9
300-499	6.0	6.2	0.6	3.9
500-999	5.1	2.8	1.7	5.8
1000+	0.7	0.9	2.4	—
Mean Cost Per User	**$129.39**	**$119.12**	**$63.53**	**$80.51**

Enrollees in Southern California Health Insurance Plans, 1967-68 [d]

Distributions of Annual Out-of-Pocket Expenses and Annual Premiums per Person

	Large Commercial	Small Commercial	Blue Cross	Blue Shield	Kaiser	Ross-Loos
$1-75	14.8%	22.7%	7.1%	12.4%	19.2%	22.9%
$75-150	46.6	36.8	34.1	37.8	62.9	48.1
$150-225	17.3	16.3	26.6	17.4	10.6	15.7
$225+	21.3	24.2	32.2	32.4	7.2	13.3
Mean	$183.32	$159.79	$234.62	$230.42	$123.61	$141.88
Coefficient of Variation	117	78	84	80	56	75

Medical Expenditure as a Percentage of Family Income

	Commercial	Provider	Group Practice
	6.6%	7.1%	3.8%

Distributions of Annual Out-of-Pocket Expenses per Family for 3-4 Person Families

	Commercial	Provider	Group Practice
$0	42.8	18.5	55.8
1-49	7.1	11.0	24.9
50-99	7.7	15.2	4.7
100-249	16.2	18.1	4.7
250-499	10.2	20.4	3.5
500-749	13.7	7.8	5.8
750-1000	1.3	7.7	0.3
1000+	0.9	1.3	0.4
Average Direct Expenses	$178	$266	$72

[a] Columbia University School of Public Health and Administrative Medicine, 1962a, pages 24, 52, 81, 113. These out-of-pocket expenditure figures are not adjusted for price differences and thus differ from those shown in Table 4-1.
[b] Wolfman, 1961, Tables 1, 3, 4. See also the note to Table 4-1 of this book.
[c] Dozier et al., 1968, pp. 66-67. These data refer to the distribution of out-of-pocket expenditures per individual and represent the combined data for employees and dependents with the exception of in-hospital care for FMC enrollees, where only data for dependents are available. The experience of annuitants in the various plans is not included. The data are only available for groupings of plans; however, the individual plans shown in Table 4-1 dominate the enrollment in each group. The BC-BS plans represent 94.6 percent of the statewide service plan beneficiaries; Cal-Western Occidental accounts for 95.9 percent of indemnity plan beneficiaries; Kaiser accounts for 84.2 percent beneficiaries, with Ross-Loos having another 9.2 percent (see page 34 in Dozier et al., 1968). See also the note to Table 4-1.
[d] Hetherington, Hopkins, and Roemer, 1975, pp. 223, 232; and Roemer et al., 1972, p. 68. See also note to Table 4-1. Note that these data do not distinguish between premiums paid by the employee or by others; the total premium cost is included in the estimates. The data in the last part of this section refer only to direct expenses, not premiums. The three categories of insurance plans are merely aggregates of the six individual plans shown above.

maximum out-of-pocket cost for a Kaiser family was less than half that of the maximum Blue Cross family.† Furthermore, only 9 percent of the Kaiser families had expenditures in excess of $400, while 22 percent of the Blue Cross families had expenditures of that magnitude. Data for out-of-pocket cost as a percentage of famly income mirror these results. For instance, only 14 percent of the Kaiser families, versus 22 percent of the Blue Cross families, had medical expenses exceeding 6.5 percent of their income.

Data for California state employees and their dependents refer only to people who used services in the specified time periods. For out-of-hospital care within a three-month period, most people have only minor out-of-pocket expenses, but 89 percent of the PGP enrollees had expenses of less than $10, a proportion nearly twice that of the other plan types. Furthermore, only 4.4 percent of the PGP users had expenses exceeding $25, in contrast to 17.5 to 26.1 percent of the other enrollees. This reflects the more extensive ambulatory coverage of the PGPs. IPA enrollees tend to have lower out-of-pocket expenses than those in the service and indemnity plans, but not as low as those in the PGPs. Distribution of expenses for IPA enrollees is also in an intermediate position. The patterns for out-of-pocket hospital expenses are even more striking; almost two-thirds of the PGP enrollees with a hospital episode had no out-of-pocket expense, in contrast to about one-tenth of the service and indemnity enrollees and one-fifth of the IPA enrollees.

These results are subject to a number of biases. The exclusion of maternity stays works against plans such as Kaiser, which have relatively complete maternity coverage. (The other PGPs have shallow maternity coverage similar to that of the other plans.) It is not known how many employees also have major medical supplementary insurance, which would cover many of their out-of-pocket expenses. Not many PGP enrollees would be expected to have such coverage. The third source of bias is that some people in plans with two-visit deductibles probably did not report these visits (Dozier et al., 1968). And although different sampling ratios were used to give samples of about the same size for each of the first three plan types, even a 100 percent sample of IPA enrollees yielded a sample that was still only one-third the size of the others (856 people). The smaller sample lowers the probability of finding people with very large expenses.

Hetherington, Hopkins, and Roemer's data for enrollees in six Southern California health plans have the advantage of offering a comparison of distributions for both families and individuals. For the total of direct expenses and premiums per person, PGPs have very few people with large expenditures. Of more interest is the rather low coefficient of variation for Kaiser enrollees, which suggests that not only are their average costs the

---

†One hundred families were interviewed for each plan, so there is an equal probability of very large expenditures.

lowest, but they have less risk of large payments as well. Comparison of distributions for families and individuals suggests that the results using the two measures are comparable. In fact, Hetherington, Hopkins, and Roemer's data give the proportions of individuals with out-of-pocket expenditures of $75 or more as 27.0, 33.1, and 6.0 percent in commercial, provider-sponsored, and group practice plans, respectively (Hetherington, Hopkins, and Roemer, 1975, p. 206). If $250+ is taken as a comparable cutoff for a family of three to four, then the data in Table 4-3 indicate proportions of 26.1, 37.2, and 10.0 percent, respectively.

In the previous chapter it was pointed out that there are no theoretical reasons to expect HMO enrollees to have lower out-of-pocket costs, although this is likely to be the case, given the usual differences in coverage. The data presented in this section support that discussion. Enrollees in both PGPs (Kaiser and Ross-Loos) and the IPAs have lower out-of-pocket costs. Not only are the average costs per person and per family lower, but the distribution of costs indicates that HMO enrollees have a substantially lower risk of large expenses. As was the case with total expenditures, the situation for IPA enrollees is not nearly as good as that for PGP enrollees, but average out-of-pocket costs, especially the risk of large costs, are substantially lower for IPA enrollees than for BC-BS and indemnity enrollees.

Again, it must be remembered that the data upon which these findings rest come from only a few plans, and many factors other than payment schemes may influence the results. They are, however, consistent with the argument that HMO enrollees can obtain substantial financial savings.

THE NUMBER AND MIX OF SERVICES

The preceding two sections demonstrated that, at least for those plans for which data are available, both total and out-of-pocket costs for HMO enrollees are lower than comparable costs for enrollees in other insurance plans. How does this cost differential arise? In Chapter 2 I predicted that the major source of the "savings" will come from fewer units of service and, in particular, less hospitalization.* It also was suggested that, whenever possible, HMOs tend to substitute less expensive care for more expensive ways of accomplishing the same end. This raises a knotty problem, because it implies that not only are some ambulatory visits potential substitutes for hospital visits, but there may be more or less expensive (or service intensive) ways to provide ambulatory and hospital visits. Thus we must examine the content as well as the mere number of visits. An overall measure of the volume of services can be obtained by using a constant index of cost to

---

*"Savings" is in quotes because it is still not known how much of the cost-utilization differential is attributable to HMO incentives and how much results from self-selection and other factors.

weight the services provided to enrollees in each plan. This is different from a total cost measure, because it uses the same weights (which need not be dollars), and thus does not confuse service mix differences with pricing differences. The choice of an index, however, is the subject of some controversy. All existing indices are based on Relative Value Studies, which in turn reflect patterns of FFS charges. These charges bear little relation to time or effort, and using them tends to give disproportionate weight to tests and procedures (Blumberg, 1977; Showstack et al., 1979).

Table 4-5 presents data from the two studies available that use a constant set of weights to compare the volume of services used by enrollees in various plans. The Anderson-Sheatsley study compares the costs and use of care by members of three trade unions and their families who had a dual choice option between Group Health Insurance, Inc. (GHI) and HIP of New York. Contrary to its name, GHI allows its members free physician choice and reimburses participating physicians on an FFS basis in accordance with a fixed fee schedule. It essentially provides Blue Shield type coverage for all kinds of physician services. HIP provides services to its members through specific group practices (see Chapter 1). Members of both plans have the same Blue Cross coverage for hospital benefits. Anderson and Sheatsley used the GHI fee schedule to value the services rendered to HIP enrollees. Their results indicate significantly lower costs for hospitalization and only slightly lower costs for physician services for HIP enrollees. Within the latter category, HIP enrollees had significantly lower utilization of surgical services but higher utilization of nonsurgical, nonobstetric services.

The Hetherington, Hopkins, and Roemer survey of enrollees in six plans includes estimates of the volume of phsycians' services. These data were drawn from the medical records of each person, and each service was translated into the units of the California Relative Value Study (CRVS). The CRVS is developed from a broad survey of physicians' fees for carefully defined procedures and is designed to measure the relative charge of each procedure with respect to a common denominator, such as a routine office visit. (See Brewster and Seldowitz, 1965; Showstack et al., 1979.) The CRVS has different scales for different types of services, such as medicine, surgery, anesthesia, laboratory, and radiology. Hetherington, Hopkins, and Roemer combine these scales using the average observed charge per unit of service. Thus their "units of medical care" approximate dollar volume of services. Excluded from the analysis are hospital room and board charges, private nurse charges, and other services not included in the CRVS. Examination of the mean number of units of care per person indicates conflicting results with respect to the two HMOs. Kaiser enrollees have the lowest per capita use (74.8) and Ross-Loos enrollees the highest (115.8). Closer examination of the data reveals substantial differences in the proportion of people with any use of the system. For people who reported some use of services, the two PGPs have the lowest volume of

Table 4-5   Comparisons of the Total Volume of Services Received by Enrollees in Various Health Insurance Plans

Members of Three New York Trade Unions, 1956-57[a]

	GHI	HIP	HIP–GHI Difference
"Gross hospital costs" per individual	$23	$13	$ –10**
"Gross physician costs" per individual	50	47	– 3
Hospitalized surgery	(11)	(5)	– 6**
Obstetrics services	(3)	(2)	– 1
Office surgery	(2)	(2)	0
Other physicians' costs	(34)	(39)	+ 5

Enrollees in Southern California Health Insurance Plans, 1967-68[b]

Units of Medical Care per Person per Year	Large Commercial	Small Commercial	Blue Cross	Blue Shield	Kaiser	Ross-Loos
None	47.8%	35.5%	33.4%	19.3%	18.8%	9.8%
1-74	20.2	25.9	27.1	54.9	47.3	51.2
75+	32.0	38.5	39.6	25.7	33.9	39.0
Mean number of units	81.9	93.4	104.8	107.5	74.8	115.8
Mean for people with services	140.7	144.8	157.4	133.2	92.1	128.4

[a] Anderson and Sheatsley, 1959, pp. 18, 90. The double asterisk (**) means that the difference in costs is significant at the .01 level.
[b] Hetherington, Hopkins, and Roemer, 1975, p. 108.

services per person. Although this adjustment is not entirely valid because the effects of the plans should be measured with respect to all people, not just users, the problem of faulty recall raises questions about the unadjusted data. If people did not report any visits in the questionnaire part of the study, the team had no way of locating the medical records for people in the nongroup plans.

The data from the Seattle Model Cities Project reproduced in Table 4-3 support the Anderson-Sheatsley findings. Although these figures are based on charges for the KCM-BC enrollees and costs for the GH enrollees, the major subsets probably approximate costs. These data indicate identical ambulatory care costs for the two enrollee groups and hospital costs for the KCM-BC enrollees that are more than twice those for the GH enrollees. Put another way, the overall per capita cost for the GH enrollees is about one-third lower, and all of the difference is attributable to the lower hospitalization costs.

In summary, then, the data suggest a lower volume of services provided to PGP members, which is independent of price differences. There are no data for IPA enrollees. The Anderson-Sheatsley and Seattle studies suggest that substantial savings accrue primarily from lower hospitalization costs and in-hospital surgeons' fees. HIP enrollees actually had more use of other physicians' services. The Hetherington, Hopkins, and Roemer results show unambiguously lower use of physicians' services for Kaiser enrollees; however, the interpretation of the use of physicians' services in Ross-Loos depends on whether services are counted per enrollee or per enrollee who used some care.

SUMMARY

This chapter is designed to set the stage for subsequent analyses of cost and utilization. As such, it addresses the general question of whether costs are lower for HMO enrollees, and if so, in what areas. It does not attempt an investigation of *why* cost and utilization might be lower. Although evidence is available from only a small number of studies, it consistently shows prepaid group practices as having the lowest total (premium plus out-of-pocket) costs. However, there is substantial variation among PGPs in relation to costs. The data also suggest that enrollees in individual practice associations have among the highest costs. Examination of out-of-pocket expenditures shows an even greater advantage for HMO enrollees. Members of both PGPs and IPAs had lower average out-of-pocket costs and substantially less variation in these costs, suggesting a lower risk of large expenditures, and consequently greater peace of mind. As was the case before, PGP performance seems to be better than that of IPAs, but the differences are not as clear.

A final examination of data from three studies indicates that the mix of services within PGPs is more heavily weighted toward ambulatory care than hospitalization. Apparent differences in total expenditures may be traced to lower hospitalization rates. The next three chapters explore this conjecture in more detail. Chapter 5 examines differences in hospital utilization, and Chapter 6 does the same for ambulatory care. Chapter 7 addresses the question of whether HMOs realize savings in producing specific types of services.

FIVE

Hospital Utilization

Both the expectations derived from theoretical considerations in Chapter 2 and the empirical evidence on the number and mix of services from Chapter 4 suggest that hospital utilization is the primary focus of HMO attempts to control costs. Because hospital utilization is measured by days of inpatient care per 1000 persons per year, it can be influenced by admission rates, length of stay (LOS) per admission, or both. If differences occur in either admission rates or length of stay, in what categories do these occur? For instance, not all admissions are equally necessary; some categories of admissions are more likely than others to be a discretionary response to patient or physician preferences. Similarly, hospitalization on the first day after a heart attack generally is less discretionary than on the twenty-first day.

This chapter first examines the data concerning total hospitalization rates for HMO enrollees and comparison groups of people in conventional systems. The second section examines the data on length of stay. The third section raises the question of what accounts for the observed differences in admission rates. Its two major subsections examine, in turn, broad categories of admissions, such as medical versus surgical, and more detailed categories of admissions that may be considered relatively discretionary. A final section offers a brief summary.

HOSPITALIZATION

The difficulty in testing the expectation that HMOs lower hospitalization rates is that it is impossible to perform controlled trials to determine whether HMOs can, in fact, reduce hospitalization rates. Instead, data must be drawn from a wide variety of natural and not-so-natural experiments that generally do not hold everything else constant. What we cannot have in pure quality, however, may be offset by a large number of comparisons between HMOs and other providers. Table 5–1 presents the results of twenty-six studies that provide a total of fifty-seven such comparisons with experience as far back as 1951. It is necessary to maintain controls over the

Table 5−1   Hospital Utilization by Type of Health Insurance Plan, 1951−1975

Study	Days/1000 Enrollees	Admissions or Discharges/ 1000 Enrollees	Average Length of Stay
A. HIP Enrollees vs. New York City Population, 1951[1] (Committee for the Special Research Project in HIP, 1957)			
HIP (quasi-HMO)	780	74	10.6
New York City, all persons	780	67	11.6
New York City, insured	540	62	8.6
New York City, uninsured	1050	75	14.0
B. Insured and Uninsured in Windsor, Ontario, 1954[2] (Darsky, Sinai, Axelrod, 1962)			
Windsor Medical Service, Ontario (FMC)	1595	186	8.6
Windsor, Ontario, other insured	1650	192	8.6
Windsor, Ontario, uninsured	762	65	11.7
C. HIP and BC-BS members, 1955[3] (Densen, Balamuth, Shapiro, 1958)			
HIP-Blue Cross	588	77 (81)[a]	7.6
Blue Shield-Blue Cross	688	96 (94)[a]	7.2
D. Union Members with dual choice, 1957 (age-sex adjusted)[4] (Densen et al., 1960)			
HIP-Blue Cross	744	70	10.4
GHI-Blue Cross	955	88	10.8
E. HIP and GHI enrollees, dual choice option (age-sex adjusted), 1957[5] (Anderson and Sheatsley, 1959)			
HIP-Blue Cross	408**	63**	6.5[b]
GHI-Blue Cross	791**	107**	7.4[b]
F. Steelworkers in several parts of the country, 1958[6] (Falk and Senturia, 1960)			
Kaiser-Permanente	570[c]	90[c]	6.3[c]
BC-BS	1032	135	7.6
Commercial insurance	1167	150	7.8
G. Members of District 65 of Retail, Wholesale and Department Store Union, dual choice enrollment (age-sex adjusted), 1958[7] (Densen et al., 1962)			
HIP (physicians), District 65 (hospital coverage)	535	64	8.3
FFS physicians, District 65 (hospital coverage)	534	64	8.4

Study	Days/1000 Enrollees	Admissions or Discharges/ 1000 Enrollees	Average Length of Stay
H. Blue Collar Union Members and Families, 1958[8] (Columbia University, 1962)			
Blue Cross-Blue Shield, New Jersey	580[b]	76[b]	7.6
General Electric Major Medical	610[b]	71[b]	8.6
Kaiser-Northern California	610[b]	79[b]	7.7
I. California State Employees and Families, dual choice (age-sex adjusted), 1962−63[9] (Dozier et al., 1968)			
Statewide Service Plans	945	130	7.3
Indemnity Plans	1005	111	9.1
Prepaid Group Practices	770	88	8.8
Foundations for Medical Care	1281	144	8.9
J. Enrollees in Southern California Health Plans, 1967−68[10] (Hetherington, Hopkins, Roemer, 1975)			
Large commercial	1150	126	4.8
Small commercial	1200	194	5.3
Blue Cross	1150	152	9.1
Blue Shield	1090	150	9.0
Kaiser	340	71	4.8
Ross-Loos	870	104	8.2
K. Enrollees in the Federal Employees Health Benefits Program, high option plans, Non-Maternity, In-Hospital Services Received Through the Plans, 1967−68[11] (Perrott, 1971) District of Columbia, Maryland, Virginia			
Blue Cross	838	83	10.1
PGP (Group Health Association) New York	379	40	9.4
Blue Cross	725	64	11.2
IPA (GHI)	661	64	10.3
PGP (HIP) California	468	43	10.8
Blue Cross	825	97	8.5
IPA (San Joaquin)	440	60	7.3
PGP	422	48	8.8

Table 5-1 (continued)

Study	Days/1000 Enrollees	Admissions or Discharges/ 1000 Enrollees	Average Length of Stay
Oregon			
Blue Cross	879	110	7.4
IPA	490	86	5.7
PGP	272	46	5.9
Washington			
Blue Cross	791	126	6.3
IPA	427	77	5.5
PGP	341	55	6.2
Hawaii			
Blue Cross	1364	183	7.5
IPA (Hawaii Medical Service)	436	59	7.4
PGP (Kaiser)	404	49	8.2
L. United Steel Workers in Sault Ste. Marie, Ontario, dual choice, 1967–68[12] (Hastings et al., 1970)			
Group Health Association; hospitalization state covered	979	109.2	8.97
Prudential, indemnity coverage; hospitalization state covered	1284	137.3	9.35
M. Medicaid enrollees aged 1–64 in Washington, D.C. 1969–72[13] (Fuller and Patera, 1976)			
Study Group experience:			
22 months before enrollment	602	109	5.5
18 months before enrollment	604	115	5.3
12 months before enrollment	593	124	4.8
12 months after enrollment	443	69	6.4
18 months after enrollment	426	76	5.6
22 months after enrollment	412	76	5.4
Medicaid universe, 1972	744	139	5.3
N. Medicare Beneficiaries in New York City (age-sex adjusted), 1969–70[14] (Jones et al., 1974)			
HIP	3439	200	17.3
Non-HIP	3896	209	18.7
O. Federal Employees Health Benefits Program Members, Washington, D.C. area, 1970: nonobstetric admissions (age-sex adjusted)[15] (Riedel et al., 1975)			
BC-BS	707.7*	99.0*	7.1
Group Health Association	390.8*	52.6*	7.4

Study	Days/1000 Enrollees	Admissions or Discharges/ 1000 Enrollees	Average Length of Stay
P. California State Employees and Dependents (nonobstetric stays), 1970−71[16] (Dozier et al., 1973)			
Indemnity	580	92 (91)	6.3
BC-BS (statewide)	737	110 (96)	6.7
Kaiser	533	74 (77)	7.2
Roos-Loos/Family Health Program (PGP)	499	64 (56)	7.8
Foundations for Medical Care	681	83 (82)	8.2
Q. Fee-for-Service and Prepaid Patients in Marshfield, Wisconsin, 1970−72[17] (Broida et al., 1975)			
1970: Population that became prepaid in 1971	413.5[b]	61.4[b]	6.73
Fee-for-service population	408.4[b]	60.4[b]	6.77
1971: Prepaid	656.5+	107.8++	6.09
FFS	464.3+	67.4	6.89
1972: Prepaid	635.4	101.5++	6.26
FFS	414.6	66.2	6.26
R. St. Louis, Missouri, randomly assigned volunteer enrollees, 1969−72[18] (Perkoff, Kahn, Haas, 1976)			
Medical Care Group	510**	73	7.0
Controls	664**	79	8.4
Results for a subgroup who enrolled in MCG during the study:			
MCG period	811[b]	78	10.0
Control period	631[b]	95	6.7
S. Families in Sault Ste. Marie, Ontario 1972−73[19] (De Friese, 1975)			
Group Health Center	1504.7	135.6	11.09
Group Health Center/Solo	2103.1	169.8	12.39
Solo	2023.6	166.8	12.13
T. Enrollees in Three HMOs in Rochester, New York—multiple choice option Medical and Surgical Services (age standardized), 1974[20] (Wersinger et al., 1976)			
Group Health (PGP)	341	54	6.3
Health Watch (IPA, but not at risk)	539	85	6.3
Rochester Health Network (PGP)	407	70	5.8
Blue Cross (1972 experience)	512	74	6.9

Study		Days/1000 Enrollees	Admissions or Discharges/ 1000 Enrollees	Average Length of Stay
U. General Motors (GM) Employees in Rochester New York: multiple choice option, age standardized medical-surgical services, cohort analysis comparing experience of the same people when in BC-BS[21] (Roghmann, Sorensen, and Wells, 1977)				
Group Health (PGP)	1974−75	361	57	6.3
Blue Cross	1972	306	65	4.7
Health Watch (IPA, not at risk)	1974−75	557	89	6.3
Blue Cross	1972	632	96	6.6
Rochester Health Network (PGP)	1974−75	466	75	6.2
Blue Cross	1972	284	74	3.8
Blue Cross stayers	1974−75	635	89	7.1
Blue Cross	1972	716	95	7.5
Non-GM Enrollees in Rochester, NY—multiple choice option, age standardized medical-surgical rates, cohort analysis comparing experience of the same people when in BC-BS during 1972 (Roghmann, Sorensen, and Wells, 1977, Table 6A.2, 6B.2)				
Group Health (PGP)	1974−75	212	34	6.2
Blue Cross	1972	385	63	6.1
Health Watch (IPA, not as risk)	1974−75	672	102	6.6
Blue Cross	1972	467	77	6.1
Rochester Health Network (PGP)	1974−75	490	85	5.8
Blue Cross	1972	395	58	6.8
Blue Cross stayers	1974−75	482	73	6.6
Blue Cross	1972	475	72	6.6
V. Medicaid (AFDC) Enrollees in HMOs and Control Populations, (Gaus, Cooper, and Hirschman,	1974−75[22] 1976)			
Group Practices		340*	46*	7.3*
Controls		888*	114*	7.7*
Central Los Angeles Health Project		210*	34*	6.4
Control		562*	90*	6.2
Consolidated Medical System		168*	26*	6.5*
Control		1316*	146*	9.0*

Table 5−1 (continued)

Study	Days/1000 Enrollees	Admissions or Discharges/ 1000 Enrollees	Average Length of Stay
Family Health Program	186*	40*	4.6*
Control	854*	142*	6.0*
Group Health Cooperative of	346*	74*	4.7
Puget Sound Control	844*	146*	5.8
Harbor Health Services	322	54*	6.0
Control	556	104*	5.4
Harvard Health Plan	358	46	7.8
Control	548	96	5.7
Health Insurance Plan of	598*	64*	9.3
Greater New York Control	1854*	114*	16.3
Temple Health Plan	522	38	13.7*
Control	564	76	7.4*
Foundation and Control:			
Redwood	630	160	3.9
Control	826	190	4.4
Sacramento	610	106	5.8
Control	546	122	4.5
W. Employees of Employers Insurance of Wausau, Wisconsin[23] (Egdahl et al., 1977, p. 392)			
Commercial Account, 1971, 3116 persons	932	126	7.4
Health Protection Plan, 1972, 3261 persons	552	121	4.5
X. Enrollees of Physicians Association of Clackamas County, average experience, 1971−75[24] (Egdahl et al., 1977, p. 393)			
Protecting Circle Plan (patients limited to participating physicians)	453	111	4.08
Medical Service Plan (about 60% of services is provided by participating physicians)	531	109	4.86
Y. Enrollees in the Seattle Prepaid Health Care Project, 1971−74[25] (Figures in parentheses exclude obstetrical days) (Diehr et al., 1976, pp. II−144, 183, 187)			
Group Health Cooperative	497 (405)	110 (78)	4.5 (5.2)
King County Medical−Blue Cross	734 (689)	140 (120)	5.2 (5.6)

Table 5–1 (continued)

Study	Days/1000 Enrollees	Admissions or Discharges/ 1000 Enrollees	Average Length of Stay
Z. Stanford University Employees in Palo Alto Medical Clinic and Kaiser, January 1972–June 1974[26] (age-sex adjusted annualized rates) (Scitovsky and McCall, 1980, pp. 30–41)			
All admissions excluding delivery:			
Kaiser	250	38	6.5
Palo Alto Medical Clinic	251	44	5.7
Deliveries per 1000 women aged 15–44:			
Kaiser	251	72	3.5
Palo Alto Medical Clinic	93	33	2.8

[a] Age-adjusted.

[b] Differences between plans *not* statistically significant at .05 level.

[c] Excludes a group with a large proportion of retirees.

* Significant at .05 level.

** Significant at .01 level.

+ Significant at .005 level.

++ Significant at .001 level.

[1] Committee for the Special Research Project in the Health Insurance Plan of Greater New York, 1957.

[2] Darsky, Sinai, and Axelrod, 1958.

[3] Densen, Balamuth, and Shapiro, 1958, p. 34. Age-adjusted data are from Donabedian, 1969, p. 12.

[4] Densen et al., November 1960, p. 1713, 1723.

[5] Anderson and Sheatsley, 1959, p. 90. GHI data excludes two persons with very long lengths of stay (48 and 205 days).

[6] Falk and Senturia, 1960, p. 89.

[7] Densen et al., November 16, 1962, pp. 62–68, 138.

[8] Columbia University School of Public Health and Administrative Medicine, 1962a, p. 152. Nonobstetrical stays in short-term hospitals. Data also exclude "free" care in government hospitals or paid for by workmen's compensation, etc.

[9] Dozier et al., 1968, pp. 53–54. Data are based on the hospitalization experience for the period July 1962–March 1963 and are adjusted to an annual basis. Maternity cases are excluded. The data include a small number of annuitants in each plan, but all figures are adjusted to the age-sex distribution of all covered persons (see p. 46). See Table 4–3 for a discussion of the plans involved in each grouping. The data also refer to discharges rather than admissions.

[10] Hetherington, Hopkins, and Roemer, 1975, p. 121, 130, 131.

[11] Perrott, 1971, Figure 4.

[12] J. E. F. Hastings et al., 1970, p. 292, with corrections reported in Hastings et al., 1973, p. 92. The data exclude newborns and are based on hospital records. Interview data provide essentially the same findings. See Mott, Hastings, and Barclay, 1973.

Table 5–1 (continued)

[13] Fuller and Patera, January 1976, pp. T–9, T–7; and Fuller, Patera, and Koziol, September 1977, pp. 705–737. The data for the study group represents cumulative experience; that is, the first line represents the full 22 months of experience prior to enrollment while the second line represents only the last 18 months before enrollment.

[14] Jones et al., December 1974, p. 11. Data are based on Medicare reimbursed services. The non-HIP group is a 5% sample of Medicare beneficiaries in the area.

[15] Riedel et al., January 1975, Tables 8, 10, 13.

[16] Dozier et al., 1973, pp. 73, 76, 84, 89. Figures in parentheses are age-sex adjusted admission rates for nonmaternity stays.

[17] Broida et al., April 10, 1975, p. 782. Medical record information was used to identify the utilization of people who opted for prepaid coverage in March 1971. The yearly data actually refer to the year before prepayment and the two years after prepayment.

[18] Perkoff, Kahn, and Haas, May 1976, pp. 437, 438. Data include psychiatry and exclude obstetrics. The differences in utilization for the subgroup are not statistically significant.

[19] DeFriese, Spring 1975, p. 139. All residents have the same financial coverage through Canadian national health insurance. Households are categorized by the predominant source of care. Those listed just as GHC were "members" and had a high or moderate use of GHC physicians; those listed as GHC-Solo were predominantly nonmembers with some use of GHC services. (DeFriese, p. 129.)

[20] Wersinger et al., September 1976, p. 33. All three plans use Blue Cross to process their hospital claims, and these claims file data are used as the basis of the statistics. Utilization data are standardized to the 1972 age distribution for Blue Cross members in Monroe County.

[21] Roghmann, Sorensen, and Wells, Table 6A.2, 6B.2.

[22] Gaus, Cooper, and Hirschman, May 1976, p. 9. These data are based on random samples of AFDC families enrolled in the designated HMO for at least six months prior to the interview. The non-HMO control families were in AFDC for at least six months, lived in the same zip codes as the HMO families, and were stratified by family size and age of household head. The one exception is the Redwood Foundation, which covers about 85 percent of the eligibles in its three counties and in which HMO membership is based on the physician's decision to participate—individuals do not enroll. In this case the control group was drawn from two neighboring counties. Hospital use is based on six month recall and results are annualized. Hospitalization data exclude pregnancy. Utilization includes any out-of-plan use.

[23] Egdahl et al., 1977, p. 392.

[24] Ibid, p. 393.

[25] Diehr et al., 1976, pp. II–144, 183, 187.

[26] Scitovsky and McCall, January 1980, pp. 30–41.

quality of the data and to use restraint in interpreting the findings; but if the results are generally consistent, we can have more confidence than if the interpretations were based on only a few, even well-designed, studies.* Most of the studies in Table 5–1 are well executed and worthy of close

*The strength of this argument depends in part on whether the results support or are contrary to our hypotheses. A few well-designed studies that produce counterintuitive results can go a long way toward rejecting a hypothesis. (See Ehrenberg, 1975; Mahoney, 1978.)

attention. The attempt in the present analysis is to present the available data without censorship. The difficulty is that we all are influenced by our expectations when examining results, and we are more likely to look for problems in studies that contradict our expectations than in those that support them. The same bias exists at the prepublication phase. Fortunately, some of the comparative data presented here come from legislatively mandated studies; however, one may still suspect some bias in the availability of data.

The best overall measure of hospital use is the number of inpatient days per 1000 enrollees per year. Total inpatient days are the product of admissions per enrollee, times the average length of stay per admission. The latter two variables are more likely to be the focus of HMO policies, because they can be affected on a case-by-case basis, while total days per year is merely the result of many individual decisions. To assist in the discussion of these results concerning hospitalization, Table 5-2 summarizes the findings for the 57 comparisons of HMO and non-HMO enrollees. In 43 of the 57 pairs, HMO enrollees had fewer hospital days than the comparison groups, and in 46 cases the admission rate was lower. The data are much more mixed with respect to length of stay. It was lower for HMO enrollees in 30 of the 57 cases, about the same in 6, and higher in 21. How should these data be interpreted? It is gratifying that about 80 percent of the cases support the predictions, but we must ask what can be learned from a careful review of the remaining 20 percent. Do these results cast substantial doubt on the findings, or do they point to special cases?

The breakdown between PGPs and IPAs provides one clue to interpretation of the data. The IPA type of HMO is much less likely to demonstrate substantial differences in admissions than the PGP type. While the IPA

Table 5—2   Summary of Findings Concerning Hospital Utilization of HMO and Non-HMO Enrollees: 57 Comparisons from 1951 to 1975

	Days per 1000 Enrollees			Discharges or Admissions per 1000 Enrollees			Average Length of Stay		
	PGP[b]	IPA[b]	Total	PGP[b]	IPA[b]	Total	PGP[b]	IPA[b]	Total
HMO enrollees < non-HMO	33	10	43	36	10	46	21	9	30
HMO enrollees = to non-HMO[a]	2	0	2	2	1	3	4	2	6
HMO enrollees > non-HMO	7	5	12	4	4	8	17	4	21
TOTAL	42	15	57	42	15	57	42	15	57

SOURCE.   Table 5–1.

[a] Includes comparisons in which rates differed by one day or discharge per 1000, or length of stay differed by .1 days.

[b] Not all cases studied involve organizations that meet all requirements of the HMO definition discussed in Chapter 1. Some of the organizations are more appropriately categorized as quasi-HMOs; however, their data have often served as the basis of HMO- non-HMO comparisons. Similarly, the PGP and IPA categorizations are somewhat approximate.

comparisons account for 26 percent of the cases, they account for 50 percent of the "unexpected results" with respect to admissions. IPAs, however, perform somewhat better with respect to length of stay, so their results for total days per 1000 are not that different from PGPs. For various reasons, which will be discussed in detail in Chapter 14, it is not surprising that IPAs appear to be less effective than PGPs in controlling hospital admission.

If PGPs are supposed to be able to control utilization, what about the remaining results? Careful examination of the studies in each category suggest reasonable explanations for most of the findings. Of the seven studies that indicate higher total utilization for PGP enrollees, two refer to plans for which there is either no financial incentive or no identification of HMO enrollees. In one of these, Study R, the medical group was not at risk (either directly or indirectly) for any of the services provided (Perkoff, Kahn, and Haas, 1976). Data from the Marshfield Clinic provide two years of evidence showing that enrollees in the prepaid plan had higher utilization (Study Q). However, enrollees could join during open enrollment periods, and physicians did not know who was a plan member and who was not (Angermeier, 1976; Broida and Lerner, 1975). Study A involves a comparison of HIP enrollees who have almost complete coverage, with the total insured population in New York City. This study has been criticized as being unreliable because it underestimates total admission rates for New York City by about 30 percent (Klarman, 1963, p. 956).

Study H (Columbia University, 1962a), shows PGP hospitalization rates between those of two conventional plans but higher than their average. It is based on a carefully conducted survey of union members in various parts of the country. The Blue Cross sample was drawn from members of the International Association of Machinists (IAM) in northern New Jersey. The major medical coverage was offered by General Electric to its employees, and the sample was drawn from IAM members in Utica, New York, about half, and Milwaukee and Cincinnati, one quarter each. There were not enough IAM members of Kaiser, so a sample was drawn from all San Francisco area blue collar union members with Kaiser coverage. The three samples were well matched by age and sex. Furthermore, the three plans all offered reasonably comprehensive coverage. This study is particularly interesting because it followed a series of published reports showing lower utilization in HIP, and the authors were surprised at their results. They expected to find lower hospitalization among Kaiser enrollees. (See Columbia University, 1962a, pp. 6, 151-152.) In fact, they devote an appendix to exploring potential problems in the survey that could account for the findings. The best answer seems to lie in the difficulty of comparing plans in vastly different geographic areas. Admission rates tend to be higher in the West than in the Northeast. For example, controlling for age, in 1957-58 there were 115 discharges per 1000 among adults aged twenty-five to sixty-four in the West versus 109 in the Northeast. On the other hand, the discharge rate for children was 50 in the West versus 63 in the East (U.S. Public Health Service, 1958, p. 15). This pattern matches that of the Columbia study, in which Kaiser had higher rates for adults and lower rates for children. Why these regional differences exist is largely a mystery.

The three remaining examples of higher PGP hospitalization rates come from Rochester, New York, with two points representing an increase in usage by people joining the Rochester Health Network. As noted in Chapter 3, enrollees in this plan were poorer and sicker than average and tended not to have a usual source of care. Sorensen et al. (1979) note that the RHN physicians were at risk only for primary care services, and RHN patients accounted for only a small fraction of the patient load. This explanation does not hold for the other Rochester anomaly, General Motors enrollees in Genesee Valley Group Health. The discussion in Chapter 3 noted, however, that these enrollees had very low preenrollment hospitalization rates.

The two studies in which PGP enrollees have about the same utilization as those in the comparison groups are also special cases. In one, Study C, the study population is composed of union members and their families, who have a dual choice between HIP and a self-insured union-sponsored plan that pays physicians on an FFS basis (Densen et al., 1962). In both cases the union provides self-insured hospitalization coverage. A key feature of this program is active education of union members and control over expenditures. It is possible that this type of control provides incentives for non-HIP patients and their physicians similar to those faced by HIP enrollees.

The second study with identical hospitalization rates, Study Z, compares Stanford employees in Kaiser and the Palo Alto Medical Clinic (PAMC). The PAMC operates largely on an FFS basis and derives only 15 percent of its revenue from prepaid enrollees; it does not own a hospital, and clinic physicians are not at risk for hospital costs. Thus the very low hospitalization rate for clinic enrollees is probably the result of organizational factors other than prepayment. This issue will be addressed in Chapter 14.

Thus, with a few exceptions, there is no evidence to reject the hypothesis that the PGP type of HMO can demonstrate lower rates of hospital days and admissions than conventional FFS situations. How strong is the evidence supporting the hypothesis? The quality of the research design varies, but in many cases it is excellent. Studies D, E, I, K, L, O, P, Q, R, S, T, U, Y, and Z all involve dual or multiple choice situations. In many of the studies (I, J, L, P, S, V, Y, and Z) the data were collected using household interviews and thus include out-of-plan utilization. In a number of these cases the interview data were checked with medical records. Out-of-plan utilization and self-selection are perhaps the major problems in comparing utilization rates. The available data suggest that out-of-plan usage is relatively low; it ranges from less than 1 percent (Gaus, Cooper, and

Hirschman, 1976, p. 6) to about 8 percent (Columbia University, 1962a). Obviously, in those cases in which such use is measured, it is not a problem in making comparisons. The issue of self-selection is more difficult to deal with, and the data are almost nonexistent. As will be discussed below, there is evidence suggesting that self-selection may account for a part of the observed differences in utilization in specific instances. However, at this point, it is fair to say that the data clearly support the prediction that admission rates and days of hospitalization are lower among HMO enrollees, especially those in PGPs.

While it is possible to develop reasonably solid evidence of *lower* hospitalization rates for HMO enrollees, the question most people ask is whether HMOs actually *reduce* hospital use. The age-adjusted figures reported in many of the studies account for some underlying differences in populations, but the self-selection issue remains. Two major cohort studies with comprehensive data are available for the three Rochester HMOs and the Seattle Prepaid Health Care Project.

Hospitalization data for enrollees in the three Rochester HMOs were presented in Chapter 3. Because the new HMOs offered much more extensive coverage for maternity and psychiatric services, the primary focus should be on medical-surgical admissions. For General Motors employees, who were typically high utilizers and accustomed to comprehensive coverage, enrollment in the two PGPs resulted in an insignificant decline in admissions (Table 5-3) and an *increase* in total hospital days (Table 3-3). For General Motors enrollees in the IPA type plan, admissions and hospital days were at first substantially below preenrollment experience; in 1975 they rose above the preenrollment rate. The latter increase is entirely attributable to a more than 50 percent increase in admissions, perhaps in anticipation of the plan's closure in mid-1976. Non-General Motors enrollees exhibit a different pattern. Those who joined Genessee Valley Group Health nearly halved their admission rate in the first year and remained at that level. People joining the Rochester Health Network experienced a substantial increase in admissions and hospital days, as did enrollees in the IPA.

The Seattle Prepaid Health Care Project includes interview data for hospitalization prior to enrollment and four years of experience within the experiment. Prior to enrollment, people who joined the KCM-BC plan had 132 admissions per 1000, in contrast to 104 for Group Health enrollees (Richardson et al., 1976, p. I-139). In the first year the rates were 147 and 99, respectively, indicating a small decrease for Group Health enrollees and an increase for KCM-BC enrollees. Both groups probably experienced a substantial increase in coverage (Diehr et al., 1976, p. II-108). Using the preenrollment experience as a measure of the selection factor reduces the apparent differential from $1.47 = (147/99)$ to $1.16 = 1.47/(132/104)$. The experience over time of enrollees in the two plans is also of interest (Table 5-4). The figures for each year show a small decline in admission rates for KCM-BC and a substantial increase for Group Health enrollees. These

Table 5−3   General Motors and Non-General Motors Utilization Rates Before and
After Joining HMOs

1972−1974−1975 Final Cohort
Admissions per 1000 Enrollee Years
Age Standardized Rates
Medical Surgical Admissions Only

	1972 (before)	1974 (1st Year)	1975 (2nd Year)	Percent Change	
				1974/ 1972	1975/ 1974
Blue Cross					
GM	95 ± 4.2	91 ± 4.1	87 ± 4.1	− 4	−14
Non-GM	72 ± .5	74 ± .5	72 ± .5	+ 3	− 3
Total	72 ± .5	74 ± .5	72 ± .5	+ 3	− 3
PGP					
GM	65 ± 7.2	52 ± 8.3	61 ± 7.1	−20	+17
Non-GM	63 ± 3.7	34 ± 3.5	34 ± 2.3	−46	0
Total	63 ± 3.3	38 ± 3.3	40 ± 2.7	−40	+ 5
Medical Foundation					
GM	96 ± 3.3	70 ± 4.9	107 ± 4.0	−27	+53
Non-GM	77 ± 3.9	98 ± 5.3	105 ± 5.4	+27	+ 7
Total	89 ± 2.5	84 ± 3.7	105 ± 3.2	+25	− 6
NHC					
GM	74 ± 16.5	75 ± 22.3	75 ± 17.0	+ 1	0
Non-GM	58 ± 6.8	80 ± 9.0	89 ± 8.3	+38	+11
Total	76 ± 6.3	80 ± 8.4	88 ± 7.4	+ 5	+10

SOURCE.   Roghmann, Sorensen, and Wells.

calendar year data, however, are confounded by enrollees who joined after
the first year. If we focus only on the original cohort, quite a different
picture emerges: there is a clear reduction in admissions for the KCM-BC
enrollees and a small, less consistent increase for Group Health enrollees,
so that after four years the Group Health enrollees actually have a slightly
higher admission rate.

Both of these studies suggest that when people must change providers to
join an HMO, as is usually the case for PGPs, a selection effect occurs
whereby people who are more likely to be high utilizers join the conventional option. Over time, the selection effect becomes less important. This
means, however, that a substantial part of the observed differences in
hospitalization rates between PGPs and conventional plans may reflect
differences in enrollees rather than practice patterns.

The crucial question remains: how much lower are HMO hospitalization
rates? The early literature, which was based primarily on the HIP studies,
quoted savings of up to 50 percent, but Klarman pointed out a number of

Table 5—4   Hospital Admission Rates for Enrollees in the Seattle Prepaid Health Care Project by Calendar Year, Tenure Year, and Plan

	All Enrollees				Enrollees Joining in 1971			
	Number of Enrollees		Admissions/ 1000		Number of Enrollees		Admissions/ 1000	
	GH	KCM-BC	GH	KCM-BC	GH	KCM-BC	GH	KCM-BC
1971	1603	3053	99	147	1603	3053	99	147
1972	1877	3879	94	141	1579	3050	92	137
1973	1689	3736	126	137	1043	2032	121	119
1974	1560	4069	122	140	677	1646	109	105

SOURCE: Paula K. Diehr et al., November 1976.

problems with such estimates, especially when attempts are made to generalize them to the population at large (1971, p. 29). To provide a convenient way of summarizing our results, Figures 5—1 and 5—2 plot data from HMOs and the comparison groups for both total days and admissions per 1000 enrollees.* Regressions through the points indicate that, within the relevant range, days per 1000 enrollees are about 5 to 25 percent lower in IPAs than in comparison groups and about 35 percent lower in PGPs than in comparison groups. Comparable results for admissions are between 10 percent higher and 20 percent lower in IPAs and 20 to 40 percent lower in PGPs.† It must be remembered that the sample sizes are small, especially for the IPAs, and that there are wide variations among plans. In fact, five of the fifteen IPAs had admission rates equal to or above those of the comparison groups. The higher hospitalization rates for IPAs relative to PGPs is also seen in other data for the age-sex adjusted utilization rates in federally qualified HMOs. For plans over three years old, the rates were 627 versus 474, while for those under three years, the rates were 660 versus 508 (Strumpf et al., 1978).

*These figures exclude data from studies B and N, which had extremely high rates for both plans. Including these points would not substantially alter our studies.

†The regression results were as follows:
Days per 1000 for 42 PGPs, HMO = $-34.07 + 0.705$ COMP $R^2 = .70$
                            (77.00) (0.074)

for 15 IPAs, HMO = $191.50 + 0.581$ COMP $R^2 = .33$
                  (203.44) (0.232)

Admissions per 1000 for 42 PGPs, HMO = $27.88 + 0.395$ COMP $R^2 = .23$
                                      (12.73) (0.115)

for 15 IPAs, HMO = $39.63 + 0.525$ COMP $R^2 = .33$
                  (26.30) (0.210)

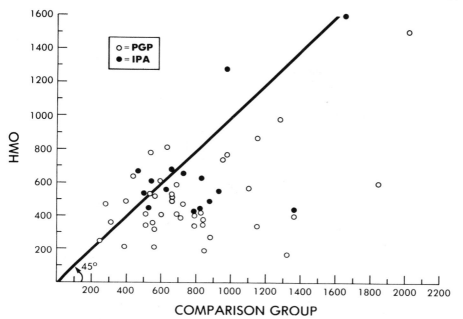

Figure 5-1   Total inpatient days per 1000 enrollees in HMOs and comparison groups.

LENGTH OF STAY

As has been pointed out above, there do not appear to be consistent differences in the average length of stay for HMO enrollees and comparison groups. In only 30 of the 57 pairs was the length of stay lower for the HMO sample. Although the subsamples are too small to support much interpretation, it is of interest that 4 of 15 IPAs had longer lengths of stay, in contrast to 17 of 42 PGPs. This suggests, perhaps, that while IPAs are less effective in keeping people out of the hospital, they can encourage their physicians to send patients home sooner than would otherwise be the case.

This points to two issues that underlie the analysis of length of stay per hospital episode. In the first place, it is reasonable to assume some latitude in the amount of time that a given person with a specific condition "should" spend in the hospital. For instance, the first seven days for a certain case might be considered necessary or good practice; longer stays become increasingly discretionary (McNeer et al., 1978). There is substantial evidence showing variations in length of stay, which apparently are related to weekly cycles, preferences for certain numbers, and other nonmedical factors. (See Donabedian, 1974; Rindfuss and Ladinsky, 1976.) Given the financial incentives faced by HMOs, we would expect them to reduce the

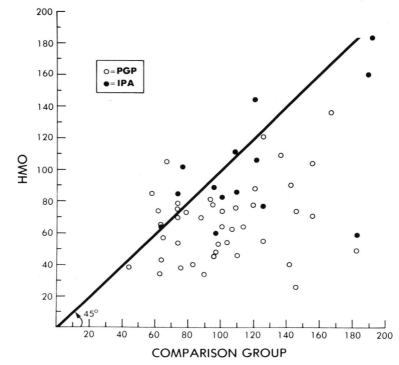

Figure 5-2   Admissions per 1000 enrollees in HMOs and comparison groups.

prevalence of such "marginal" days and thus reduce the length of stay for each type of case.

The second point that affects the average length of stay is related to how HMOs reduce admissions. It appears unlikely that admissions are reduced across the board; some categories of health problems are much more likely to require hospitalization than others, and HMOs are less likely to reduce admissions of the former. This point will be discussed in more detail in the context of discretionary admissions. At this time, we need only point out that if an HMO reduces admission rates for some diagnoses more than for others, this change in case mix is likely to alter the average length of stay, regardless of whether treatment patterns for specific cases (once admitted) are changed. In particular, if less serious (more discretionary) cases tend to require shorter stays, then reducing the proportion of such cases will tend to increase the average length of stay in HMOs. In the remainder of this subsection we will examine the influence of case-mix on length of stay, and in the next subsection specific diagnoses and procedures will be examined to gain insight into the types of cases that account for lower admission rates in HMOs.

One simple way to address the length-of-stay question is to examine the distribution of cases by length of stay for California state employees in various plans, as in Table 5-5. Rates are given in terms of cases (admissions)

Table 5–5   Number Hospital Stays per 1000 Persons by Length of Stay: California State Employees and Dependents, 1970–71 (Basic Only)

	Indemnity	Statewide Service	Kaiser	Ross-Loos/ FHP	IPAs
Admissions per 1000	101	119	87	76	107
Days of stay					
1 day	10.5	8.7	11.4	10.1	6.7
2	15.9	17.7	6.4	2.3	17.4
3	16.0 } 52.7	16.5 } 62.7	21.8 } 47.4	12.4 } 45.2	21.0 } 61.9
4	10.3	19.8	7.7	20.4	16.8
5	13.8	9.6	7.9	8.0	13.8
6	6.4 } 25.9	9.2 } 25.2	4.8 } 16.1	1.1 } 14.8	4.6 } 20.5
7	5.7	6.4	3.4	5.7	2.1
8–15	16.0	22.3	16.7	9.2	15.6
16+	6.3	8.7	7.1	6.8	8.8
Average length of stay	5.8	6.5	6.4	7.0	6.6

SOURCE: Dozier et al., 1973, derived from pp. 79, 81, 87. Supplement to Medicare not included.

per 1000 enrollees, rather than as a percentage of cases within the plan. This enables us to focus on what changes in the pattern appear to be associated with differential admission rates. At the high end of the scale, all the plans have about six to eight cases per 1000 enrollees that use sixteen or more days in the hospital. It is likely that only the more serious conditions require such long stays, and the relative uniformity across plans is as expected. In the eight- to fifteen-day category all three HMOs have lower case rates than the service plans, but their rates are comparable to that of the indemnity plan.* Admission rates in PGPs for cases in the five- to seven-day category are substantially below those of the indemnity and service plans, while IPAs are in an intermediate position.

It is among very short stays (one to four days) that patterns change substantially. The high admission rates in IPAs and service plans appear to be attributable to cases with short stays. One frequent claim about HMOs is that they reduce the number of brief hospital stays designed for laboratory tests and other diagnostic procedures. This would lead to a prediction of a lower rate of one-day stays in HMOs, especially in PGPs, which are supposed to be better equipped to do such procedures on an outpatient basis. Instead, the opposite is true; PGPs have the highest admission rates

*The rather low rate of eight- to fifteen-day cases in the indemnity plan may be a reflection of its coverage, which allows full payment for the first $600 of in-hospital services and 75 percent of the next $1000, exclusive of basic room and board. This includes charges for drugs, supplies, operating room, X-ray, and laboratory (Dozier et al., 1973). It is likely that by the second week in the hospital, the patient's out-of-pocket costs begin to mount rapidly.

for one-day stays and IPAs the lowest. The clue to this puzzle is in the rate for two-day stays, which is extremely low for PGPs and about the same for the other three plans. For one and two-day stays combined, the PGPs have substantially lower admission rates, while the IPA rate is comparable to that of the traditional plans. One interpretation of these findings is that PGPs do, indeed, reduce very short-stay admissions, and if someone does require admission for a minor procedure, it can generally be done in one day rather than two. For instance, rather than checking in the night before scheduled surgery, patients may be asked to arrive early on the morning of the operation (Klitsner, 1976).

This interpretation can be tested more directly with the data presented in Table 5-6, which categorizes admissions in each plan by the reason for the hospital stay. If two categories—diagnosis of illness/injury and X-ray/laboratory test—are combined, it is apparent that PGPs have markedly lower admission rates for such minor procedures. The IPA rate is between those of the indemnity and service plans. Admission rates for treatment of injury are reasonably similar, as would be expected for a group of conditions that tend not to be discretionary. The wide differentials in maternity stays reflect self-selection among enrollees for the better maternity coverage in HMOs (Hudes et al., 1979). The particularly high rate for IPAs may help to explain their high rate of short-stay cases, because most deliveries involve less than four days in the hospital.

Riedel et al. (1975) provide the most detailed diagnostic data available concerning admission rates and length of stay. These are drawn from PGP and BC-BS members of the Federal Employees Health Benefits Program in Washington, D.C. Data are available for forty-five specific diagnoses and an "other" category (Table 5-7). The overall length of stay for Group Health

Table 5–6   Number of Hospital Stays per 1000 by Reason for Stay: California State Employees and Dependents, 1970–71 (Basic Only)

	Indemnity	Statewide Service	Kaiser	Ross-Loos FHP	IPAs
All Reasons	101	119	87	76	107
Maternity	9.9	6.4	11.7	11.8	23.4
Surgery	44.4	47.4	34.2	35.3	44.2
Treatment of illness	13.9	25.1	15.8	8.1	11.4
Treatment of injury	5.2	4.9	5.3	3.7	4.6
Diagnosis of					
Illness/Injury	6.0	9.2	2.5	3.2	10.1
X-rays/Lab Tests	2.8	5.5	2.8	—	—
Diagnosis or Tests	(8.8)	(14.7)	(5.3)	(3.2)	(10.1)
Other	18.8	20.6	14.6	13.9	13.3

SOURCE: Dave Dozier et al., 1973, derived from p. 79. Supplement to Medicare not included.

Association (GHA) members is 6.6 days, almost the same as that of BC-BS members, 6.5 days. If the two diagnoses for which coverage differs (diseases of the oral cavity, salivary glands, and jaw and psychotic and psychoneurotic disorders) are excluded, the pattern remains—6.56 and 6.44, respectively. However, the GHA admission rate is nearly half that of BC-BS—68.8 per 1000 versus 118.4 per 1000. (All of these data are age-sex adjusted.) Is it possible that GHA both reduces the length of stay for patients it admits and excludes "unnecessary" admissions with shorter "normal" stays, resulting in canceling effects? This question may be answered by recomputing the length of stay for GHA patients with the admissions mix of BC-BS patients. The resulting figure is 6.46, scarcely different from the other two figures. Thus, at this level of detail, the equality in overall length of stay between the two plans is not attributable to consistent differences in case mix.

Several points are worth discussion in connection with these unexpected results. First, as hinted above, the forty-five diagnostic categories may be too crude to capture fine differences in severity and "true" case mix. Thus it is possible that within each category the GHA patients were "sicker," and their requirements for more care just balanced the incentives to reduce length of stay. However, it is unlikely that such a fine balancing would occur. Second, the "nonresults" are not attributable to the similarity in case mix between GHA and BC-BS. Admission rates in the latter range from 8.0 to 0.7 times those of GHA. Third, there is substantial variation in how long each program treats specific diagnoses. The proportionate difference in length of stay [computed as $(LOS_{BC-BS} - LOS_{GHA})/LOS_{GHA}$] ranges from +53 percent to −34 percent. All of these factors suggest that if true differences were present, they could be seen in these data. Instead the observed variations in length of stay appear to be nonsystematic, and the diagnoses that have lower admission rates in GHA include both long and short-stay cases. For the forty-three diagnoses with comparable coverage, the correlation between the ratio of the adjusted admission rates (column 3) and the length of stay for Blue Cross enrollees (column 4) is only −.21. A final factor should be mentioned; 65 percent of the GHA admissions were to university hospitals, in contrast to 10 percent of the BC-BS admissions (Riedel et al., 1975, p. 14). The style of care in university hospitals is different from that in nonteaching hospitals, and this often appears as a longer length of stay. (See Slee and Ament, 1968.) On the other hand, Schroeder and O'Leary (1977) found the length of stay for patients in the major teaching hospital used by GHA to be somewhat lower than the length of stay for patients admitted to a community hospital by the same group of physicians. Data from the Seattle Prepaid Health Care Project provide a counter example. (Diehr et al., 1976) For women in GH the length of stay was 4.16 versus 5.51 days for women in KCM-BC. Using sixteen diagnostic categories, if the GH length-of-stay is weighted by the KCM-BC admissions, the length of stay is 4.64. This suggests that about

Table 5-7   Admission Rates per 1000 Member Years and Average Length of Stay for Selected Diagnostic Categories in Blue Cross—Blue Shield and GHA (Age/Sex Adjusted)

Selected Diagnostic Categories+	Admission Rates per 1000			Length of Stay Age/Sex Adjusted		
	Age/Sex Adjusted		Ratio of Adjusted Rates++			(BC-GHA/ GHA)(100)
	BC-BS	GHA		BC-BS	GHA	
1. Diseases of oral cavity, salivary glands, and jaw**	2.1	0.2*	10.5	2.0	3.4*	−41
2. Disorders of menstruation	2.4	0.2*	8.0	3.2	3.1	3
3. Acute respiratory infections	1.7	0.3*	5.7	4.0	3.0	33
4. Hypertrophy of tonsils and adenoids, chronic tonsillitis	5.9	1.5*	3.9	1.5	1.6	−6
5. Arthritis, rheumatism, gout	0.9	0.3*	3.0	14.0	12.1	16
6. Pneumonia	1.2	0.4*	3.0	7.5	7.7	−2
7. Bronchitis, emphysema, and other diseases of the respiratory system	1.4	0.5*	2.8	9.1	7.0	30
8. Spirochetal, parasitic, and other infectious diseases	1.1	0.4*	2.8	6.4	6.0	7
9. Other diseases of breast and female genital system	8.9	3.4*	2.6	5.5	6.0	−8
10. Selected diseases of the urinary tract	7.5	2.9*	2.6	5.0	5.1	−2
11. Diseases of skin and subcutaneous tissue	2.4	1.0*	2.4	5.0	6.5	−23
12. Diseases of liver and pancreas	0.7	0.3*	2.3	14.0	11.4	23
13. Diseases of thyroid and other endocrine glands	0.9	0.4*	2.3	8.2	6.5	26
14. Chronic cystic breast disease	1.1	0.5*	2.2	3.0	2.6	15
15. Psychotic and psychoneurotic disorders**	1.3	0.6*	2.1	19.2	12.6*	52
16. Other diseases of circulatory system	3.3	1.6*	2.1	10.0	9.0	11
17. Diabetes mellitus	1.0	0.5*	2.0	11.0	10.2	8
18. Selected diseases of upper respiratory tract	1.0	0.5*	2.0	3.0	4.0	−25
19. Selected diseases of the heart	1.3	0.7*	1.9	12.0	11.8	2
20. Diseases of upper gastrointestinal system	2.1	1.1*	1.9	9.3	10.1	−8
21. Diseases of gallbladder and biliary ducts	1.1	0.6*	1.8	12.1	9.4*	29
22. Other diseases of intestines and peritoneum	2.0	1.1*	1.8	7.3	8.0	−9
23. Hyperplasia of prostate and prostitis	0.7	0.4*	1.8	7.1	10.0*	−29
24. Diseases of the eye	1.8	1.0*	1.8	4.5	5.0	−10
25. Infectious diseases caused by viruses	0.9	0.5*	1.8	8.7	5.7*	53
26. No classifiable diagnosis or no illness	4.0	2.4*	1.7	6.0	6.0	0
27. Osteomyelitis and other diseases of bone and joint	1.7	1.0*	1.7	12.0	10.0	20
28. Other diseases of musculo-skeletal system	1.0	0.6*	1.7	4.3	6.0	−28
29. Arteriosclerotic and other heart disease	1.6	1.0*	1.6	13.2	17.2*	−23

Table 5—7 (continued)

Selected Diagnostic Categories+	Admission Rates per 1000			Length of Stay Age/Sex Adjusted		
	Age/Sex Adjusted		Ratio of Adjusted Rates++			
	BC-BS	GHA		BC-BS	GHA	(BC-GHA/ GHA)(100)
30. Injury to internal organs	1.8	1.1*	1.6	6.4	5.0	28
31. Appendicitis	1.1	0.7*	1.6	5.4	6.3	−14
32. Fibromyoma of uterus	1.8	1.2	1.5	8.5	8.2	4
33. Delivery	17.9	13.0*	1.4	4.0	4.3*	−7
34. Allergic disorders	0.8	0.6	1.3	5.5	6.0	−8
35. Fractures, dislocations, and sprains of selected sites	3.4	2.6*	1.3	9.3	12.0*	−22
36. Diseases of the ear	1.0	0.8*	1.3	2.7	4.1*	−34
37. Inflammatory and other diseases of the central nervous system	0.8	0.5*	1.3	8.3	10.3	−19
38. Other diseases of appendix, hernia, and intestinal obstruction	4.6	3.8*	1.2	6.0	5.5	9
39. Malignant neoplasms	1.6	1.4*	1.1	13.0	12.6	3
40. Complications of pregnancy	5.0	4.4	1.1	3.0	3.2	−6
41. Congenital anomalies	1.4	1.3	1.1	7.0	6.2	13
42. Birth injuries and diseases of early infancy	0.9	1.0	0.9	11.0	13.1	−16
43. Other diseases of male genital organs	1.4	1.6	0.9	4.0	4.0	0
44. Adverse effects of chemical substances and other trauma	0.7	0.8	0.9	5.0	7.3*	−32
45. Wounds and burns	1.0	1.5*	0.7	7.0	5.1	37
46. All other diagnoses	13.6	7.3	1.9	9.9	9.6	3
47. All diagnoses	121.8	69.6	1.8	6.5	6.6	−9

SOURCE: Riedel et al., January 1975, pp. 21, 23.

+ Categories with fewer than 30 admissions in either plan excluded.

++ BC-BS/GHA.

* BC-BS/GHA difference in rates significant at .05 level. (For admission rates these are computed from the unadjusted data.)

** Categories with differences in benefit structure between the two plans. These are excluded from the analysis.

one-third of the apparent difference in length of stay is attributable to case mix.

In summary, our predictions concerning length-of-stay in HMOs were mixed, as were the empirical results. On the one hand, HMOs have an incentive to reduce stays of patients for whom an extra day in the hospital will make little difference in outcome. On the other hand, HMOs also have an incentive to reduce admissions of those who do not really need hospitalization. Everything else being equal, the average HMO hospital patient probably has a more serious health problem, and this could lead to a longer length of stay. It does appear that HMOs, especially PGPs, have substantially fewer admissions that last only a few days. There is evidence too that at least part of this differential is attributable to lower admission rates for diagnosis and testing. Of the two sets of diagnosis-specific comparative data, one suggests that even though there are wide differences in admission rates and lengths of stay for specific diagnoses, the PGP in question did not have an overall effect on length of stay, controlling for case mix. The other study does indicate a PGP effect on length of stay, controlling for case mix.

WHAT ACCOUNTS FOR DIFFERENCES IN ADMISSION RATES?

The previous section provides evidence that the overall number of hospital days is lower for HMO enrollees and that this occurs primarily through lower admission rates, rather than consistently shorter length of stay. The questions arise: do these reduced admission rates occur differentially by diagnosis? And if so, do HMOs reduce admissions of those cases that appear to be less in need of in-hospital care? To answer these questions we will first examine some theoretical arguments concerning differential admission rates of what might be termed "discretionary admissions." Then data will be examined concerning HMO and non-HMO admission rates for broad categories of care and for specific diagnoses and procedures that have been questioned as being "unnecessary."

Some differences in economic incentives between HMOs and non-HMOs may help to predict what types of admissions might be differentially affected, if we examine reasons for hospitalization. One obvious reason is to provide services that cannot be performed elsewhere. Between the two broad categories of treatment, medical and surgical, the latter is more likely to be dependent on hospital facilities, although new ambulatory surgical centers allow many outpatient operations (Rosenberg, 1970; Thurlow, 1971). Even without a separate surgical center, many hospitals use their operating rooms for patients who are not admitted as inpatients. As will be seen below, this is a major factor for some HMOs. A second consideration is that a much larger proportion of a surgeon's income, if paid on an FFS basis, comes from performing in-hospital services (operations), than is the case for internists. Thus, if the FFS system has incentives to provide more care than would be the case under a fixed payment system, we would expect to find a greater differential among surgical than among medical admissions. Of course, this incentive can be at work without an effect on admissions, if patients are operated on a nonadmit basis.

A third reason for admission is to perform various diagnostic tests that also could be done on an outpatient basis. Incentives to hospitalize for such procedures will depend, in part, on the patient's insurance coverage for in-

and outpatient tests and the relative profitability of performing the tests. For example, even if the patient has full insurance coverage for inpatient and outpatient care, an FFS physician may choose not to perform tests on an outpatient basis if more money can be made through other services. HMOs will have an incentive to use the least expensive means of providing the services. If the HMO is a PGP, there may be a sufficient volume of tests to warrant offering them on an ambulatory basis. However, if the HMO is an IPA and its patients are widely dispersed, there may be too few people at any one location to offer alternatives to inpatient care.

A fourth reason to hospitalize patients is that it is easier for a physician to see more patients per hour in the hospital than in the office. For instance, in 1973 internists saw 3.1 patients per hour in the hospital versus 2.7 in the office; comparable figures for surgeons were 4.2 and 3.6, respectively (American Medical Association, 1974, pp. 174, 183, 184). More importantly, the net revenue per hospital visit is almost certainly higher than for an office visit. Fees for follow-up hospital visits ($14.65 for internists and $15.30 for surgeons) are between those of initial ($20.34 and $17.59) and follow-up ($11.13 and $10.34) office visits, but the physician has no overhead (rent, nurses, secretaries, and so on) for the hospital visit (American Medical Association, 1974, pp. 209, 211, 212). Professional expenses amount to about 40 percent of a physician's gross revenue, and it is reasonable to expect them to try to shift as many expenses as possible to other entities, such as hospitals. If HMOs can make their physicians sensitive to the costs incurred by the hospital, then they may attempt to reduce "hospitalization for convenience."

Differences in Broad Categories of Admissions

These considerations lead us to a number of predictions. First, it is reasonable to expect that HMOs will achieve a disproportionate share of their "reductions" in admissions through reductions in surgical admissions. This is based on the assumption that the large surgical fee would serve as a greater incentive for surgeons to operate in a questionable situation than for internists to hospitalize. Second, although the optimal surgery rate cannot be specified, it is reasonable to expect HMOs to achieve greater "reductions" when there is a relatively high rate of surgery in the community. (See Pauly, 1979). Third, because IPA physicians are paid on an FFS basis by the organization, in contrast to the situation in most PGPs, it is likely that IPAs will be relatively less effective than PGPs in "reducing" surgery. Fourth, it may be expected that HMOs "reduce" admissions for diagnosis and laboratory tests when possible.

Table 5-8 presents data concerning total and surgical admissions for twenty-five comparisons of HMO enrollees with other populations. Variations in both sets of data are substantial, with differences in total admissions per 1000 from −21 to +120 and in surgical admissions from −12 to +44.

Table 5–8   Admission Rates in HMOs and Comparison Groups for All Reasons and for Surgery

Study[a]	Total Admissions per 1000			Surgical Admissions per 1000			Surgical Admissions as % of Total	
	Comparison	HMO	Difference[b]	Comparison	HMO	Difference[b]	Comparison	HMO
C. HIP vs. BC-BS members	96	77	19	50	41	9	52%	53
D. HIP vs. GHI	88	70	18	62	49	13	70	70
E. HIP vs. GHI	110	63	47	76	43	33	69	68
F. Kaiser vs. BC/Commercial	143	88	55	66	33	33	46	38
H. Kaiser vs. Blue Cross/GE Major Medical (Adult only)	74	95	-21	46	58	-12	62	61
L. Group Health vs. Prudential Indemnity (Sault Ste. Marie) 42	137	109	28		62	46	16	45
M. Medicaid Enrollees in GHA—After vs. Before	109	76	33	33	18	15	30	24
P. Kaiser vs. Indemnity/Blue Cross	110	87	23	46	34	12	42	39
Ross-Loos vs. Indemnity/BC	110	76	34	46	35	11	42	46
FMCs vs. Indemnity/BC	110	107	3	46	44	12	42	41
R. MCG group vs. Controls	79	73	6	43	50	-7	54	68
Dilution group—After enrollment vs. before	95	78	17	49	49	0	52	63
T. Group Health vs. Blue Cross (unstandardized)	74	52	22	50	38	12	68	73
Health Watch vs. BC (unstandardized)	74	81	-7	50	53	-3	68	65
Rochester Health Network vs. BC (unstandardized)	74	58	16	50	37	13	68	64

V. Medicaid Enrollees

Consolidated Medical System vs.

Control	146	26	120	64	20	44	44	77
Family Health Program vs. Control	142	40	102	46	14	32	32	35
Group Health Cooperative of Puget Sound vs. Control	146	74	72	84	50	34	58	68
Harbor Health Services vs. Control	104	54	50	42	28	24	40	52
Harvard Community Health Plan vs. Control	96	46	50	44	24	20	46	52
HIP vs. Control	114	64	50	36	16	20	32	25
Temple Health Plan vs. Control	76	38	38	36	20	16	47	53
Redwood FMC vs. Control	190	160	30	120	82	40	63	51
Sacramento FMC vs. Control	106	122	−16	72	66	6	70	54
Z. Stanford Employees Kaiser vs. PAMC	44	38	6	32	25	7	73	66

a For sources and qualifications concerning the data, see Table 5−1.
b Difference = Comparison rate − HMO rate.

But the base or comparison admission rates vary so much (from 74 to 190 for total admissions and 33 to 120 for surgical admissions) that just examining the differences is very confusing.

One way to test the first three predictions mentioned above is to compare the proportion of total admissions in each plan accounted for by surgery, as shown in the last pair of columns and in Figure 5-3. This at least partially controls for the wide variations, which probably are due to differences in population characteristics. Surprisingly, none of the hypothetical relationships are supported by the data. Of the twenty-five pairs, thirteen show a lower proportion of surgery in HMOs, and eleven show a higher proportion, with one pair having exactly equal rates. Furthermore, the scatter suggests a tight clustering around the 45° line, with one exception—a very high surgery proportion in an HMO. This indicates that HMOs reduce admissions equally in surgical and nonsurgical categories. Second, if HMOs were to find it easier to achieve reductions in surgery the higher the relative rate is in the community, the scatter should have a slope of less than 45°.

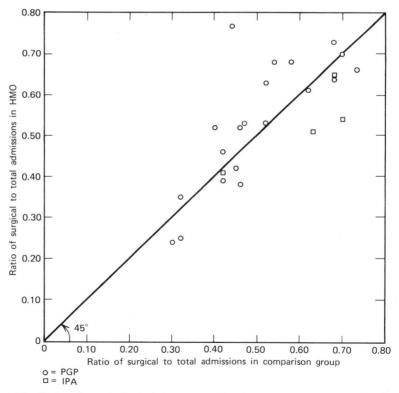

Figure 5-3 Ratio of surgical admissions to total admissions in 25 pairs of HMOs and comparison groups. The 45° line represents an equal proportion of surgical admissions in HMOs and comparison groups.

The difference between regression through the scatter and the 45° line is not statistically significant, indicating that regardless of the proportion of surgical admissions in the control group, HMOs tend to retain about the same proportion. Apparently, surgery is no easier to reduce when it accounts for 70 percent of the admissions than when it accounts for 30 percent. Third, our predictions were that IPAs, with their FFS payments to surgeons, would find it more difficult to reduce surgery than would PGPs. The scanty data that are available directly conflict with this expectation; all four of the IPAs had a lower proportion of surgery than their comparison groups, in contrast to only ten of the twenty-one PGPs.

These surprising findings warrant some discussion about potential biases in the data that could account for these results. Obviously, surgical and medical admissions account for a substantial fraction of total admissions, but we must ask whether other admissions systematically change within HMOs to bias the results. The two main categories that are omitted are obstetrical and diagnostic admissions. HMOs tend to have a somewhat higher rate of obstetrical admissions than comparison groups, in both relative and absolute terms. (This is due largely to differences in coverage.) Thus some of the data presented above are biased by the inclusion of maternity cases in the total admissions figures. However, this will tend to bias upward the estimate of the HMO's effect on surgery, making the proportion of admissions attributable to surgery lower than would be the case if there were no differential in maternity rates. For diagnostic admissions, the bias works in the other direction, to reduce the apparent affect of HMOs on surgical admissions. The data in Table 5-6 provide the best evidence available on these issues. The two PGPs have substantially lower rates of admissions for diagnosis, X-ray, and laboratory tests, but the admission rate in the IPA plan is about equal to the average of the comparison groups. These differentials are reduced if they are considered in terms of the proportion of all admissions. The data in Table 5-9 are derived from Table 5-6 and indicate, at least in that sample of four plans, that the biases are not substantial, and the various measures give basically the same results. In fact, to the extent that any shifts are apparent, they are

Table 5-9   Relative Importance of Surgery Using Different Bases for Total Admissions

	Comparison	Kaiser	Ross-Loos	FMCs
Surgery ÷ Total	42%	39%	46%	41%
Surgery ÷ Total − Maternity	45	45	55	52
Surgery ÷ Total − (Diagnosis/ Lab/X-ray)	47	42	48	46
Surgery ÷ Total − (Diagnosis/ Lab/X-ray − Maternity)	50	49	58	60

SOURCE.   Table 5-6.

toward raising the concentration of surgery admissions in HMOs relative to the comparison group.

One relatively recent change in the delivery of surgical care is the use of the operating room for patients who otherwise are not admitted to the hospital. This is comparable to the procedures performed in ambulatory surgical centers and is to be distinguished from the very simple surgical procedure commonly performed in a physician's office. Comparative data exist for only one setting, Scitovsky and McCall's Kaiser-PAMC study. They found that Kaiser performed 32 percent of all surgical procedures on a nonadmission basis, in contrast to 14 percent for the PAMC. A sense of the rapid growth of this type of care can be drawn from Kaiser Portland, where the proportion of "do not admit" surgery increased from a very low proportion in 1966 to 35 percent in 1974 (Greenlick et al., 1978). Similar increases have been documented in British Columbia (Shah and Robinson, 1977). Even within a single Kaiser region, such as Southern California, differences in the use of outpatient surgery accounts for 14 percent of the substantial variation in patient days per 1000 population across medical centers (Klitsner, 1976, p. 26).

Thus the available data do not support three of the four hypotheses concerning differential admission patterns in HMOs for broad groups of cases. Instead, HMOs appear to have equally lower admission rates in both surgical and nonsurgical categories. This equality appears to hold regardless of whether surgery accounts for a large or small proportion of admissions. Contrary to our expectations, IPAs appear to have a more consistently lower relative rate of surgery than do PGPs. The data do support the prediction that PGPs attempt to reduce the admission rate for diagnosis, laboratory tests, X-rays, and minor surgery.

Discretionary and Nondiscretionary Admissions

There is increasing debate in both medical and lay literature about what constitutes necessary medical care. (See Fuchs, 1974; Illich, 1976; Bunker, 1970; Powles, 1973; Pauly, 1979; U.S. House of Representatives, 1975, 1976.) When the question is posed in this fashion, it is inevitable that more heat than light is generated in the ensuing debate. Instead, let us assume that there is some scale concerning the degree to which an admission or procedure is discretionary and that we consider, not one particular case, but 100 cases with the same diagnosis. Most people agree that some categories of cases either (a) have a higher proportion of discretionary cases or (b) have a higher average value on the discretionary index. For example, most people would probably rate plastic surgery to reduce the size of one's nose as more discretionary than plastic surgery after third-degree burns.

Direct evidence that at least some admissions are considered discretionary by the recommending physician is provided by Anderson and Sheatsley (1967). They interviewed physicians concerning the necessity and urgency for hospitalization of a sample of their patients. For 30 percent of these cases hospitalization was not deemed "absolutely necessary," and for half of these the physician indicated that the alternative was treatment on an ambulatory basis (1967, p. 87). When asked about the usual handling of "this kind of patient," the proportion of "absolutely necessary" cases fell by about 10 percent. Of course, limiting the sample to patients who were actually hospitalized and asking their physicians about the necessity of admission probably results in an overestimate of "necessity." In fact, when asked about the appropriateness of then current (1960-61) practice, 52 percent of the physicians believed there was too much hospitalization, in contrast to 5 percent who felt there was not enough (Anderson and Sheatsley, 1967, p. 98).

It is important to distinguish two aspects of the discretionary index: urgency and necessity for hospital care. Cases that fall into the urgent category require immediate treatment. For example, most trauma would be considered urgent. However, it should be recognized that some of these cases could be treated equally well on an ambulatory basis. Nonurgent cases can be postponed, and thus may be scheduled at the patient's and physician's convenience. The second aspect of discretion is the necessity of hospital care. In some cases hospitalization is the only way to provide treatment, while in other cases treatment could be provided on either an inpatient or outpatient basis. The alternatives to hospital care may vary from aggressive ambulatory medical treatment to a wait-and-see approach, in the hope that the problem will resolve itself. It is important to recognize that some necessary procedures, such as repair of a detached retina or correction of orthopedic impairments, are nonurgent and can be scheduled when convenient.

It might be expected that the two aspects of discretionary care will have different implications for the comparison of admissions by HMOs and non-HMOs. Both systems have an incentive to schedule nonurgent cases when it is most convenient. If HMOs operate with a tighter bed supply, then the waiting period for cases that can be postponed is likely to be longer, and a somewhat higher fraction of HMO patients may recover without hospitalization. This latter effect is unlikely to be large. The major differences between HMOs and non-HMOs should appear in those cases for which hospitalization is discretionary.

The problem of course, is in determining what types of admissions fall in the "relatively discretionary" category. It is unusual to find an authoritative pronouncement in medical literature that a certain list of diagnoses should not be treated on an inpatient basis. Instead, there have been two approaches, one general and one specific, both of which rely on empirical studies. Rafferty (1971; 1972; 1975) uses a weighted index to compare types of admissions. The weights are merely the average length of stay for each diagnosis, using a constant data base. He argues that discretionary cases tend to have shorter lengths of stay. Therefore, if a hospital's case mix shifts toward cases with shorter stays, it tends to be treating more discretionary cases. (In this analysis the actual length of stay in question is not at issue.) Evidence for the relationship between discretionary admissions and length of stay comes from Anderson and Sheatsley (1967) and is presented in Table 5–10. It is apparent from the distributions that shorter stays were more common for those patients for whom hospitalization was not absolutely necessary. However, it is not clear that the relationship is sufficiently close to allow us to use "short length of stay" as a proxy for "discretionary." Overall, 46 percent of the admissions were zero to five days; for "absolutely necessary" conditions, 61 percent of the patients stayed longer than five days, but even for those for whom "hospitalization might be a good idea," 39 percent stayed that long. Thus, although there is some relationship, a great many necessary admissions last only a few days, and a great many discretionary admissions have long stays.* However, even with this limitation, Rafferty's index approach provides a useful summary measure.

The specific approach is based on a comparison of hospitalization rates for certain diagnoses and procedures across geographic areas. If large variations are found and there is no evidence of comparable differences in the underlying prevalence of the disease, then it is inferred that, at least for some of the cases in the high-rate areas, hospitalization was discretionary. These arguments are buttressed by two additional sets of data, one indicating that differences in procedure rates appear directly related to the availability of medical personnel to perform the services, and the second indicating few differences in mortality or morbidity across regions (Bunker, 1970; Wennberg and Gittelsohn, 1973, 1975; Wennberg, Gittelsohn, and Soule, 1975; Vayda, 1973; Roos, Roos, and Henteleff, 1977). Although the authors of these studies generally refrain from using the terms "necessary" and "unnecessary," it is reasonable to expect those procedures that have a wide variation in occurrence to include a greater proportion of discretionary cases than those that appear to be relatively insensitive to variations in the supply variables. For our purposes, the primary problem with these studies is that they tend to be limited to specific surgical procedures with high rates of frequency. Table 5–11 presents these data along with data concerning surgery rates per 100,000 population by procedure. The problem of selectivity is not as important as would first appear to be the case. Comparative data are available for twelve of the eighteen most common operations, and these twelve account for over

---

*Anderson and Sheatsley also provide the data for a comparable table relating length of stay to the amount of elapsed time from the start of the problem until admission (1967, p. 34). For these "postponable" admissions, the relationship is even less clear. Of those admitted the same day as their "starting date," 37 percent had stays of less than six days, while for those admitted six months or more after the "starting date," 57 percent had stays of less than six days. But Anderson and Sheatsley do not provide a cross classification of admissions that contrasts "postponability" with "necesssity."

Table 5—10   Length of Stay by Degree of Necessity for Hospitalization According to Recommending Physician: Massachusetts, 12 Months, 1960—61

Physician Said:	Length of Stay								Total	
	0—1	2—3	4—5	6—7	8—14	15—21	22—30	31+	%	N
Hospitalization absolutely necessary	8.5	18.8	12.1	14.6	25.9	8.3	5.6	6.1	99.9	1139
Patient much better off in a hospital	11.9	28.7	16.2	11.3	22.9	5.2	2.4	1.2	99.8	327
Hospital might be a good idea	5.9	35.3	19.6	12.7	15.7	5.9	2.9	2.0	100.0	102
Did not recommend at all	15.4	35.9	17.9	5.1	10.3	5.1	5.1	5.1	99.9	39

SOURCE.   Anderson and Sheatsley, 1967, p. 88.

one-third of all operations. The focus on surgical procedures is a more difficult problem. It appears that there is much less consistency in assigning medical diagnoses, so that it is more difficult to categorize patients clearly. This is in contrast to the relatively uniform classification of surgical procedures. The proportion of discretionary medical admissions may be above average in such diagnostic categories as upper respiratory infections.

Although some procedures are clearly identified in the literature as being in the relatively discretionary category and therefore should show substantial variations across areas, it is important to determine whether such variations also occur in the relatively nondiscretionary categories. Table 5—11 provides only partial confirmation of the predicted stability for nondiscretionary procedures. For instance, appendectomies are performed at about the same rate in the United States, Canada, England, and Wales; yet there is more than a twofold variation among areas within Vermont. Thus, even for appendicitis, there may be a substantial degree of discretion involved in whether a person with a given set of symptoms should be immediately operated upon or watched carefully and treated medically. A preference for the latter practice pattern could result in substantially lower appendectomy rates (Neutra, 1977). Large variations also are evident for procedures such as reduction of fracture and mastectomy. Overall comparisons provide only partial confirmation. For 1965-66, 1.96 times as many operations were performed in the United States as in England and Wales (Bunker, 1970, p. 136), and of the discretionary procedures, five were above that ratio, four were below, and two were

Table 5–11   Number and Rate of Operations with Large Frequencies Performed for Inpatients Discharged from Short-Stay Hospitals, by Sex: United States, 1971, and Comparison of Procedure Rates in Various Areas (Excludes Newborn Infants and Federal Hospitals)

Surgical Operation and ICDA Code[a]	Both Sexes[b]	Male	Female	USA/England and Wales[d] Male	USA/England and Wales[d] Female	Canada/England and Wales[e] Male	Canada/England and Wales[e] Female	13 Vermont Service Areas[f] Highest 2/Lowest 2
	(rate per 100,000 population)							
All operations[a]	7,805.3	6,333.4	9,151.0					
+*Tonsillectomy with or without adenoidectomy 21.1–21.2 5.2	478.3	457.0	496.4	2.0	2.0	2.0	2.0	
+Dilation and curettage of uterus, diagnostic 70.3	380.5	...	734.0					
Biopsy A1–A2	373.9	244.9	492.9					3.5[g]
+*Hysterectomy 69.1–69.5	282.0	...	544.1					
*Repair of inguinal hernia 38.2–38.3	241.5	446.5	50.0	—	2.4	—	2.2	2.2
Excision of lesion of skin and subcutaneous tissue 92.1–92.2	203.4	187.8	216.3	1.7	1.8	1.8	2.1	1.4
+*Cholecystectomy 43.5	184.6	88.0	273.6	2.9	3.0	5.0	7.0	2.9
Oophorectomy; Salpingo-oophorectomy 67.2–67.5	161.7	...	311.9					
+Appendectomy[c] 41.1	157.3	167.7	146.5	1.0	0.8	1.0	0.9	2.4
Closed reduction of fracture without fixation 82.0	154.1	180.3	128.7					
Operations on muscles, tendons, fascia, and bursa 88–89	135.6	146.2	125.5			2.0[h]	2.4[h]	
Reduction of fracture with fixation 82.2	130.1	117.3	141.6					

108

Dilation and curettage after delivery or abortion 78.1	129.1	...	249.1					—[g]
Mastectomy 65.2–65.6	125.7	11.8	231.2	1.9	1.6	3.2	1.4	2.3
+*Extraction of lens 14.4–14.6	120.3	102.3	136.6	1.4	1.2	2.0	2.1	
Ligation and division of fallopian tubes, bilateral 68.5	105.5	...	203.5					
*Hemorrhoidectomy 51.3	105.4	114.2	96.8	2.7	4.4	1.9	3.0	3.6
*Prostatectomy 58.1–58.3	102.5	212.9	...			2.5	—	2.8
Cesarean section 77.0	95.9	...	185.1			—	1.2	
Repair of obstetrical laceration 78.2–78.3	93.3	...	180.0					
*Excision and ligation of varicose veins 24.4	51.5	23.6	76.9			1.0	2.1	4.0

[a] Includes data for surgery not shown in table. Source: U.S. National Center for Health Statistics (Blanken, Gary E.), 1974, p. 4.

[b] Includes data for sex not stated.

[c] Limited to estimated number of appendectomies excluding those performed incidental to other abdominal surgery.

[d] Source: Bunker, 1970, p. 137. Rates are for USA (1965) and England and Wales (1966).

[e] Source: Vayda, 1973, p. 1226. Rates are age-adjusted, for Canada (1968) and England and Wales (1967).

[f] Source: Wennberg and Gittelsohn, December, p. 1105. Rates are the average of the highest and lowest two hospital service areas of the 13 in Vermont.

[g] Includes all dilation and curettage procedures.

[h] Includes all fractures.

* Identified as elective–discretionary by Vayda.

+ Identified by the American Association of Professional Standards Review Organizations as "common procedures that . . . have a significant potential for inappropriate utilization," 1978.

equal to it. For 1967-68, there were 1.6 times as many nonobstetrical operations for women and 1.8 times as many for men in Canada as in England and Wales (Vayda, 1973, p. 1225). These age-adjusted data clarify the results; the sex-specific ratio for twelve of the fourteen elective procedures is above that of the sex-specific ratio for all procedures.

Thus our search for empirical measures of discretionary admissions has resulted in two methods, each of which is less exact and discriminating than is ideal. However, given the limitations in methodology, what can be said about the extent to which HMOs differentially reduce discretionary admissions? Broida (1975) provides the case-mix index data for the Marshfield Clinic experiment. He develops the length of stay weights from the experiences of enrollees in the prepaid plan and matched samples of nonenrollees during the year before the plan began operation. Using this index, he found that prior to enrollment, the prepaid population had an index value of 94.85, which indicates a mix of admissions weighted toward those of a shorter length of stay (which is taken to mean more discretionary). In the three years after enrollment, the index rose slowly (95.41, 95.53, 98.66), suggesting small case-mix changes in favor of those with longer stays. On the other hand, the FFS sample showed substantial variation in their indices over the four-year period (103.75, 95.78, 99.34, and 103.86). So it is not at all clear that the slight trend for the prepaid sample is meaningful. Furthermore, given the particular characteristics of the Marshfield experiment and the experience of a substantial increase in admissions after prepayment, it is difficult to interpret these data.

The index number test should be more fruitful when applied to the data in Table 5-7, which compares GHA with BC-BS using age-sex adjusted data. The average length of stay for people in the two plans was used as the weight in this analysis. With the overall admission rates for the combined sample, the computed length of stay is 6.596 days. If the same weights are used with the GHA admission mix, the computed length of stay is 6.695, yielding an index value of 101.5 and indicating a slight shift toward longer length of stay (less discretionary?) cases in GHA. However, these results are hardly substantial. Instead, they suggest that the 43 percent reduction in admissions for GHA (relative to BC-BS) is not selectively achieved in short-stay admissions.

A more direct test of the hypothesis that HMOs differentially reduce discretionary admissions is presented in Table 5-12. If HMOs are able to screen out the more discretionary cases, we would expect them to show larger relative reductions in the admission or procedure rates for such cases than for all cases combined. The data are sparse, but in general they provide only limited support for the hypothesis. Only twenty-five of the forty-one entries in the table are lower than the overall rates, a finding unlikely to differ from a random sample. However, these data are hardly a random sampling from the same universe; they come from a wide range of studies of varying quality. A few patterns emerge that are of interest. With the exception of Study R, the HMOs seem to have low rates of tonsillectomies, even when considered relative to their overall surgery rates. This is not surprising, because for quite some time tonsillectomies have been prime examples of discretionary procedures. It would not be surprising if they were considered poor form in the PGPs.* Furthermore, substantial changes in tonsillectomy rates have been occurring in the FFS sector. Perrott notes a 25 percent reduction over the period 1961 to 1968 in the rates for people with the BC-BS option of the Federal Employees Health Benefits Program (1971, p. 262). There was also a 50 percent reduction in tonsillectomies between 1969 and 1976 (Bear, 1977). Even more striking is the large rate change in Vermont following feedback to physicians of Wennberg and Gittelsohn's initial results (Wennberg and Gittelsohn, 1975, p. 130). Thus it appears that tonsillectomy rates are particularly poor indicators of performance. The data for the remaining seven discretionary procedures are about evenly split between those above and those below the overall ratios.

How these data are to be interpreted is not entirely clear. It is evident, however, that most of the previous discussions of hospital utilization in HMOs have focused on only part of the story. Even as careful an observer as Donabedian notes:

The one thread that runs with absolute uniformity throughout all the comparisons given . . . is the tonsillectomy rate, which is always lower in prepaid group practice. This, plus the observation that surgical hospitalization rates are lower in the three major HIP studies (Studies C, D, and E), would lead one to believe that unjustified surgery tends to be less frequent in prepaid group practice. Further evidence is offered . . . which shows hospital admission rates for conditions that often require surgery as reported in several comparative studies which involve comparisons of HIP with an alternative plan (1969, p. 14).

It is true that HMOs exhibit markedly lower surgery rates than their comparison groups (Table 5-8), and also that PGPs have low rates for specific discretionary procedures. However, the rates for nonsurgical admissions tend to be equally low, and the discretionary rates, with the exception of tonsillectomies, are not consistently lower than the rates for all surgery. Whether these lower surgical rates are too low will be discussed in Chapter 9. Furthermore, the data concerning the whole mix of admissions lend little support to the hypothesis that HMOs differentially reduce discretionary or short-stay admissions. Nor do diagnostic-specific data support the differential admissions hypothesis. For the GHA-Blue Cross

*The results in Study R are based on very small samples and control populations that have unusually low surgery rates. Thus the lack of differences between the two groups is not surprising. Furthermore, as has been discussed in Chapter 2, the MCG physicians had no financial incentives to reduce hospitalization.

Table 5–12 Comparison of Rates for Selected Procedures in HMOs and Comparison Plans

	Ratio of HMO Admission Rates to Control Groups (see notes below)									
	T/A	Hyste-rectomy	Hernia	Cholecy-stectomy	Cataract	Hemorr-hoidectomy	Prosta-tectomy	Varicose Veins	All Surgery	All Admissions
	1	2	3	4	5	6	7	8		
Study C (pp. 25–26)[a] HIP/BC-BS (age-sex adjusted) (BC-BS with medical-surgical coverage)	0.56[b]	1.10[e]	1.16[i]	1.09[l]	—	0.53[o]	1.06[q]	0.93[s]	0.83	0.79
Study D (pp. 1717, 1719) HIP/GHI (males, age-adjusted)	—	—	0.69[i]	0.92[l]	—	0.11[o]	2.08[r]	—	0.95	0.93
HIP/GHI (female, age-adjusted)	0.46[b]	0.65[e]	1.30[i]	0.74[l]	—	0.71[o]	—	0.41[s]	0.76	0.76
Study G (p. 66) HIP/Union Plan	0.69[c]	0.76[e]	0.77[i]	0.87[l]	—	0.95[p]	—	0.88[s]	—	0.98
Study H (pp. 155–157) Kaiser/BC-BS+GE	0.35[b]									1.08
Study K (p. 19) High Option: Group Practice/Blue Cross	0.35[b]	0.52[f]	0.71[j]						0.45	
Study L (p. 294) Group/Indemnity	0.32[b]	—[g]							—[t]	0.80
Study O (Table 4–9 above) GHA/BC-BS	0.25[d]		0.83[k]	0.55[l]			0.57[q]			0.53
Study R MCG/Control[u]	1.35[b]	0.73[h]	1.30[j]	1.14[m]	0.49[n]	—	—	—	1.14	0.92

Study Y [v]								
GH/KCM-BC	0.17 [c]	0.16 [h]	—	0.59 [m]	—	—	—	0.65
Study Z [w]		1.71 [h]			—	—	—	0.70

Procedures—Diagnoses

[a] See Table 5–1 for a detailed description of the studies

[b] Tonsillectomy with or without adenoidectomy

[c] Coded as ear, nose, throat disorders in children under 15 years of age.

[d] Hypertrophy of tonsils and adenoids

[e] Diseases of the female genital tract

[f] "Female surgery," which includes mastectomy, dilation and curettage (nonmaternal), and hysterectomy.

[g] Of the following seven diagnoses—"other operations on uterus and cervix; operations on vagina; other operations on female genital organs, excluding obstetrical; operations inducing or assisting delivery; operations after delivery or abortion; Caesarian section and other obstetrical operations; and certain operations of the uterus and supporting structures—all but the last showed lower rates in GHA (J. E. F. Hastings et al., 1973, pp. 94, 103).

[h] Hysterectomy

[i] Inguinial hernia

[j] Repair of inguinal hernia

[k] Coded as "Other diseases of Appendix, Hernia, and Intestinal Obstruction."

[l] Gallbladder disease

[m] Cholecystectomy

[n] Coded as "Ophthalmologic Surgery."

[o] Hemorrhoids

[p] Coded as rectal disorders.

[q] Hyperplasia of the prostate

[r] Diseases of the prostate

[s] Varicose veins of lower extremity

[t] Of the 26 groups of operations with 20+ cases, 16 (including the 6 mentioned in note g) were less frequently performed in GHA, and 10 were performed more frequently.

[u] See Perkoff et al., May 1975, p. 621. These data are adjusted to rates per person year. There were a total of only 139 admissions for each group (MCG and Control).

[v] See LoGerfo et al., January 1979, p. 4.

[w] The "Hysterectomy" figures include all female genital system and maternity-related procedures except deliveries. Scitovsky and McCall, January 1980.

113

data presented in Table 5-7, 37 percent of the lower GHA admission rate is attributable to four diagnostic categories, but these four represent 33 percent of the Blue Cross admissions and 30 percent of GHA admissions. If GHA differentially reduced admissions in a few diagnostic categories, the first figure would be substantially larger than the other two. Similarly, the four diagnostic categories accounting for 22 percent of the differences in days between the two plans represent 21 and 20 percent of each plan's days. Also, contrary to expectations, IPAs appear to have somewhat proportionately lower surgery rates than PGPs. The one prediction concerning the source of the HMO utilization savings that was supported is the lower rate of admissions for diagnosis and tests in PGPs.

SUMMARY

HMO enrollees have lower hospitalization rates than do comparable people in the conventional medical care system. For enrollees in prepaid group practices evidence supporting this statement is overwhelming. For enrollees in individual practice associations the results still hold, although they are less clear. Overall, HMO enrollee hospitalization rates are about 30 percent lower than those of conventionally insured populations. There is relatively little consistent difference in patterns of overall average length-of-stay for patients admitted to the hospital. This lack of difference, however, seems to be the result of some offsetting factors, rather than identical stays in various settings for specific categories of patients. The overall differences in hospital days per 1000, therefore, are primarily attributable to lower admission rates for HMO enrollees. Much of the existing literature suggests the lower surgery rates in HMOs and low rates for selected discretionary procedures as potential explanations for the lower admission rates. If this were true, the case in favor of HMOs would be substantially strengthened by the argument that not only do they reduce utilization of expensive services, but that reduction comes in categories that are known to be medically unnecessary. Unfortunately, the data are inconclusive on this point and seem to provide at least as much support to the hypothesis that HMO admission rates are lower in all categories, or at least that there is no differential with respect to necessary-unnecessary treatment.

This is obviously an important statement, and it cannot stand without further qualification. As has been discussed, the measures of discretionary care in this section are blunt tools used to identify what might be fine distinctions in patient care. However, until better measures are developed and applied to comparisons of HMOs and non-HMOs, it seems wiser to remain skeptical than to confuse theory and rhetoric with evidence. A more important point is that the designation of certain categories of cases as discretionary tells us little about the other cases. Most of the emphasis in the literature has been on "unnecessary" surgery, but it is possible that surgeons have fallen victim to the fact that if they remove some tissue that is later found by a pathologist to be healthy, then the procedure may be termed "unnecessary." In fact, the question is whether, prior to the operation, surgery was the best decision. Internists, on the other hand, rarely can be faced with evidence that their patients would have recovered without the specific treatment that they ordered. Thus truly unnecessary or discretionary admissions may be just as common in the "all other" category, but it is difficult to determine if this is the case. The fuzziness of admitting medical diagnoses and differences in patterns of diagnosis across regions and institutions further complicates an analysis.

This observation leads to three alternative, but not mutually exclusive, interpretations of the existing evidence. In the first place, there may be some discretionary cases in all categories, and an effective HMO develops ways of preventing such patients from being admitted. It need not limit itself to cases identified in the literature as "discretionary." Second, self-selection may be an important factor in explaining the differences in admission rates—that is, HMO enrollees may be basically healthier or may merely prefer less hospital care, and this factor may account for the relatively low rates in "nondiscretionary" categories. Third, HMOs may "undertreat," or the traditional providers "overtreat," nondiscretionary cases. Few good outcome studies have been done to determine the appropriate level of treatment, instead of just identifying the "standard community practice." Until these and other, more detailed studies are done to identify how HMOs really obtain their savings, it is important to recognize the substantial variations in performance within HMOs, and it is best to move cautiously and carefully to separate rhetoric from evidence.

SIX

Ambulatory Care

Ambulatory care plays a prominent role in the logic behind health maintenance organizations. Ambulatory visits can substitute for inpatient care, for example, when diagnostic tests can be performed on either an inpatient or outpatient basis. Ambulatory visits also may be used to identify and treat problems before they become serious enough to warrant hospitalization. HMOs encourage ambulatory care by offering complete or nearly complete coverage for such visits, which eliminates financial barriers to their use. But there are countering incentives for HMOs to discourage all but "necessary" care, be it inpatient or ambulatory. Thus, if one observes higher ambulatory utilization in an HMO, it is often impossible to determine whether this is because it is encouraging preventive visits, substituting outpatient for inpatient care, or is faced with greater consumer demand because of its relatively low price. Furthermore, if contrasted with a conventional reimbursement plan with extensive ambulatory coverage, the HMO might even provide fewer ambulatory visits.

Not only are relative utilization rates difficult to predict on theoretical grounds, but the empirical testing of these predictions is fraught with problems. It is likely that more people will use out-of-plan services for ambulatory care than for hospital care because of the cost differential. This leads to a strong preference for interview data over plan or insurance company records. However, there is a substantial body of evidence indicating that people tend to forget about physician visits (U.S. National Center for Health Statistics, Series 2, Numbers 7, 41, 45, 49; 1965, 1971, 1972, 1972). This recall problem can be partially overcome by using short time periods, say one month, but this eliminates the possibility of examining utilization patterns of people who use no services within a long time period, as well as of those who are consistently high utilizers of care. Data problems are further complicated when one attempts to define an ambulatory visit. For instance, are only physician visits counted, or does one also include visits to an allied health professional? How does one count a visit to a physician that is followed by a series of laboratory tests and X-rays performed by different people in the same office? The same building? In three different buildings? It should be apparent that comparisons of ambulatory utilization are particularly subject to error and that they must be interpreted with care. This chapter first will examine the number of ambulatory visits of various types. The second section will examine differences in the content of ambulatory visits. A final section offers a brief summary. (Efficiency in the provision of ambulatory care will be treated in the next chapter.)

THE NUMBER AND TYPE OF AMBULATORY VISITS

Table 6-1 presents statistics for both the average number of visits per person per year and for the proportion of people with one or more visits. The data for visits per year for HMOs and comparison groups are plotted in Figure 6-1, thus controlling for differences in populations and study designs. It is apparent that in twenty-one of the thirty-three pairs the utilization rate for HMO enrollees is higher than the rate for the comparison group. In a few cases the study methodology suggests that there may be potential biases leading to an underestimate of utilization in the non-HMO group because of a reliance on claims data (studies L, Q, R, and AA). However, elimination of these data would not substantially alter the findings—eighteen of the remaining twenty-nine pairs show higher rates in the HMO group. There are only seven observations of IPAs in our data, and six of these show substantially higher ambulatory care rates than their comparison groups. This is consistent with the FFS payments to IPA physicians, which lead to less of an incentive to reduce visits than is the case for salaried physicians in PGPs. It also implies that for the PGPs with reliable data (that is, not claims forms), only eleven of the nineteen cases show higher ambulatory visit rates, hardly evidence of a consistent difference.

Regressing the number of visits in the HMO on the number in the comparison group yields the following equation:

$$y = 2.28 \qquad .569\,x$$
$$\underline{(0.56)* + (0.132)*}$$
$$R^2 = .37$$

This implies that HMO enrollees have more ambulatory visits when the comparison enrollees have visit rates in the low to moderate range. There is a crossover, however, and when comparison enrollees have more than 5.3 visits per year, HMO enrollees have fewer visits.

Careful studies of utilization behavior recognize that it is important to distinguish among at least three types of visits: (1) preventive use, which is not undertaken in response to particular symptoms; (2) the initial visit for an illness episode; and (3) follow-up visits. (See Kasl and Cobb, 1966; Hershey, Luft, and Gianaris, 1975; Dutton, 1976; Berki and Ashcraft, forthcoming.) The important distinction, for our purposes, has to do with

---

*The figures in parentheses are standard errors. Both coefficients are significant at the .01 level.

Table 6–1   Ambulatory Visits by Type of Health Insurance Plan, 1951–1975

Study	Physician Visits per Year	Percent with 1+ Visit
A. HIP Enrollees vs. New York City Population, 1951		
HIP	—	70.3%
New York City, all persons	—	58.4
B. Populations in Windsor, Ontario, 1954		
Windsor Medical Service (FMC)	4.16	68
Other Insurance	2.58	58
No Insurance	2.68	50
E. HIP and GHI Enrollees, dual choice, 1957 (nonsurgical, nonobstetrical doctor visits in home, office, or hospital)		
HIP	5.5	75
GHI	6.0	74
H. Blue Collar Union Members and Families, 1958 (Office and home visits, excluding free care)		
Blue Cross-Blue Shield-New Jersey	4.1	68
General Electric Major Medical	4.6	74
Kaiser-Northern California	5.9	77
I. California State Employees and Families (dual choice), 1962–63 (age-sex adjusted, out-of-hospital physician visits)		
Statewide Service Plan	3.7	—
Indemnity Plans	3.7	—
Prepaid Group Practices	4.5	—
Foundations for Medical Care	4.7	—
J. Enrollees in Southern California Health Plans, 1967–68 (Data drawn from medical records; data from questionnaires refers to 3 months and is in parentheses.)		
Large commercial	2.77 (.51)	52.6 (38.6)
Small commercial	4.26 (.73)	60.9 (47.9)
Blue Cross sponsored	3.94 (.96)	66.8 (50.8)
Blue Shield Sponsored	4.09 (.46)	80.7 (30.6)
Kaiser	4.70 (.79)	81.2 (65.9)
Ross-Loos	4.61 (.81)	90.2 (48.2)
L. United Steel Workers in Sault Ste. Marie, Ontario, dual choice, 1967–68		
Group Health Association	6.2	68.9
Prudential Indemnity Coverage (see note L at end of Table)	(4.2)	65.2
M. Medicaid Enrollees aged 1–64 in Washington, D.C., 1969–72		
Study Group experience		
22 months before enrollment	4.16	—
22 months after enrollment	3.54	—
Medicaid universe, 1972	3.91	—

Table 6–1 (continued)

Study	Physician Visits per Year	Percent with 1+ Visit
O. Federal Employees in Washington, D.C., 1972–74		
Group Health Association	5.44 (6.29*)	79 (81*)
Blue Cross-Blue Shield	5.52 (4.90*)	79 (75*)
P. California State Employees and Dependents, 1970–71		
(Outpatient hospital and physician visits, age-sex adjusted)		
Indemnity	4.57	—
Blue Cross-Blue Shield (statewide)	4.41	—
Kaiser	5.09	—
Ross-Loos/Family Health Plan	5.56	—
Foundations for Medical Care	5.20	—
Q. Fee-for-Service and Prepaid Patients in Marshfield, Wisconsin, 1970–72		
1970—Population that became prepaid in 1971	1.84+	—
FFS	1.34+	—
1971—Prepaid	3.69++	—
FFS	1.49++	—
1972—Prepaid	3.68++	—
FFS	1.73++	—
R. St. Louis, Missouri, Randomly Assigned Volunteer Enrollees, 1969–72		
(Office visits, consultations, ambulatory surgery, outpatient psychiatric visits)		
Medical Care Group (clinic records)	3.56*	—
Controls (interview recall)	2.12*	—
U. GM Enrollees in Three HMOs and Blue Cross in Rochester, New York, 1974–1975		
Survey 1—1974		
Genesee Valley Group Health/Rochester Health Network (PGPs)	6.0	91%
Health Watch (IPA)	4.2	98
Blue Cross	4.4	84
Survey 2—1975 HMO enrollees compared with their own 1974 experience under BC-BS		
GVGHA/RHN—1975	3.6	88
BC-BS—1974	2.7	82
Health Watch—1975	5.4	90
BC-BS—1974	4.5	94
V. Medicaid (AFDC) Enrollees in HMOs and Control Populations, 1974-75		
Group Practice	3.96	—
Control	4.04	—
Central Los Angeles Health Project	3.84	—
Control	4.56	—

Table 6−1 (continued)

Study	Physician Visits per Year	Percent with 1+ Visit
Consolidated Medical System	3.91	—
Control	3.86	—
Family Health Program	3.44	—
Control	3.64	—
Group Health Cooperative of Puget Sound	5.14	—
Control	6.06	—
Harbor Health Services	4.36	—
Control	2.92	—
Harvard Health Plan	2.74	—
Control	2.53	—
Health Insurance Plan of Greater New York	4.43	—
Control	4.61	—
Temple Health Plan	3.13	—
Control	3.95	—
Foundation and Control		
Redwood	5.17	—
Control	4.51	—
Sacramento	6.34	—
Control	4.69	—
Y. Low-Income Enrollees in the Seattle Prepaid Health Care Project, 1971−74		
Group Health Cooperative of Puget Sound	4.46	80%
King County Medical/Blue Cross	4.32	71[++]
Z. Stanford University Employees, 1973−74		
Kaiser	3.59	74%
Palo Alto Medical Clinic	3.83	82
AA. Aged Welfare Recipients in New York City, 1962−64		
Year prior to enrollment:		
HIP enrollees	—	63
Non-HIP enrollees	—	55
Study year:		
HIP enrollees	5.3	70
Non-HIP enrollees	5.4	55
BB. Kaiser vs. California, Physician Visits, 1965		
Kaiser-Permanente	4.50	—
California	4.42	—
CC. Medicaid Populations in Two Counties, Oregon, 1971		
Clackamas County (FMC)	—	80.3
Washington County (FFS billing)	—	85.1

Table 6-1 (continued)

Identifying letters correspond to those used in Chapter 5.
* Difference significant at p < .05
+ Difference significant at p < .005
++ Difference significant at p < .001

SOURCES:
A. Committee for the Special Research Project in the Health Insurance Plan of Greater New York, 1957, p. 52.
B. Darsky, Sinai, and Axelrod, 1958, pp. 72–73.
E. Anderson and Sheatsley, 1959, p. 37.
H. Columbia University School of Public Health and Administrative Medicine, 1962a, pp. 160, 163.
I. Dozier et al., 1968, p. 52.
J. Hetherington, Hopkins, and Roemer, 1975, p. 92.
L. J. E. F. Hastings et al., March-April 1973, pp. 96–98. It is pointed out that the data source for the people covered by Prudential (claims) could lead to a substantial underestimate of the number of physician visits.
M. Fuller, Patera, and Koziol, September 1977, p. 718.
O. Meyers et al., November 1, 1977. Figures in parentheses are adjusted for the substantial racial differences in enrollment. Before adjustment plan differences are not significant, but after adjustment they are statistically significant at the .05 level.
P. Dozier et al., 1973, p. 89.
Q. Broida et al., April 10, 1975, pp. 780–783.
R. Perkoff, Kahn, and Haas, May 1976, p. 439.
U. Ashcraft et al., January 1978, pp. 14–32. Note that these are annualized data based on six-month recalls. The figures in the second column, concerning percent with 1+ visits refer to families, not individuals.
V. Gaus, Cooper, and Hirschman, May 1976, p. 10. Data for Central Los Angeles Health Project and control refer only to physician contacts, not all ambulatory visits. All data are annualized rates based on a one-month period.
Y. Paula K. Diehr, personal letter dated February 25, 1980. These data are for people enrolled at least 12 months. Comparable findings for all enrollees are published in Diehr et al., 1976, pp. II. 30, 37, 38.
Z. Scitovsky, Benham, and McCall, May 1979.
AA. Shapiro et al., May 1967, pp. 785–786. About one-third of New York City's caseload of people receiving Old Age Assistance (OAA) in 1962 were enrolled in seven HIP groups in an effort to provide better continuity of care than was available through the existing panels of physicians and outpatient clinics. Data were drawn from welfare and HIP records.
BB. Klarman, May 1971, p. 30. The Kaiser data are adjusted to account for out-of-plan visits by Kaiser members, and both sets of data are then adjusted to account for nonphysician contacts.
CC. Berkanovic et al., 1974, p. 34.

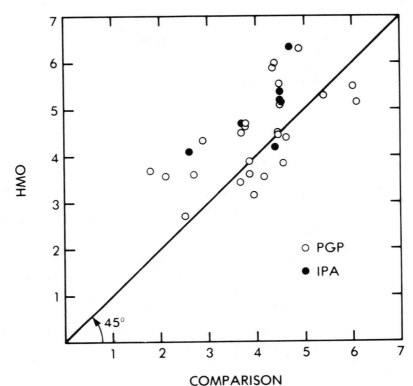

Figure 6-1 Ambulatory visits per person per year in 33 pairs of HMOs and comparison groups. The 45° line represents equal utilization in the HMO and comparison group. Data are drawn from fifteen studies covering the period 1951–1975.

the patient's relative amount of control in each situation. For preventive and initial visits, the patient has the greatest degree of control, although the physician may encourage or discourage visits for specific purposes. Physicians tend to have the most control in determining the number of follow-up visits. (See, for instance, Richardson, 1971; Gertman, 1974.) In combining these distinctions concerning control with previously discussed incentives, we can make the following predictions. The lower costs for ambulatory care in HMOs should reduce financial barriers to seeking care for both preventive and illness-episode care and thus should increase the relative number of patient-initiated visits. For follow-up care, incentives for the provider are different in the two settings. The HMO has an incentive to provide a minimum of follow-up visits, while the FFS provider may offer more. Of course, the different patient coverages must also be considered. The HMO patient may press for more follow-up visits in order to allay anxiety, while in the traditional setting, the cost of additional visits may lead the patient to decide not to return, even when requested to do so.

There are a number of ways to test these predictions with the data at hand. The rather fragmentary data in Table 6-1 indicate that, with only three exceptions (studies U4, Z, and CC), a greater proportion of HMO enrollees have at least one ambulatory visit per year. This suggests that barriers to initiating care are lower in HMOs. (There is, of course, the recall problem, and someone who has insurance coverage with a deductible may well be less likely to remember small numbers of visits because they are not reimbursable.) It also implies that the differential in the average number of ambulatory visits is partly the result of the fact that there is a larger fraction of people in non-HMOs with no visits. The other side of the coin is that among users of services, HMO and non-HMO enrollees will be more likely to use about the same number of services.

Figure 6-2 summarizes and rearranges the data from Table 6-1 to demonstrate the importance of the insurance coverage held by the comparison group. When the comparison population must pay out-of-pocket for all or most of its ambulatory care, they almost always utilize fewer such services, and they are less likely than are the HMO enrollees to utilize any ambulatory services. The picture is different when insurance coverage is nearly complete; then a majority of comparisons show lower utilization by HMO members.

The data provided by Gaus, Cooper, and Hirschman (study V) offer direct evidence concerning the influence of HMOs on patient and physician-initiated visits (1976). With the exception of the two IPAs that

	Insurance Coverage for Ambulatory Visits under Comparison Plan	
Annual Visits		
HMO > Comparison	Ⓑ, H, I1, ⑫, J1, J2, L, O, P1, P2, ⓟ₃, Q, R, U1, U3, Ⓤ₄, BB	V2, V5, V6, Ⓥ₉, Ⓥ₁₀
HMO = Comparison	—	Y
HMO < Comparison	Ⓤ₂, Z	E, M, V1, V3, V4, V7, V8, AA
Proportion of Enrollees With Visits		
HMO > Comparison	A, Ⓑ, H, J1, J2, L, O, U1, Ⓤ₂, U3	AA, Y
HMO = Comparison		E
HMO < Comparison	Ⓤ₄, Z	ⒸⒸ

Figure 6-2. Summary of ambulatory visit data by financial incentives facing the comparison population. (Source: Table 6-1. Letters refer to studies referenced in Table 6-1. Circled studies indicate IPA-HMOs.)

had substantially higher rates of ambulatory visits than the controls, there was essentially no difference in the average total number of visits between HMOs and controls. These data are of particular interest because Medicaid enrollees (who form the samples in all of these comparisons) have essentially complete ambulatory coverage. Table 6-2 presents annualized patient and physician-initiated ambulatory physician contacts for the nine HMOs and their control populations. There is no pattern in the *proportion* of visits that are patient-initiated. In only five of the nine cases did HMO enrollees initiate a larger fraction of the visits. The actual visit rates tell a different story. In seven of the nine pairs HMO enrollees initiated a larger *number* of visits than was the case for their control groups. The differential is particularly evident for IPA enrollees, while it is less clear for PGP enrollees. These data also allow a comparison of nonpatient-initiated visits. With comparable coverage for enrollees, it would be expected that HMOs have fewer follow-up visits than FFS providers. However, there are no such patterns in the average follow-up visit rates, with the possible exception of higher rates for IPA enrollees. As will be discussed below, financial incentives are only some of the many factors that help to determine practice patterns.

Focusing only on people who use ambulatory services, we can ask if there is evidence that there are different distributions with respect to the number of services per person. That is, do HMOs reduce the proportion of people who use a great many services? This is of particular interest because a small fraction of high utilizers account for a large proportion of the total services rendered. (See Densen, Shapiro, and Einhorn, 1959.) Comparative data on the distribution of visits are available for only a limited number of studies. In the first HIP comparison, study A, it appears that not only does the New York City sample include a much larger proportion of people with no visits in a year, but among those with visits, a substantially higher proportion have many visits than is the case among HIP enrollees. In the New York City sample 7.4 percent had 20+ visits versus 5.8 percent in HIP, and 35.1 percent had 5+ visits versus 31.8 percent in HIP. Of course, the New York City sample included a great many people with no coverage, and there was no matching by age, sex, and income. The comparison of HIP and GHI enrollees, study E, showed not only identical proportions of people with visits, but the distributions of visits were also identical. The Hetherington, Hopkins, and Roemer study of six Southern California plans, study J, only provides a breakdown by 0, 1 to 3, and 4+ visits per year. Within this context, there are no differences in the distributions for users. Even cruder breakdowns in study CC (0, 1 to 2, and 3+) indicate a slightly larger proportion of high utilizers in the non-IPA county, 65 percent versus 61 percent. A substantially different pattern arises from the more careful analysis of Windsor, Ontario, study B. Not only did a larger fraction of IPA enrollees have some visits, but Windsor Medical Service (WMS) users were much more likely to have a larger (19+) number of visits

Table 6−2   Outpatient Physician Contacts per Year for Medicaid Enrollees in HMOs and Controls by Type of Visit (Patient or Physician Initiated)

	Annualized Rates			Percent Patient Initiated
	Total	Patient Initiated	Other	
Group Practices	3.48	1.95	1.53	56%
Controls	3.60	1.98	1.62	55
Consolidated Medical System	3.48	1.98	1.50	57
Control	3.48	1.77	1.71	51
Family health program	3.00	1.89	1.11	63
Control	3.24	1.82	1.42	56
Group Health Cooperative Puget Sound	4.08	2.20	1.88	54
Control	4.80	2.11	2.69	44
Harbor Health Services	3.84	2.07	1.77	54
Control	2.88	1.90	0.98	66
Harvard Health Plan	2.52	1.46	1.06	58
Control	2.16	1.12	1.04	52
HIP	3.96	2.14	1.82	54
Control	4.20	2.48	1.72	59
Temple Health Plan	2.88	1.47	1.41	51
Control	3.72	2.08	1.64	56
Individual Practice Associations				
Redwood	4.08	2.16	1.92	53
Control	3.84	1.96	1.88	51
Sacramento	5.16	2.58	2.58	50
Control	3.96	2.10	1.86	53

SOURCE: Derived from Gaus, Cooper, and Hirschman, May 1976, Table 5.

(5.2 percent) than enrollees in other insurance plans (2.8 percent). The same pattern holds for relatively high users, with 23.8 percent of the WMS users having 8+ visits versus 14.2 percent of "other insured."

The Seattle Prepaid Health Care project offered complete coverage to enrollees in both the prepaid group practice and KCM-BC plan (study Y). Because the KCM-BC physicians were paid FFS and were not at risk, it is not surprising that a larger proportion of KCM-BC enrollees had very high visit rates—more than 20 visits per year (Diehr et al., 1976, pp. II.37-38). The comparison of Stanford employees in Kaiser and the PAMC yields a different story (study Z). Kaiser enrollees were more likely to have no visits, 26 percent versus 18 percent, but the two groups had essentially identical proportions of users in the 7 to 10, 11 to 15, and 16+ categories (Scitovsky, Benham, and McCall, 1979, Table 3).

The HIP experimental enrollment of Old Age Assistance recipients, study AA, provides valuable data concerning the apparent effect of the HMO on utilization of ambulatory care (Shapiro et al., 1967, p. 787). As indicated below, those people who had no ambulatory visits in the year prior to enrolling in HIP substantially increased their visit rates, while those with a great many visits reduced their rates. Although this type of change is often associated with regression toward the mean, a standard statistical problem when there is random variation, the data for non-HIP enrollees suggest that there is a real "HIP effect."* If one is willing to assume that the two groups are comparable, then it appears that HIP enrollment resulted in 1.8 more visits per year for previous nonusers and a reduction of 5.6 visits for the highest users.

Visits in Year Prior to the Study Year				
	None	1−3	4−9	10 or more
Average Number of Physician Visits in Study Year				
HIP enrollees	3.1	4.6	6.7	9.1
Non-HIP enrollees	1.3	3.0	5.6	14.7

THE MIX OF SERVICES

The range of services delivered in an ambulatory visit can cover a wide spectrum, and unless such variation is taken into consideration, comparisons may be meaningless. For instance, Bailey (1970) has shown that many of the differences in internist "output," which had been considered reflective of economies of scale, actually were attributable to physicians in larger groups performing more in-house laboratory procedures. Among the things to consider in this area is the type of visit—doctor office visit (DOV) versus telephone consultation, referrals, follow-up visits, and the use of various tests.

One major problem in analyzing the data is the lack of comparability in the coding of various items from provider to provider. Thus it is useful to examine the Hetherington, Hopkins, and Roemer data, which were drawn

*"Regression to the mean" occurs whenever there is random variation in the variable in question, such as visits per year, and the groups being observed were chosen at a particular time because they had particularly high or low values, such as the 0 and 10+ groups. Even if there is absolutely no experimental effect, one would expect some of the people in the lowest group to increase their visits and some in the highest group to reduce theirs. Thus the average of 1.3 visits for the non-HIP enrollees may well be due to this random movement. Shapiro et al. (1967) do not present the average value for the 10+ groups in the first year, but for the non-HIP enrollees it was probably more than 14.7.

from medical records and are uniformly coded (Table 6-3). The number of visits per year varies markedly across plans, with the two PGPs having the highest average visit rates, and the apparent content of the visits also seems to vary. A substantially higher proportion of visits to PGPs indicated a physical examination, and these examinations were relatively more complete.* Kaiser patients are more likely to have laboratory or X-ray services during a visit (29.9 percent) than patients in either Ross-Loos (21.6 percent) or any of the other plans (21.9 to 24.2 percent). This finding is mirrored in the frequencies with which specific results are reported. It is of some significance that the greatest differences are found in chest X-rays, for which the two PGPs have in-house facilities and offer the most complete coverage. Urinalyses are simple and can generally be done in a physician's office with a minimum of equipment; thus it is not surprising that relatively high rates are found for all patients.

Hetherington, Hopkins, and Roemer use relative value scales to measure the quantity of services provided. The data indicate little variation in the units of laboratory and X-ray services per visit in which they were used; in fact the PGPs seem to have a lower average "intensity." Thus the variation in diagnostic services stems from the proportion of people who receive such services, not how much is done to each. Overall, there is evidence that ambulatory visits to PGPs are more likely to result in a thorough physical examination and laboratory and X-ray procedures. Some of this difference, however, may be a reflection of different coverage levels. In the Seattle Prepaid Health Care Project, for example, the rate of X-rays for GH enrollees was only 60 percent that of KCM-BC enrollees. These issues will be addressed more completely in Chapter 9 on preventive care.

These data may be placed in perspective by comparing them with the content of all office practice visits (Table 6-4) as reported in the National Ambulatory Care Survey for 1973-74 (U.S. National Center for Health Statistics, De Lozier, 1975). In contrast to the national data, the proportion of visits involving physical examinations in the Hetherington, Hopkins, and Roemer systems (58 to 80 percent) is relatively high, suggesting that this refers to substantially less than a complete physical examination. Patients in the six California plans had laboratory or X-ray services in 22 to 30 percent of their visits. This is consistent with the national data showing that nearly 20 percent of all visits include some laboratory work, and 7 percent include X-rays. The national data also indicate that almost 19 percent of all office visits involve an injection or immunization. Thus, while the rates reported by Hetherington, Hopkins, and Roemer are high, they are not unreasonable, particularly if patient visits are weighted toward those specialties more likely to perform injections. The data for Kaiser, however, indicate that

---

*As is the case with all data drawn from medical records, these data must be interpreted with care. They represent only those physical examinations that are recorded and thus may merely indicate that PGP physicians keep better records.

Table 6–3 Content of Ambulatory Care under Various Health Plans

	Large Commercial	Small Commercial	Blue Cross	Blue Shield	Kaiser	Ross-Loos
Doctor visits per person per year	2.77	4.26	3.94	4.09	4.70	4.61
Percent of visits with physical examination recorded	57.9	58.2	62.0	57.5	80.3	75.1
Completeness of exam, range 0–3	1.35	1.48	1.34	1.29	1.66	1.49
Percent of visits with lab and radiology services	23.7	24.2	24.1	21.9	29.9	21.6
Mean number of units per visit with use	2.82	3.05	3.00	2.80	2.71	2.85
Lab and X-ray results reported per 1000 patients						
CBC	66	80	60	69	94	82
Urinalysis	112	91	108	88	139	102
Serology	8	18	9	18	17	8
Chest X-ray	1	29	17	29	52	38
Percent of visits with injections (excl. immunizations)	28.0	25.8	17.9	25.6	4.0	26.9
Mean injections per patient per year	1.26	1.82	1.40	2.26	0.17	1.39
Referrals to specialists:						
Percent of visits with referral	1.6	1.6	1.4	1.5	6.6	3.5
Percent of patients with 1+ referrals within the year	20.3	10.2	7.5	11.4	34.7	20.0
Referral to a paramedical worker						
Percent of visits with referral	0.4	1.6	0.3	0.7	1.2	1.2
Percent of patients with 1+ referral within year	0.6	3.7	0.9	6.5	5.7	12.6
Percent of visits with follow-up requested (or end of illness noted)	42.0	45.9	49.2	40.7	49.1	50.7
Percent of visits that were follow-up visits	46.8	50.0	53.9	41.1	49.2	61.9

SOURCE: Hetherington, Hopkins, and Roemer, 1975, pp. 92, 169, 182, 188.

Table 6–4   Treatments and Services Rendered and Disposition of Visits, Office Visits, United States May 1973 – April 1974

| | | Medical Specialties | | | Surgical Specialties | | | | |
	All Specialties	General and Family Practice	Internal Medicine	Pedi-atrics	Other Medical Specialties	General Surgery	Ob/Gyn	Other	Psy-chiatry	Other
Number of visits, in thousands	644,893	260,310	74,693	53,659	40,964	44,846	50,715	88,227	20,300	11,180
Percent of Visits With Treatment and Service Ordered or Provided[a]										
General history and exam	35.9	36.3	43.7	49.8	25.1	28.7	43.6	29.0	11.1	43.8
Lab Procedure or test	19.6	17.4	35.1	19.5	16.8	13.0	41.5	9.5	*	16.0
X-rays	7.1	5.3	15.4	3.0	8.1	7.8	1.7	12.2	*	*
Injection or immunization	18.6	24.8	14.6	29.7	33.4	10.6	4.0	5.1	10.3	14.0
Drug therapy (prescription or nonprescription)	49.4	58.8	57.8	45.2	50.2	29.7	41.4	33.2	36.6	57.6
Percent of Visits by Disposition of Visit[a]										
No follow-up planned	12.7	16.1	10.0	13.9	8.4	11.2	4.6	13.7	4.9	*
Return at specified time	61.2	54.8	67.0	48.1	77.0	61.9	76.1	60.9	84.3	63.5
Return if needed	21.4	25.8	17.7	32.5	10.9	17.1	14.4	18.9	7.1	20.9
Other	9.4	6.6	14.1	12.4	8.4	13.9	9.8	10.8	*	14.3
Telephone follow-up planned	(2.9)	NA	NA	NA	NA	NA	NA	NA	NA	NA
Referred to other physician	(2.7)	NA	NA	NA	NA	NA	NA	NA	NA	NA
Returned to referring physician	(1.1)	NA	NA	NA	NA	NA	NA	NA	NA	NA

SOURCE.   U.S. National Center for Health Statistics, De Lozier, October 1975, pp. 39, 42, 43.

[a]More than one service and disposition could be recorded for each visit. Furthermore, some items have been omitted in this table.

*Figure does not meet standards of reliability or precision.

only 4 percent of visits involved an injection, a rate matched only by Ob/Gyn visits in the national data. This suggests that there is some data or interpretation problem in the Hetherington, Hopkins, and Roemer study.

There are conflicting predictions concerning the effects of PGPs on referral rates and requests for follow-up visits. On the one hand, under a capitation system physicians are no longer concerned about losing a patient who is referred to a specialist. On the other hand, if a physician is overloaded with work, a referral is often an easy way to move the patient on (Freidson, 1975, p. 66; Mechanic, 1976, p. 90). Note that in the first case the observed PGP referral rate is "correct," and the FFS rate is "too low," while in the second case the PGP rate is "too high" and the FFS rate is "correct." Of course, no one knows the correct rate of referrals. The same argument holds for the use of more tests in order to ease the immediate patient load (Freidson, 1975, p. 61). Mechanic (1976) also points out that FFS physicians recognize that patients may be suspicious of excessive follow-up requests. On the other hand, financial incentives facing PGP physicians tend to discourage the use of excessive tests, procedures, and physician time. Which of these two sets of incentives dominates will depend on the specific situation in question.

The Hetherington, Hopkins, and Roemer data in Table 6-3 indicate that only 1.4 to 1.6 percent of the visits by non-PGP enrollees resulted in a referral to a specialist, in contrast to 6.6 percent of the Kaiser visits and 3.5 percent of the Ross-Loos visits. The non-PGP rates are somewhat lower than the national data for referrals (Table 6-4) but are consistent with them. The differences among provider types are not nearly as striking for referrals to paramedical workers. These data suggest that the "fear of losing the patient" effect is more important than the "overload" effect. If the overload effect dominated, PGP physicians would have a high referral rate to paramedical workers, as well as to specialists. This does not appear to be the case. The rate of requests for follow-up visits is somewhat higher in the two PGPs. Unfortunately, Hetherington, Hopkins, and Roemer include "end of illness" in these data, so the figures are not exactly comparable. Even with this inclusion, the rates are lower than those reported nationally. There is little evidence of a pattern in the proportion of follow-up visits.

Contrary data are presented by Hirsch and Bergan (1973) concerning three ambulatory care systems: a union clinic (PGP), an FFS group, and a network of solo FFS practitioners. The PGP physicians tended to have much higher rates of scheduled follow-up visits than the solo FFS physicians, while the FFS group was in an intermediate position. The same pattern was present for referrals. However, this was not an indication of "patient churning" by overloaded PGP physicians. The average weekly visit rate for solo practitioners was nearly four times that of PGP physicians, and there are clear indications that the latter were underworked. The data with respect to laboratory utilization are fairly clearcut: 20 percent of the PGP visits resulted in laboratory use, in contrast to 40 percent for the FFS group and 32 percent for the solo FFS providers. The latter two figures are high in comparison with the national data. Hirsch and Bergan (1973) suggest that the high rate for the FFS group was due to its ownership of a laboratory and its ability to charge for such services. Little additional information is available about the three sites or the methods used in collecting the data.

Perkoff, Kahn, and Haas (1976) report a substantially higher rate of laboratory and X-ray services per person year for the experimental MCG group than for the control group. The differential is much less dramatic when examined on a per visit basis. There were 14.4 X-ray services per 100 visits for MCG members versus 11.2 per 100 control visits. Both figures are higher than any reported in the national data, with the exception of the rate for internists. The figures for laboratory services are 38.4 per 100 for MCG members and 32.3 per 100 for the controls, again at the high end of the scale. Eisenberg et al. (1974) report on the practice patterns of the four pediatricians who served the MCG and practiced in their own FFS setting. A key difference was that the MCG was located in the Washington University Medical Center, with all the necessary facilities and available consultants, while the FFS setting was several miles from other providers and did not include laboratory or X-ray facilities. An additional difference was the use of a registered nurse at the MCG; in 18 percent of the cases, the nurse was the only provider to see a patient. The FFS group employed medical technicians who were never the only person to see a patient. An average of 1.10 laboratory tests were performed per MCG visit versus 0.66 per FFS visit. A routine hematocrit for well children at the MCG accounts for a 0.20 test per visit difference. However, differences in test rates of from 16 to 100 percent occur for all five other tests. These do not appear to be related to convenience or to whether the test was billed separately. There also was a significantly higher referral rate for the MCG children. These differences are difficult to interpret because of the small size of the patient groups, the differences in ages of the children, and other factors. They do suggest that the organizational setting may influence the practice pattern of even the same physicians.*

Table 6-5 provides an indication of the wide variation in the use of various paramedical services across ten PGPs. The rate of laboratory tests per enrollee ranges from 2.35 to 4.56, and the ratio of tests per ambulatory visit shows about the same two-fold variation. Given the relative paucity of data, it is useful to consider the extent of variability within a given practice. Kaiser-Permanente in Portland, Oregon maintains an extensive data base and has published a series of reports that offer a view of practice patterns

---

*It is also of interest that the pediatricians terminated their association with the MCG at the end of the experimental phase, suggesting that there was some dissatisfaction with the arrangement.

Table 6−5   Numbers of Paramedical Clinic Services (A) per 100

Services	Plan 1		Plan 2		Plan 3		Plan 4	
	A	B	A	B	A	B	A	B
Laboratory tests	137	456	73	233	108	352	95	348
X-ray investigations	16	58	18	60	14	45	10*	35*
Optometry	8	26	5	17	—	—	—	—
E.K.G.	3	12	2	7	2	6	—	—
Physiotherapy	9	30	2	8	—	—	—	—

SOURCE.   Jocelyn Chamberlain, June 1967, Table 3.
* Plan 4 uses a different definition for X-ray counts.

within a single PGP. One source of variation is the change in patterns over time. In 1949 the plan provided 4461 doctor office visits, 2534 laboratory services, and 482 radiology services per 1000 members (Saward, Blank, and Greenlick, 1968, p. 239). By 1971 these rates had changed to 3483 doctor visits, 4050 laboratory services, and 967 radiology services (Saward, Blank, and Lamb, 1973, p. 37). Thus within this period there appears to have been a substitution of ancillary services for doctor office visits. (Some of these trend data will be examined in Chapter 8.) Substitution also may have resulted from increased emphasis on use of the telephone. Greenlick et al. (1973) point out that the average Kaiser Portland enrollee had one phone call per year to medical personnel during 1969. This is about twice the number reported in the National Health Interview Survey for the same year (U.S. National Center for Health Statistics, Wilder, 1972). A breakdown of the Kaiser calls indicates that 40 percent concerned prescriptions or test results. An additional 47 percent concerned symptoms, and of these, 42 percent resulted only in discussion; 38 percent of the callers were given a prescription, and only 20 percent were told to come in. Although similar breakdowns for the non-Kaiser population are not available, it is conceivable that Kaiser encourages telephone calls for symptom reporting and follow-up as alternatives to office visits. A comparison of federal employees in Group Health Association of Washington, D.C. and in BC-BS indicates that, after adjusting for race, GHA enrollees have significantly more telephone calls to the doctor's office, excluding those for appointments (Meyers et al., 1977, p. 31).

A second source of variation is across physicians within the group. All Kaiser Portland physicians are board-eligible or board-certified and practice full-time for the plan. One would expect a substantial degree of homogeneity in their practice patterns, but this is not the case. With respect to telephone use, among twenty-two physicians in the Department of Medicine, the ratio of calls per doctor office visit ranged from 0.21 to 1.26, and the proportion of physician-initiated calls ranged from 1 to 28 percent. Similar variations occur in the manner in which individual physicians handle patient-initiated calls dealing with symptoms. For example, one

Ambulatory Physician Services, and (B) per 100 Persons Covered per Annum

Plan 5		Plan 6		Plan 7		Plan 8+		Plan 9+		Plan 10+	
A	B	A	B	A	B	A	B	A	B	A	B
64	235	38	176	79	260	72	235	67	235	97	387
15	53	8	39	15	49	15	49	16	56	14	57
8	30	—	—	—	—	5	15	5	16	3	11
—	—	—	—	2	5	—	—	—	—	—	—
5	18	1	4	—	—	7	22	5	17	5	21

+ Data apply only to one contract group within the plan.

internist requests that 50 percent of the callers come in, while two ask only 4 percent of their callers to make a visit. However, these two deal with the remaining 96 percent of their call-in patients in very different ways; one prescribes medication to 89 percent of them, while the other prescribes for only 49 percent (Greenlick et al., 1973, p. 133).

The variation in practice patterns occurs in other areas as well. The data in Table 6-6 show the distribution of Kaiser Portland internists by their ratio of laboratory services-DOV for the six-month periods beginning January 1967 and January 1970.* This suggests that while the overall rate of laboratory services-DOV has increased, there remains a substantial spread in practice patterns. Freeborn et al. (1972) also point out that patterns of laboratory use tend to be consistent from year to year, with correlations ranging from .62 to .84.

Pineault (1976) examined the use of various types of services within the group for patients with acute diseases and undiagnosed diseases—two broad categories with different degrees of ambiguity, which together accounted for 40 percent of the internists' office visits. He examined clinical services (physician visits and telephone calls) and technical resources (X-rays and laboratory tests) separately, with the specific services rendered weighted by a relative value scale. The coefficients of variation for the average clinical services rendered per episode by each physician were relatively small: 7 for acute diseases and 18 for undiagnosed diseases. A less comprehensive but more dramatic picture is given by the range of weighted services across the thirty-four physicians: 14.3 to 20.2 for acute diseases and 7.0 to 18.9 for undiagnosed diseases. The results for the use of technical services are much more striking. The ranges are 2.3 to 15.0 and 6.1 to 31.6, with coefficients of variation of 42 and 37, respectively, for the two disease categories.

An obvious question arises: how representative are these data from the Kaiser Portland setting? Fortunately, there are some data bearing on

---

*Six-month data are used, because there appears to be a seasonal variation in the distributions. The patterns are essentially the same if the last six months of each year are considered.

Table 6−6   Ratio of Laboratory Services per Doctor Office Visit, Kaiser-Oregon

	1.00	1.00−1.49	1.50−1.99	2.00−2.49	2.50+	All Physicians in the Department of Internal Medicine
January 1, 1967− June 30, 1967	17.6%	58.9%	17.6%	5.9%	0.0	100.0%
January 1, 1970− June 30, 1970	0.0	10.7	28.6	35.7	25.0%	100.0

SOURCE.   Freeborn et al., 1972, p. 848.

variations in practice patterns within other settings. Schroeder et al. (1973) report on variation in laboratory and drug costs for patients of faculty internists at the General Medical Clinic, George Washington University Medical Center; and Lyle et al. (1974, 1976) report on various aspects of the office practice of eight internists practicing in a North Carolina FFS group. These data are presented in Table 6-7. If anything, they suggest that the Kaiser Portland experience exhibits even less variation than other settings.

Several aspects of these data are of interest. There appears to be less variation per episode or per visit in the use of physicians' services than in the use of technical services, such as laboratory and X-ray. This tends to follow from various practices, such as appointment scheduling, which constrain the amount of physician time per visit, while the constraints on the use of ancillary services must be more subtle. Pineault (1976, p. 126) argues that Kaiser physicians have incentives to substitute physicians' services for "technical" services and that this behavior increases with the time a physician has served in the medical group. But neither his theoretical nor his empirical arguments are convincing, and he does not present evidence concerning whether technical services are used as substitutes for physican time.

The 1973 Schroeder et al. study indicates the highest degree of variation in practice patterns, but more importantly, it suggests that not all of the variation is unavoidable.* After the results of the initial audit were presented to the physicians, a second audit was performed, which indicated significant reductions in laboratory costs, although there was a slight increase in drug costs. A breakdown of the changes in patterns by physicians who were low, medium, and high users is revealing. As would be

---

*In part, the very high coefficients of variation in this study may be attributable to using as the unit of observation annualized costs per patient based on a three-month time period. If some physicians request follow-up visits within a shorter period of time (perhaps because they are full-time rather than part-time), then such data would identify them as "high cost," even though they may use no more services in the full course of treatment.

Table 6-7 Variations in Practice Patterns within Specific Settings

	Range	Mean	Coefficient of Variation*
Kaiser-Oregon[a]			
(34 internists; 12 months)			
Physician visits and telephone calls (weighted/episode)			
Acute diseases	14.3-20.2	17.40	7
Undiagnosed	7.0-18.9	13.38	18
Technical services			
Acute diseases	2.3-15.0	8.11	42
Undiagnosed	6.1-31.6	14.04	37
George Washington University-General Medical Clinics[b]			
(31 internists, part time, 3 months)			
First Audit			
Lab costs (annualized per patient)	$ 8-174	$71.84	49
Drug costs (annualized per patient)	$28-158	$85.00	41
Second Audit			
Lab costs	$ 1-162	$50.87	80
Drug costs	$29-180	$90.41	39
George Washington University-General Medical Clinics[c]			
(13 internists treating hypertensives)			
Lab costs per patient (annualized)	$ 8-161	$54	78
Internists in an FFS Group-North Carolina[d]			
(8 physicians)			
Disposition of visits			
Return appointment to physician	33%-64%	46%	21
Refer to outside consultant	3.0%-8.7%	5.4%	19
Procedures and Treatments per 100 visits (8 physicians)			
Lab tests	15.2-35.8	28.2	24
X-Ray	9.0-24.1	20.3	25
ECG	3.4-17.5	12.2	37
Drugs	51.1-65.1	58.4	8
Diet	5.9-15.2	10.7	30
Average procedure charge per encounter	$13.61-19.48	$16.10	15
Average professional charge per encounter	$12.66-14.61	$13.55	4
Total charge per encounter (including professional fees)	$27.06-34.09	$29.65	9
Palo Alto Medical Clinic[e]			
Visits per day-6 general and family practitioners	21.0-26.9	24.3	9
7 internists	10.7-14.2	12.3	10
Duration of visits (minutes)			
6 GP-FPs	15.2-18.4	16.4	8
7 internists	25.1-34.5	29.3	10

Table 6−7 (continued)

	Range	Mean	Coefficient of Variation*
Physician-generated revenue per hour (professional fees, tests, and procedures)			
6 GP-FPs	$81.73−106.01	$91.28	10
6 internists	$72.15−110.82	$91.53	19
Physician-generated revenue per visit			
6 GP-FPs	$22.61−27.21	$24.77	7
6 internists	$38.42−54.59	$45.36	15

[a] Pineault, February 1976, pp. 130−131.
[b] Schroeder et al., August 20, 1973. These data were computed from a scatter diagram presented on page 970. The calculated means were all within 3% of the published means.
[c] Daniels and Schroeder, June 1977, pp. 482−487.
[d] Lyle et al., May 1976, pp. 596, 598, 599.
[e] Roney and Estes, March-April 1975, pp. 128, 131.
* The coefficient of variation = (Standard deviation/Mean) * 100

expected, those physicians who were in the high cost group showed the greatest reduction by the second audit, a 42 percent decrease in laboratory costs, and a 4 percent decrease in drug costs. However, those physicians in the lowest cost group showed nearly as large a percentage reduction in laboratory costs (−41 percent); this was more than offset by a 36 percent increase in drug costs, resulting in a small (2 percent) net increase in overall costs per patient. The middle cost group had a small reduction in laboratory costs, which was almost exactly balanced by an increase in drug costs. These results suggest that some services ordered by the very high users may be clinically unnecessary, and this is recognized when questions are raised about wide variations. They also suggest that at the low end of the scale, laboratory tests and drugs may be seen as partial substitutes whereby extensive testing could be done to decide upon a treatment, or a reasonable guess could be made upon less data, and the patient's response to a particular therapy would be more carefully monitored. (See Bombardier, 1976.) The question of substituting one type of ambulatory service for another obviously is important in comparing productivity and costs in different settings. Of particular interest is a follow-up study by Schroeder, Schliftman, and Piemme (1974), which showed no correlation between costs and rankings of clinical competence. A third study indicated negative but insignificant correlations between cost and outcomes in treating hypertensives, as well as no relationship between laboratory costs and two measures of physician productivity (Daniels and Schroeder, 1977).

Data from the eight-person group practice in North Carolina (Lyle et al., 1976) indicate substantial variation in practice patterns within even such a small, homogeneous group. The proportion of visits ending in a return appointment, referral to a consultant, and laboratory tests or X-rays all closely coincide with the data presented in Table 6-3. This lends further support to the argument that for ambulatory care PGP practice patterns are not unlike practice patterns in other (group) settings. The experience of primary care physicians within the PAMC also supports the findings of less variation in physician visits than in tests, procedures, and so on, and shows that there is substantially more variation in such use by internists than by family or general practitioners.

SUMMARY

Predictions concerning the expected effects of HMOs on ambulatory care were composed of several parts: higher visit rates because of better coverage and substitution of outpatient for inpatient care, and lower rates because of incentives to economize. The fragmentary data reflect these conflicting incentives. The evidence is consistent on one point: a larger proportion of HMO enrollees have at least one visit per year than is the case for nonenrollees. Data for matched groups with the same ambulatory coverage (such as Medicaid enrollees) suggest that it is largely the result of the differential coverage. Data concerning ambulatory visit rates are particularly sensitive to problems in study design and data collection. If we exclude four studies with particularly questionable methodology, in nearly two-thirds of the twenty-nine comparisons, HMO enrollees have a larger number of visits. If this is broken down by HMO type, enrollees in six of seven IPAs had more visits than the comparison populations, while PGP enrollees had about the same chance of having more or fewer visits as their control populations. If we control for the extent of third-party coverage for ambulatory care, it is apparent that HMO enrollees might use fewer services than people with relatively complete coverage seeing FFS providers.

A key distinction in ambulatory care is between those visits over which the consumer has the greatest control—the initial visit in a series—and those over which the physician has the greatest control—follow-ups. Data concerning Medicaid recipients suggest that HMO enrollees initiate more visits than the control groups, and this is particularly apparent in the IPAs. Follow-up visits for the Medicaid populations show no consistent pattern. Other studies suggest that PGPs tend to reduce the proportion of people with large numbers of visits, while IPAs are less effective in doing this.

In terms of the mix of services, the data suggest that the content of HMO ambulatory visits is not particularly different from that in the average FFS visit. There is some evidence of more complete physical examinations and slightly higher rates of laboratory tests and X-rays in the most complete study available, but these patterns do not appear to be consistent. Instead, one can find comparisons in which HMO enrollees have higher and lower test rates. There also appears to be no consistent pattern with respect to referrals or follow-up visits. In fact, although formal tests are difficult to undertake, it is unlikely that the available data would enable one to reject the null hypothesis that ambulatory visits in HMOs are no different from ambulatory visits in FFS practice. Adding to the difficulties in making comparisons between provider types is the wide variation in practice behavior among physicians within a single setting. This may well be an indication that medicine is more art than science; it certainly suggests that there is no such thing as "standard practice." The wide internal variation means that the selection of particular practitioners to join a group may have a substantial influence on the average observed behavior within a setting. Furthermore, the fact that HMOs appear to have no less variability within their settings than do FFS groups suggests that these differences in practice have not been especially responsive to the special financial or organizational incentives unique to HMOs. Or more precisely, there is no evidence to indicate that such incentives have resulted in more homogeneity of HMO practice patterns.

SEVEN

Efficiency in Producing Medical Services

There is little reason to expect HMOs to have particular advantages in the efficiency with which they produce specific types of medical care services. The primary advantages of the generic HMO relevant to efficiency are its knowledge of the population it serves, its ability to plan so that only the necessary facilities and staff are maintained, and the presence of financial incentives to minimize excessive medical care inputs. We would expect HMOs to have fewer excess or underutilized resources at any point in time. Empirical testing of this proposition is difficult, because it is often argued that, at least within the observable range, additional physicians and beds are rapidly utilized to near capacity (Roemer and Shain, 1959; M. Feldstein, 1971; Fuchs and Kramer, 1972). Thus a finding that HMO and non-HMO hospitals have the same occupancy rates does not necessarily imply that there are no differences in their true efficiency. It would be preferable to examine staffing patterns and the use of specialized equipment in order to determine if the potential advantages of planning are realized. Also a wide variety of organizational forms are included within the HMO concept, and many of the questions concerning technical efficiency are relevant only to particular types of HMOs. Thus organizations that purchase inpatient services from community hospitals are not likely to have as much impact on the cost of such services as HMOs that completely control their hospitals. Similarly, the efficiency of producing ambulatory care services is likely to be dependent on the specific method of organizing such services (solo, small group, large group, and so on). With these caveats in mind, we will first examine data concerning inpatient care; then we will consider the ambulatory care data.

THE PROVISION OF INPATIENT CARE

Examination of the costs of providing inpatient care must be restricted to those HMOs that control their own hospitals. This is the case only with a limited number of PGPs. (Note that the HMO need not own the hospital; it can maintain effective power if it merely accounts for a substantial fraction of the hospital's patients.) One could also consider the performance of hospitals in areas served almost entirely by an IPA, but such data generally are unavailable. Even within the constraints of the available data, it is not clear how to interpret cost differences. As has been shown above, there is overwhelming evidence that HMO enrollee admissions rates are substantially below those of people with traditional insurance coverage. Although theoretical expectations and the prevailing rhetoric argue that these apparent reductions occur in the less necessary categories, there is little evidence to support the argument. Nor do the data indicate a clear pattern with respect to differences in length of stay.

These same arguments bear upon the predicted cost relationships; if HMOs screen out the less serious cases, then their inpatient mix will be sicker and require more services. A similar argument holds for length of stay: the last few days of any case tend to be the least expensive; if HMOs discharge people sooner, then they will have higher average costs per day, even though their costs per case may be lower (Blumberg and Gentry, 1978). This leaves us in a partial quandary. If HMOs have higher costs, then they could be less efficient, or they could be treating sicker patients. On the other hand, lower HMO costs might be suggestive of greater efficiency, unless it can be shown that the HMO hospital is treating less expensive cases. One must be careful in such a comparison to make sure that both hospital groups have similar responsibilities. For instance, an HMO hospital could have much lower costs than its neighbors if it sent all of its complicated cases to other hospitals. Note that this is true even if the HMO pays for such care, as is usually the case, and it includes such cost and utilization in its per-member data. It is also important to remember that the utilization studies outlined in Chapter 5 refer to comparable, usually employed populations. Overall, HMOs have a much lower proportion of the elderly and unemployed, who tend to be higher users of hospital services.

One study in the mid-1960s compared the average daily cost of hospitalization in Kaiser Northern California ($56.06) with that of all short-term, voluntary, nonprofit hospitals in California ($63.48) (National Advisory Commission on Health Manpower, 1967, p. 209). But these data may be questioned because of the very broad scope of hospitals included in the comparison group. More recent data from the California Health Facilities Commission show average daily costs during the period 1970-76 for Kaiser hospitals to be about 80 to 90 percent of non-Kaiser hospital costs. For costs per admission the ratio is generally 70 to 80 percent, which reflects the shorter length of stay in Kaiser hospitals (Carter and Allison, 1978).

Table 7-1 presents substantially more detailed data for 1974 concerning Kaiser hospitals in California and Oregon and the Group Health Cooperative of Puget Sound hospital. For each HMO hospital a community hospital in the area was selected, matching on the basis of size (number of beds) and

Table 7–1 "Performance" Measures for HMO-Controlled Hospitals and Matched Community Hospitals, 1974

	Northern California		Southern California		Oregon		Washington	
	K-P	Community	K-P	Community	K-P	Community	GHCPS	Community
Number of hospitals	11	11	7	7	1	1	1	1
Number of beds in sample	1,966	1,966	1,722	1,707	250	220	260	259
Average number of beds per hospital	179	179	246	244	250	220	260	259
Admissions per bed per year	41.6	40.2	51.2	38.6	60.8	54.6	62.2	60.0
Births per bassinette per year	58.1	35.1	60.3	34.8	72.4	63.1	78.8	53.3
Length of stay	5.9	6.7	6.0	6.7	5.0	5.7	4.9	5.0
Occupancy rate (percent)	67.7	73.7	84.4	70.5	84.0	85.0	82.2	82.6
Average daily census (ADC)[a]	1,449	1,500	1,569	1,244	232	198	236	233
Expense per patient day	$168	$159	$165	$171	$139	$127	$103	$140
Expense per admission	$912	$1,018	$917	$1,092	$652	$686	$474	$660
Personnel per bed	1.83	2.44	2.29	2.74	4.09	3.25	2.64	3.30
Personnel per ADC	2.48	3.20	2.52	3.75	4.41	3.62	2.96	3.65
Payroll per bed	$22,358	$23,415	$25,765	$22,646	$27,832	$23,895	$20,442	$29,386
Payroll per ADC	$30,335	$30,689	$28,277	$31,074	$30,108	$26,551	$22,521	$32,665
Average wage (payroll/personnel)	$12,224	$9,584	$11,241	$8,276	$6,808	$7,342	$7,748	$8,912
Payroll as a percent of total expense	49.6	52.8	46.8	49.7	59.2	57.2	60.0	63.9

SOURCE. American Hospital Association, *Hospital Statistics, 1975 Edition.*
[a] Computed using an estimated length of stay of 2.8 days per birth.

type of teaching affiliation. In this manner it was possible to control for regional variations in practice patterns and prices, as well as for the use of major teaching hospitals for complex (and expensive) cases. Although there are data from four regions, the Oregon and Washington data are each based on only one pair of hospitals, while the California regions include seven and eleven pairs and thus are subject to less random error. It should be noted, however, that substantial variation occurs within Kaiser regions. Hester (1979) refers to 55 percent variation in age-sex adjusted hospitalization rates across the seven medical centers in the Kaiser Southern California region. (See also Klitsner, 1976.)

The data with respect to expenses per patient day are inconclusive; in two cases the HMO hospital costs are higher, and in two they are lower. In all four cases length of stay in HMO hospitals is shorter, and this results in lower costs per admission. These "cost savings" range from 5 to 28 percent.* It may be argued that the cost data could be arbitrary because of differences in accounting procedures and variability in data reported by individual hospitals. One partial control for this is to examine the underlying factors that may contribute to these observed cost differences. One factor that does *not* appear to account for the differences is occupancy rate. It is nearly identical in two cases, substantially higher in one, and lower in the other. In fact, the 67.7 percent rate in Kaiser Northern California is surprisingly low and may be attributable to the smaller average hospital size in that region. Small hospital size generally is associated with lower average occupancy, partly because of the importance of specialized beds within the hospital and the inability to substitute beds in the short run (for example, pediatric and coronary care unit beds are not equivalent). Another factor is that hospitals such as Kaiser, with shorter lengths of stay, tend to have lower occupancy rates (Gould, 1978). HMO hospital administrators often contend that AHA figures do not accurately reflect occupancy based on fully staffed beds. That is, as the census fluctuates, they adjust their staffing. Administrators in conventional hospitals are likely to behave similarly. (The 1974 occupancy rate for Northern California Kaiser hospitals, however, is substantially lower than that for either prior or succeeding years.) HMOs do appear to utilize their existing nursery capacity more efficiently (more births per bassinette).

Labor costs are a key component of hospital expenses, and different staffing patterns can lead to substantially different costs. One issue in examining labor costs is whether they should be considered as fixed costs, like beds, or as variable costs, like medical supplies. This becomes important when one considers the normal variation in hospital occupancy—the more flexible a hospital's staffing, the greater its potential cost savings (Hershey, Abernathy, and Baloff, 1974). Thus two measures of staffing ratios will be examined: personnel per bed, which is a fixed cost measure,

*As before, "cost savings" is in quotation marks because it is impossible to determine whether the observed differences are due to HMO savings or to other factors.

and personnel per average daily census (ADC), which controls for occupancy rate differences. Both measures yield approximately the same results. With the exception of Kaiser Oregon, the HMOs have substantially lower (16 to 33 percent) staffing ratios than do the matched hospitals. However, with the exception of GHCPS, their personnel costs per bed, or per ADC, are not very different from those of the matched hospitals. The explanation for this lies in the substantially higher average wages paid by the Kaiser hospitals in California. Although this may be the result of some artifact of the data, it is possible that those Kaiser hospitals choose to employ fewer, but more highly skilled and paid personnel. Because of Kaiser's early focus on union enrollment, Kaiser hospital employees were unionized long before most other area hospitals.

Despite the limitations of using data from a single site, the cost information from the Seattle Prepaid Health Care Project is extremely valuable. Table 7-2 presents various short-term hospital cost data for GH and KCM-BC enrollees. The substantially higher costs per person for KCM-BC enrollees (76 percent) are largely due to higher utilization rates. Of secondary importance are longer stays and costs per day. The costs per day for KCM-BC enrollees are only 15 percent greater, and this is attributable to higher costs for ancillary services such as drugs, laboratory tests, and X-ray. Thus the basic costs of medical care do not appear to be very different.

Another expected source of savings in HMO-controlled hospitals might be realized through more efficient patterns in admissions and length of stay. For instance, it is often observed that admission rates are lower during

Table 7-2 Seattle Prepaid Health Care Project per Person, per Admission, and per Diem Short-Term Hospital Costs by Sex and Plan, 1971–1974

Item	GH	KCM/BC	Ratio KCM/BC:GH
Costs per person[a]	$ 58	$102	1.76
Costs per admission[a,b]	$535	$723	1.35
Average length of stay[b]	4.6	5.3	1.15
Costs per day[b]	$118	$136	1.15
Room	74	71	0.96
OR/delivery	28	21	0.75
Drugs	6	12	2.00
X-ray	3	5	1.67
Laboratory tests	5	13	2.60
Other	3	13	4.33

SOURCE. McCaffree et al., 1976, p. III–31.

[a] Costs for KCM/BC are taken directly from statements issued by the hospital and do not reflect the Blue Cross discount of 3 percent. Costs also exclude the administrative fee charged by KCM-BC.

[b] Excludes four cases with lost records at GH, and fifty-five admissions for KCM-BC for which detailed statements are not available.

weekends; this may reflect the extra costs associated with overtime or bonus payments for weekend staff. However, a Michigan study demonstrated that patients admitted on Saturday or Sunday had an average stay of 8.5 days versus 6.8 days for those admitted on weekdays (Blue Cross and Blue Shield of Michigan, 1977). It appears that little was done for the weekend admissions until Monday, and in fact, the differential stay was larger for surgery patients. Given the financial incentives for HMOs, it is perhaps surprising that Kaiser Portland patients admitted on weekends stayed 5.4 days, while those entering on weekdays stayed 4.98 days. As in the Michigan data, the differentials were larger for surgical than medical admissions (Hurtado, Marks, and Greenlick, 1977, pp. 36-37).

A major means by which HMOs increase their technical efficiency is by avoiding duplication of facilities. Community hospitals often compete for physicians by purchasing specialized equipment that is used at far less than capacity (Salkever, 1978; Lee, 1971; Harris, 1977). HMO-controlled hospitals should not face this problem. The Kaiser-Permanente plan emphasizes centralization of certain types of care. The program's 1975 annual report states:

> To eliminate or minimize overlapping or duplication of expensive technological services, Kaiser-Permanente centralizes many activities within an area or Region, or utilizes community resources. For example, in the Northern California Region, which operates 11 medical centers and four detached outpatient facilities, neurosurgical procedures are centralized at one hospital; newborn deliveries are limited to eight locations; and open heart procedures are referred to the special team at the medical center of one of the nation's leading medical schools. In the Southern California Region, radiotherapy and open heart procedures are conducted within the Program, and are centralized at the Los Angeles Medical Center. Laboratory services for the entire Region also are centralized. Activities with the same objectives—the most efficient allocation and use of resources—also occur in the other Regions of the Kaiser-Permanente Program. (Kaiser Foundation Medical Care Program, 1976, p. 8)

In addition, the 1968 annual report emphasized the appropriate use of modern, clinically effective and cost-saving equipment (Kaiser Foundation Medical Care Program, 1969). On the other hand, an external review body reported few differences between Kaiser and community hospitals with respect to innovations in personnel and technology (National Advisory Commission on Health Manpower, 1967).

One crude test of whether the Kaiser plan utilizes a different mix of facilities and services than do community hospitals can be obtained by comparing availability of services in the two California regions with a set of matched hospitals. The American Hospital Association annual *Guide to the Health Care Field* includes information on the presence of forty-six special facilities and services, but these data must be interpreted with caution. As can be seen in Table 7-3, while some categories are specific, others, such as an occupational therapy department, are less meaningful. For example, a hospital may provide occupational therapy services without maintaining a specific department for that purpose.

A more important factor that influences data interpretation involves the contexts within which the two sets of hospitals operate. The Kaiser plan has the expressed intention to provide almost all hospital services required by its population. Therefore, we can consider the Kaiser hospitals in a given region to be a relatively self-contained unit. In the Northern California region eleven hospitals serve a population of about 1.2 million people. In about the same area, approximately 3.5 million non-Kaiser enrollees are served by nearly 100 community hospitals. Thus the ratio of hospitals to population is about three times as great for the non-Kaiser enrollee, suggesting that the average travel time to the nearest hospital will be less than that for the Kaiser enrollee. This has direct implications for the allocation of specific facilities. For example, most health planners agree that highly specialized facilities, such as open heart and burn care units, should be highly centralized and that travel time is not a major issue.

Other services should be available at nearly every moderately sized hospital. There is an intermediate group of facilities that is unnecessary to have at all hospitals that are located close together, but as hospitals become more widely dispersed, it is reasonable to have more such facilities. As an extreme example, a 100-bed hospital serving an isolated rural region should have a substantially wider range of services than the same size hospital in a densely populated urban region. If the analogy holds, and if the average Kaiser enrollee travels farther to a Kaiser hospital, then we might expect that Kaiser hospitals will have more of certain types of facilities than a comparable set of community hospitals. An informal survey of health services analysts was used to identify those facilities and services that are likely to be sensitive to such density issues (Table 7-3). Thus, if the planning and control aspects work in the Kaiser system, we would expect to find relatively fewer facilities in the "centralized" category, the same number in the "decentralized" category, and somewhat more in the "density sensitive" category.

Table 7-3 presents the number of facilities and services available in the eighteen California Kaiser hospitals and a group of eighteen community hospitals, which were matched for size, location, and teaching status. Excluding five services that are difficult to classify or are based on special programs, the Kaiser hospitals averaged 16.28 services and the comparison group 16.33. Examining specific types of services reveals some differentiation between the two groups. Although the Kaiser hospitals collectively have only four of the "highly centralized" services, in contrast to ten for the community hospitals, almost all of this difference is attributable to psychiatric inpatient units. Community hospitals recently increased their psychiatric units in response to major cutbacks in the state hospital system.

Table 7-3   Presence of Special Facilities and Services in Kaiser and Non-Kaiser Community Hospitals Northern and Southern California, 1974

	Number of Hospitals with Facility	
	Kaiser	Non-Kaiser
"Facilities that should be centralized"		
Open heart surgery	1	2
Organ bank	0	0
Burn care unit	1	1
Rehabilitation inpatient unit	1	1
Psychiatric inpatient unit	1	6
"Facilities that might be sensitive to density"		
Intensive care unit (cardiac only)	11	7
Intensive care unit (mixed)	16	18
Premature nursery	12	9
X-Ray therapy	5	7
Cobalt therapy	1	3
Radium therapy	6	7
Electroencephalography	12	14
Renal Dialysis (inpatient)	4	6
Renal Dialysis (outpatient)	1	5
Occupational therapy department	2	8
Rehabilitation outpatient unit	1	2
Psychiatric outpatient unit	8	4
Psychiatric emergency unit	7	8
Organized outpatient department	7	4
Abortion Service (inpatient)	12	11
Abortion Service (outpatient)	5	8
Abortion (inpatient or outpatient)	(12)	(13)
Speech therapy services	3	8
Diagnostic radioisotope facility	13	16
Therapeutic radioisotope facility	9	10
Inhalation therapy department	14	18
Self care unit	0	0
Extended care unit	1	3
Psychiatric partial hospitalization program	1	4
Psychiatric consultation and education services	6	4
Clinical psychology services	6	5
Emergency department (24-hour staffing)	18	16
Genetic counseling service	3	0
Podiatric services	5	4
"Facilities that should be available at nearly every hospital"		
Physical therapy	18	18

Table 7–3 (continued)

	Number of Hospitals with Facility	
	Kaiser	Non-Kaiser
Social work department	18	9
Postoperative recovery room	16	18
Pharmacy with registered pharmacist (full or part time)	18	17
Histopathology laboratory	15	15
Blood bank	15	8
"Indeterminant or Dependent on Specific Coverages and Programs"		
Dental services	1	9
Family planning service, organized clinic	2	1
Home care department (administered by the hospital)	15	0
Hospital auxiliary	0	18
Volunteer services department	13	9
Total facilities per 18 hospitals	324	341

SOURCE. American Hospital Association, *Guide to the Health Care Field, 1975 Edition.*

In the "density sensitive" category, the "average service" is offered by 6.75 Kaiser hospitals, in contrast to 7.46 community hospitals. This is contrary to our discussion concerning the potential influence of density on planning. Examination of specific services and facilities reveals some interesting patterns. The greater number of premature nurseries in the Kaiser system is perhaps not surprising, given that Kaiser has a disproportionate share of births. Also Kaiser uses only fourteen (of eighteen) hospitals for obstetrics, as opposed to fifteen in the community sample (American Hospital Association, 1975). Other services that are more likely to be present in Kaiser hospitals are ambulatory services—psychiatric outpatient, outpatient, psychiatric consultation and education, clinical psychology, emergency, genetic counseling, and podiatry. Two exceptions are of interest: intensive care units and abortion services. Kaiser has more intensive cardiac care units; this may represent increased specialization. However, there are also two Kaiser hospitals with only coronary care units and no mixed intensive care facilities. Surprisingly, Kaiser seems to avoid outpatient abortions, except for five Kaiser hospitals offering outpatient abortions in Southern California. This difference in practice style reflects the substantial degree of independence afforded each medical group. In Northern California abortions are performed using inpatient facilities on a same-day basis. Patients are not hospitalized unless complications develop.

The only major differences in local facilities and services appear in social work departments and blood banks. The blood bank differences may be partly attributable to differences in interpretation of the term. Perhaps the only other difference of importance is the clear emphasis in Kaiser hospitals on home-care departments. However, this may well be a reflection of the integration of services in Kaiser, rather than a differential availability of services. The community hospitals may utilize independent home-health agencies.

The above results are based on a comparison of Kaiser hospitals and community hospitals of similar size. An alternative comparison would treat the Kaiser hospitals as a single system and compare their performance as a model for rational regional planning with the "system" of all other hospitals in the same area. This second approach is closer to a population-based comparison, but it cannot control for the facts that Kaiser has different populations enrolled and may utilize certain specialized resources in the community. Other factors that must be considered are the smaller average size of Kaiser hospitals, which leads to fewer facilities, and distances among hospitals. In a study that controlled for size, type of hospital control (Kaiser, county, proprietary, university, district, and other), and distance to the nearest hospital with alternative facilities, it was found that San Francisco Bay Area Kaiser hospitals tended to have fewer specialized facilities than nonprofit community hospitals (Luft and Crane, 1979). This was particularly evident for the more technology-intensive and competitive facilities, such as inhalation therapy departments, intensive care units, electroencephalographs, and diagnostic radioisotope units. When Kaiser hospitals had those facilities and services, they were more likely to be in larger hospitals than was generally the case for nonprofit hospitals. Kaiser was more likely to have certain other facilities; these tended to be noncapital-intensive and outpatient-oriented facilities, such as psychiatric partial hospitalization, social work, occupational therapy, and home care.

There is also evidence that Kaiser hospitals have consistently lagged behind others in the introduction of new facilities, apparently adopting a "wait and see" attitude. For example, Kaiser had contracted for computerized tomography and open heart surgery at local hospitals, but now is requesting permission to open its own units. In part, this may be because its volume is now sufficient to achieve substantial economies of scale (McGregor and Pelletier, 1978; Finkler, 1978). Since there is substantial excess capacity in the community units, it is also argued that, while Kaiser could negotiate favorable contracts, it may face internal pressures by its medical staff for in-house facilities. (West Bay Health Systems Agency, 1978). Thus Kaiser management may be able to delay and limit, but not eliminate, the technological imperative in medicine.

While these data concerning overall costs and facilities are highly fragmentary, data concerning the finer details of inpatient care are almost entirely lacking. Radiologic and laboratory services are becoming major factors in hospital costs, and it is often argued that FFS physicians and hospitals have little incentive to reduce utilization of such services because of their high profitability (Schroeder and Showstack, 1977; Fineberg, 1977). One study suggests that physicians within an HMO do not automatically lower their usage of ancillary services, and in fact, are somewhat resistant to special educational programs (Federa, 1978).

There is only one comparative study of the inpatient use of such services. Hastings et al. (1973) indicate that the use of radiologic services per discharge was 7 percent higher for GHA patients than for those covered by the indemnity plan, while GHA patients had 28 percent more laboratory services. (The lower admission rate for GHA members suggests that those who were admitted might have been sicker.) Of course in both cases hospital costs were borne by the provincial insurance plan. Hurtado, Marks, and Greenlick (1977) report substantial increases in the use of laboratory services in the Kaiser Oregon plan. From 1969 to 1974 the number of tests per discharge increased 20.4 percent, while the number of tests per patient day rose 38.9 percent. Again, we do not know if the rate of increase or the absolute levels are higher or lower than is the case in non-HMO hospitals.

Another important potential efficiency is the use of ambulatory-surgical facilities, that is, the elimination of hospital admissions for patients requiring only minor surgery. Kaiser Portland reports that "do-not-admit" surgery rose from a very small portion of all procedures in 1966 to 35 percent of all procedures performed in the operating room in 1974 (Greenlick et al., 1978). However, in British Columbia hospitals with an FFS reimbursement system, the proportion of "not-admitted" surgeries rose from 7.4 percent in 1968 to 22.1 percent in 1974 (Shah and Robinson, 1977). Since the latter figures are provincial averages, it is likely that a number of hospitals match the Kaiser performance. Comparable data for the United States do not exist, but ambulatory surgical centers have been growing rapidly (Jaggar et al., 1978; Kirkman, 1978).

This review of data concerning the efficiency of inpatient care suggests that when an HMO controls its own hospital some savings are generated in the delivery of services. Although the costs per day present a mixed pattern, shorter lengths of stay result in 5 to 28 percent lower costs per case in the HMO hospitals. Except in the case of newborns, the increased efficiency is not related to higher occupancy rates. HMO hospitals tend to use different staffing patterns, with fewer personnel who are often more highly paid. This may reflect an increased reliance on more highly skilled personnel. A comparison of the facilities and services offered suggests that the Kaiser plans do not have a greater degree of regionalization for the most highly specialized facilities, but they do tend to provide the intermediate range of services, especially those that are technology-intensive, with proportionately fewer facilities than community hospitals.

This discussion of relative efficiency must be understood within the realities of a hospital market that has placed little premium on efficiency. Recent health planning legislation and federal cost containment guidelines have led to more regionalization among community hospitals (Chambers and Russell, 1978; Lewis, 1974; Neumann et al., 1978) and efforts to control costs (Kirchner, 1978; Maxwell, 1978; Sorensen and Saward, 1978; DiPaoli, 1978). At the same time, this is likely to put more pressure on HMOs to maintain a competitive cost advantage by improving efficiency. For instance, there is much unexplained variation in HMO performance. In the question and answer period at a conference for HMO medical directors, it was mentioned that Harvard Community Health Plan had a four-day obstetrics stay, while GHCPS had a three-day stay. Given the importance of obstetrical admissions in HMOs, it is surprising that such a difference was not commented upon. Furthermore, the GHCPS stay had remained constant for about a decade, while the length of stay in all Seattle hospitals had fallen from 5.0 to 5.5 days to 2.5 to 2.6 days (Dorsey, 1976, p. 35).

The changing health care environment in the 1980s is likely to see many more innovations and efforts to promote efficiency, and it is difficult to predict the relative performance of HMOs and conventional providers.

THE PROVISION OF AMBULATORY CARE

There are two major issues concerning technical efficiency in the provision of ambulatory services: (1) whether HMOs can realize economies of scale; and (2) whether HMOs are more likely to use various types of allied health personnel to substitute for physician time. As outlined below, the question of economies of scale relates primarily to group practices, regardless of whether they are prepaid or FFS. The potential for using allied health personnel is partly related to the question of scale, but it may also reflect certain characteristics unique to prepayment. People may choose an HMO because its good financial coverage is more important to them than the more personalized care that an independent practitioner may offer. FFS physicians, however, may lose part of their attractiveness if they begin to substitute physician assistants in place of themselves. If HMO enrollees value the physician-patient relationship less highly, they may be more receptive to such substitution.

Economies of Scale and Production Efficiencies

The question of whether group practice leads to economies of scale has long been a subject of debate (Fein, 1967; Klarman, 1970; Roemer and Shonick, 1973). It is important to recognize that the issue here has little to do with HMO performance as a unique organizational form. The economies of scale, if they exist, should be equally obtainable by FFS and prepaid groups. In fact, if HMO groups tend to have a more complicated patient mix (for which there is little evidence), then their apparent productivity will be lower than that of FFS groups. The measurement of productivity is also biased by the financing system. FFS payment provides direct incentives to produce easily measured, billable units of service. Capitation incentives may lead physicians to perform equal or more effective services, such as careful history taking, that, because they take more time, appear to lower productivity. The quality question also makes comparisons difficult. Not all patient visits are alike, and any evaluation of economies of scale should control for a constant level of quality. In addition, it is important to have a clear understanding of what is meant by economies of scale and productivity. Bailey points out:

Productivity—a rate concept—is concerned with the question of how much output can be obtained from a unit of input. Since the physician is usually viewed as the scarce resource in the production of medical services, (the) analysis will focus upon average physician productivity specifically (1970b, p. 43). The concept of economies of scale deals with inputs and outputs but in a broader fashion than the concept of physician productivity because it includes how *all* input factors are combined in firms of various size to produce the final output(s). The key point is this: it is to be expected that the *proportions of factors* used will differ in firms of different scale producing the same type of good or service, primarily because of the indivisibility of certain factors which cannot be acquired in all sizes with similar efficiency characteristics (1970b, pp. 44-45).

The problem, of course, is in the empirical implementation of the theoretical measures. There are no agreed-upon measures of outputs or inputs, and the available data are far from ideal, even given a specific set of measures. Thus it is not surprising that the available literature is mixed on the presence or absence of economies of scale. Roemer and Shonick (1973) provide a good summary of the literature up to 1973. In brief, Boan (1966) offered some rather simple data showing higher ratios of ancillary personnel and lower salary costs per physician in group practice than in solo practice, coupled with higher average net incomes for the group physicians. Yett (1967) used cross-sectional data on total expenses per physician as a function of the volume of patient visits per physician and found definite economies of scale. However, this does not speak to the question of whether costs per unit fall as the number of physicians per office increases. Reinhardt and Yett (1972) estimate a series of production functions relating patient visits per week (or gross patient billings) to practice inputs, such as personnel, equipment, supplies, and physician time. Their results indicate that physicians in single specialty partnerships or groups tend to process 4 to 13 percent more patient visits per week than do solo practitioners, at any given level of factor input. Furthermore, they point out that these results are less than would be expected from the crude comparisons of output, because group physicians tend to work more hours per week and employ more aides. These results must be interpreted with caution, because less than 5 percent of the physicians were in groups of four or more, far below the usual size of PGPs.

There is also a body of literature presenting data suggesting that either there are diseconomies of scale or there is no relationship between scale and productivity. Bailey (1970a) has presented data from a detailed survey of thirty-one office practices of internists in the San Francisco Bay Area. His findings indicate that while the use of assistants and gross revenues per physician *increase* with the size of practice, the number of office visits per physician time with patient *tends to fall* with scale. The extra paramedical hours appear to be used in the production of technical products, such as EKG, laboratory, and X-ray, which account for a larger fraction of the gross revenues as the practice increases in size. Thus Bailey argues that there are no particular economies of scale in the production of physicians' services, and that the gross data really represent a different product mix, with larger practices directly providing more technical services. Small physician practices can achieve similar results by sending their laboratory work out to other firms. Although this study is based on a small sample, it does raise important questions about the need to hold constant the mix of services when testing for economies of scale.

More broadly based evidence indicating the absence of economies of scale is found in a national survey of 5799 pediatricians by Yankauer, Connelly, and Feldman (1970). Their findings indicate that the number of physician visits per unit of time bears almost no relationship to the size of the group practice. A series of studies by Kimbell and Lorant utilize data from the American Medical Association's periodic survey of physicians and medical groups (Kimbell and Lorant, 1972, 1973; Lorant and Kimbell, 1976). Their findings are consistent with others in that the most important factor in determining physician visits is the amount of physician time. However, for group practices they found decreasing returns to scale—a 10 percent increase in inputs results in only an 8 percent increase in visits, although in terms of gross revenues there are constant returns to scale.

While these results are apparently contradictory, the wide differences in data sources and methods of analysis make it conceivable that all are correct, given the specific issues each addresses. The relatively small size of most groups in the United States also makes interpretation of data relating to group size particularly difficult. For instance, in 1975 over half of all groups had only three to four physicians, and only 7 percent had sixteen or more physicians (Goodman, Bennett, and Odem, 1976). The distinction between single and multispecialty practice also is important, because different types of physicians have very different rates of visits. As would be expected, single specialty groups are heavily weighted toward the small end of the size distribution.

Some illustrative measures of physician productivity in 1973 are given in Table 7-4 in order to provide a framework for our summary.* Physicians in solo practice in every specialty spend fewer hours per week in direct patient care and see fewer patients than do physicians in partnerships and groups. Furthermore, they see fewer patients per hour, an indication that their productivity is lower, if we assume that the patient visits are comparable. Closer examination of the data, however, suggests that the greatest work effort (in terms of hours per week) and productivity (visits per hour) tends to occur in the smallest of the nonsolo practices—offices with two to four physicians. Thus both these unadjusted data and most of the more detailed studies are consistent with the view that there may be economies of scale as practice size increases, but these economies reach a maximum at a relatively low scale, about two to five practitioners. Whether productivity per physician remains constant or even declines beyond that point is difficult to evaluate.

A crude but more comprehensive measure that serves to supplement these data is the ratio of total expenses to gross revenue by practice size. The available data indicate that this ratio rises steadily as the group size increases from three to five to thirty or more physicians (McFarland and Odem, 1974). This suggests that even if larger groups do have more patient visits per physician hour, this increased productivity may be obtained by increasing the relative use of other inputs. In particular, managerial inputs tend to become more important as size increases (Scheffler, 1975).

There are no precise data available to test whether HMO physicians are more efficient providers of ambulatory services than FFS practitioners. Some data, however, can be used for "order of magnitude comparisons." The number of patient visits per week reported in Table 7-4 can be combined with the average number of weeks worked per year by physicians in practices of various sizes. This results in total patient visits per physician per year. However, all the HMO data refer to ambulatory or office visits, and unfortunately, the AMA data provide only a breakdown of office visits by specialty, not practice size. If the overall proportion of total office visits (71.1 percent) is applied to the total figures, we have the following rates of visits per physician per year:†

		Size of Practice					
Total	Solo	2	3	4	5−7	8−25	26+
4698	4456	5654	5234	4812	4529	4556	4032

*More recent data are available (Gaffney, 1979), but these 1973 statistics will be used for comparison purposes later and are chosen to reduce the impact of the declining trend in productivity (Owens, 1978).

†American Medical Association, *Profile of Medical Practice, 1974,* pp. 178, 180, 182, 183.

Table 7−4 Measures of Physician Productivity by Type of Practice and Specialty, 1973

Type of Practice	Total**	Specialty					
		General Practice	Internal Medicine	Surgery	Obstetrics− Gynecology	Pediatrics	Psychiatry
Average Number of Total Patient Visits per Week, 1973							
Total	140.0	190.3	129.8	130.2	135.0	160.5	53.8
Solo	132.5	177.0	126.6	120.4	113.1	145.9	51.5
2 physician	167.4	244.8	139.0	148.3	152.4	169.9*	72.1*
Group:							
3 physician	156.3	215.1	144.4	140.7	163.6	197.0*	73.9*
4 physician	143.7	238.8*	110.7	138.8	149.9*	167.8*	39.2*
5−7 physician	136.1	180.4*	135.3*	126.8	177.4*	208.1*	49.2*
8−25 physician	137.8	181.3*	148.8	160.2	117.1*	161.3*	N.A.
26 and over	121.7	170.2*	115.9	132.5*	132.0	111.3*	N.A.
Average Number of Hours of Direct Patient Care per Week							
Total	46.6	47.8	48.4	47.9	49.2	45.3	41.6
Solo	45.3	46.8	47.2	46.1	47.2	43.4	41.5
2 physician	49.4	51.7	47.3	51.5	51.5	47.7	38.5
Group:							
3 physician	49.3	51.5	51.1	50.0	51.0	47.4	46.1*
4 physician	48.8	52.3*	51.8	48.0	54.8*	45.6*	NA
5−7 physician	46.0	48.3	52.7	45.2	50.0*	41.1*	40.4*
8−25 physician	48.7	45.5*	50.7	54.2	48.1*	50.8*	45.0*
26 and over	45.9	38.8*	47.0	51.7	48.3*	44.7*	NA

Average Number of Patient Visits per Hour

Total	3.00	3.98	2.68	2.72	2.74	3.54	1.29
Solo	2.92	3.78	2.68	2.61	2.40	3.36	1.24
2 physician	3.39	4.74	2.94	2.88	2.96	4.13*	1.87*
Group:							
3 physician	3.17	4.18	2.83	2.81	3.21	4.16*	1.60*
4 physician	2.94	4.57*	2.14	2.89	2.74*	3.68*	NA
5–7 physician	2.96	3.73*	2.57*	2.81	3.55*	5.06*	1.22*
8–25 physician	2.83	3.98*	2.93	2.44	2.43*	3.18	NA
25 and over	2.65	4.39*	2.47	2.56*	2.73*	2.49*	NA

SOURCE.   Derived from the American Medical Association, *Profile of Medical Practice, '74*, pp. 173, 182. Reprinted with permission from the American Medical Association.

* Based on fewer than 30 observations.

** Physicians reporting radiology, anesthesiology, and other specialties are included in this total column.

Note: Fewer physicians reported patient visits than hours of care, so that the first two tables are not exactly comparable. The third table, which is based on the first two, should therefore be interpreted with care.

There is a rather consistent pattern showing the highest volume of visits per year in two-physician practices with a steady decline as the practice gets larger. Solo practitioners have a yearly office visit volume that is between that of the eight to twenty-five and twenty-six or more practitioner groups.

Comparable data for ambulatory visits per physician in a number of PGPs are given in Table 7-5. The first set of data, from the mid-1960s, does not identify the plans, but it is notable for the low volume of visits per year and the wide variation in visit rates. Data are available for four Kaiser regions for various years, and they exhibit substantial variation.* The mean for the 10 Kaiser data points is 4352, a figure that is comparable to the results found for the largest groups in the AMA data. Although the number of Kaiser physicians in the medical group in each region can be large, in some cases exceeding 1000, the number who practice in any one set of offices can range from two to 200+ (Kaiser-Permanente Medical Care Program, 1976). Given the crudeness of these data, it appears that for the Kaiser plans physician productivity is comparable to that of average large group practices in the country, which in turn is lower than that of small groups.† One way to interpret these results is through the assumption that physicians who choose to work in relatively large groups desire certain benefits, such as longer vacations, more time for educational leave, and less pressure in terms of patients per hour. There is some evidence to support the idea that different types of physicians are attracted to solo, small group, and large group practices. (For more discussion of this issue, see Chapter 12.) The data are thus consistent with the hypothesis that the unique financial incentives of HMOs have little influence on physician productivity above and beyond the effects of group size.

One additional comment should be made about these data. The figures in Table 7-5 suggest that the Hawaii and Oregon regions have substantially higher physician productivity. Williams also notes that the Oregon program has consistently maintained the highest level of earnings with the lowest level of expenses and revenue of any region. He suggests that this

*The coefficient of variation for the first set of data is 11.3, while for the 10 Kaiser data points it is 10.8

†Several points should be noted in this comparison. First, the AMA figures are adjusted to represent only office practice visits and thus should be comparable to the HMO data. Second, there is substantial evidence that HMOs use less hospital care for their enrollees. If this results in a corresponding decrease in the amount of time that physicians work in the hospital, then PGP physicians should be able to see more outpatients per week. Third, the issue of out-of-plan use of ambulatory services is not relevant to this productivity question; the only issue is the number of patients seen by each physician. It is relevant, however, to include visits by people who are not members of the health plan. The Saward, Blank, and Lamb figures in Table 7-5 include such an adjustment. For inpatient services, nonplan admissions were only about 5 percent of the total. The use of ambulatory services is likely to be even lower. It is not known if the other data are adjusted for nonmember use. Fourth, although these data are presented as visits per physician, it must be recognized that in some cases patients are treated primarily by a paramedic worker. This may also be the case in FFS practices, and the only substantive question is whether PGPs utilize more such workers.

Table 7–5   Measures of Physician Productivity in Prepaid Group Practices

	Physicians per 1000	Ambulatory Services per 1000 Members per Year	Services per Physician per Year
Herbert[a]			
Plan 1	0.992	3340	3367
2	1.062	3220	3032
3	0.900	3260	3622
4	0.919	3880	4222
5	0.900	3130	3478
6	0.869	3300	3794
Kaiser–Oregon[b]			
1969	0.73	3191	4397
1970	0.75	3383	4502
1971	0.77	3483	4502
Kaiser–Southern California[c]			
1968	0.91	3750	4120
1969	0.90	3650	4055
1970	0.93	3675	3950
Kaiser–Northern California, 1970[d]	0.992	3900	3950
Kaiser–Hawaii, 1970[d]	0.870	4300	4950
Kaiser–Northern California, undated[e]	NA	NA	3827
Kaiser–Hawaii, undated[e]	NA	NA	5266

[a] Herbert, September 1972, pp. 5, 10.
[b] Saward, Blank, and Lamb, 1973, p. 37.
[c] Somers, 1971, pp. 63, 67.
[d] Harvard Business School, 1972, p. 76.
[e] Williams, February 1971, p. 41. These two figures were quoted as extreme rates within Kaiser.

might be attributable to "somewhat lower utilization and considerably higher productivity, but the reasons have not been intensively studied" (1971, p. 64). A potential explanation is that the Hawaii and Oregon regions are by far the smallest and most centralized of the four major, stable Kaiser regions. The relatively small size may lead to better control and more group effort to be efficient. (See Newhouse, 1973, and Sloan, 1974.) A recent study of federally qualified HMOs supports the idea that any economies of scale are attained at relatively small enrollment levels (Bothwell and Cooley, 1979).

Yet mere counts of the number of visits per physician are only the first step in evaluation of HMO effects on productivity. The content and style of the actual visits must be examined to determine whether quantity is achieved at the expense of quality. Mechanic (1975) offers data concerning practice patterns of pediatricians and internists in solo practice, group practice, and prepaid group practice. He admits that the definition of the original population is ambiguous and that selection is evident among the respondents. Many groups use internists to provide most of their adult medicine, so the role of general practitioners is unclear. In spite of these shortcomings, the data are suggestive on a number of important points. The PGP physicians tend to work fewer hours per week, but they also see fewer patients, with the exception of the PGP general practitioners, who seem to have a much higher visit rate. The PGP physicians are less likely to perform certain commonly used procedures, but this may well be due to greater specialization of functions. (Thus patients may see different providers within the group for various services, so the average visit may have the same content.) Mechanic suggests that the PGP physicians respond to increased patient load by processing patients more rapidly, rather than extending their work hours. Not having enough time to deal with each patient leads these physicians to perceive their patients as having relatively trivial problems, and this feeds physician dissatisfaction. This may also result in lower quality of care. (These issues will be more fully addressed in later chapters.)

Somewhat contradictory findings are offered by Watkins, Hughes, and Lewit (1976), who compare the time utilization of general surgeons in a PGP with a population of FFS general surgeons in community practice. The former were able to maintain twice the operating load with 50 percent more practice time. This greater productivity was the result of (1) restricting the practice to a single geographic setting, (2) seeing only surgical patients, (3) reducing unproductive office waiting time, and (4) utilizing paraprofessional personnel for selected operating assistance. Although the PGP surgeons worked more hours per week, the evening schedules were designed to be as convenient as possible. The PGP surgeons spent more time per patient visit and had widely varied operating loads. Watkins, Hughes, and Lewit (1976) point out, however, that the PGP patient load is high even in comparison to other PGPs, so these specific findings may not be generalizable. Moreover, the ratio of enrollment to surgeon for the plan was at a historical high, and the plan subsequently added another general surgeon. The reasons they give for higher productivity relate to improved location, scheduling, and use of paraprofessionals, rather than to longer working hours alone. These improvements could probably be obtained in a well-run FFS group.

Roemer and Shonick present the case that the evaluation of physician productivity in terms of office visits may be illusory, because FFS physicians, especially those in solo and small group practices, can "run up physician visit 'scores' by hospitalizing freely" (1973, p. 297). In contrast, the larger, better-equipped group practices are expected to do more diagnostic work on an outpatient basis and thus spend more time with each patient. However, the available data on the types of services rendered do not support the argument that there are substantial differences in ambulatory care practices across provider types. (See also Baker, 1978.)

The Use of Allied Health Personnel

The primary means by which larger practice size is expected to affect physician productivity is through the use of more allied health professionals (AHPs). It is argued that an AHP can assume responsibility for the routine aspects of care at lower cost than if the same services are provided by a physician. The discussion often is confused by the fact that two distinct groups of personnel assist physicians. The first group consists of traditionally trained nurses, nurses' aides, laboratory and medical technicians, and clerical staff. The second group is composed of people with specially designed skills, who undertake specific tasks that were traditionally performed by physicians. There are many names for the people in this latter group: physician's assistant, primary care associate, nurse practitioner, Medex, and nurse midwife, to name just a few. In fact, it sometimes seems as though there are nearly as many job titles as there are such people— about 10,000. There are well over 400,000 traditionally trained personnel in physicians' offices.

Table 7-6 presents data on the average number of traditional personnel in physicians' offices. In some cases the number of one specific type of aide per physician increases with practice size, and in others it falls. The apparent economy in the use of clerical personnel is reasonable. As practice size increases, there seems to be a reduction in the use of nurses and nurse's aides per physician, although the greatest drop-off occurs in small practices. This suggests that task delegation levels off when one reaches a scale of about four physicians. Empirical studies suggest that physicians could profitably hire more personnel of this type, and yet they have not done so except when pressured by excess demand (Reinhardt and Yett, 1972; Reinhardt, 1972; Yankauer, Connelly, and Feldman, 1970). One argument given for this resistance is a fear of malpractice costs. Kehrer and Intriligator (1975) strongly suggest that increased malpractice premiums cannot account for this resistance, although the psychological stress related to the fear of being sued because of the actions of one's employees may be an important influence. An additional factor is that while an AHP can substitute for a physician in standard office practice cases, any substantial increase in practice size is accompanied by an increase in emergency calls that cannot be covered by the AHP.

The staffing pattern of the Southern California Kaiser group is reasonably consistent with the AMA survey. This group appears to have about

Table 7—6 Average Number of Selected Types of Full-Time Personnel per Physician by Type of Practice, United States, 1973, and Kaiser—Southern California, 1970

	Selected Types of Personnel				
Type of Practice	Registered Nurses	Licensed Practical Nurses	Nurses' Aides	X-Ray Lab and Medical Technicians and Assistants	Secretaries Receptionists Clerks
Total	0.59	0.31	0.38	0.93	1.15
Solo	0.66	0.33	0.42	0.68	1.24
2 person	0.52	0.34	0.34	1.04	1.09
Group:					
3 person	0.48	0.31	0.30	1.13	1.08
4 person	0.44	0.28	0.28	1.12	0.96
5—7 person	0.60	0.27	0.53	1.65	1.02
8—25 person	0.50	0.27	0.22	1.13	0.90
26 person and over	0.37	0.20	0.33	1.17	0.69
Southern California Kaiser, 1970	0.46	0.44		0.72	1.19

SOURCES. American Medical Association, *Profile of Medical Practice, '74*, p. 217 (reprinted with permission from the American Medical Association); Somers, 1971.

the same number of nurses and aides per physician as the average physician group of twenty-six or more, but it has a somewhat greater emphasis on highly trained registered nurses. On the other hand, the relatively low ratio of laboratory and medical technicians and the high ratio of clerical personnel in Kaiser are surprising. Little more can be said from but one observation.

In their study of pediatricians, Yankauer, Connelly, and Feldman (1970) emphasize the value of the ability to delegate patient care, as opposed to technical-clerical tasks. It is in this area that the greatest gains are expected, and the more highly trained, "new" AHPs come to the fore. A number of studies outline the potential gains from such task delegation (Golladay, Miller, and Smith, 1973; Smith, Miller, and Golladay, 1972; Zeckhauser and Eliastam, 1974; Golladay, Manser, and Smith, 1974). Some empirical studies suggest that potential gains often are not achieved in practice (Hershey, Kropp, and Kuhn, 1978; Hershey and Kropp, 1979). Many reasons have been put forward to explain this failure, but two are of particular interest to us: (1) there may be real indivisibilities in the use of AHPs because of their specialized skills, so that only large groups can use them efficiently; and (2) most of the projections have not considered the implementation problems related to physician acceptance and role definition. The first issue is fairly self-evident; the second is neatly described by Record and Greenlick (1975). In brief, the Kaiser Portland group hired physicians' assistants, pediatric nurse practitioners, and certified nurse midwives, but only the first group was fully accepted by the physicians. After three years it seems that the internists were able to define complementary practice areas for the physicians' assistants. This enhanced the physicians' patient care activities by allowing them to focus on more complex cases. On the other hand, the pediatricians and Ob/Gyn specialists felt that the AHPs would take over certain functions they preferred to do themselves. The success or failure did not appear to be related to the physicians' work overload or to the external market. While this situation may represent only the particular circumstances in the Kaiser Portland setting, it does suggest that working relationships are important factors to consider. (See Fottler, Gibson, and Pinchoff, 1978; Connelly and Connelly, 1979; Sullivan et al., 1978; Burkett et al., 1978.) Chapter 12 examines physician satisfaction in more detail.

This leads to two sets of expectations with respect to the use of AHPs in HMOs. First, to the extent that there are indivisibilities associated with task delegation, large group practices will be better able to employ AHPs efficiently, although PGPs are unlikely to have particular advantages over FFS groups. Second, potential differences in the working relationships within FFS and prepaid groups may lead us to expect greater acceptance of AHPs in the PGP. At a superficial level, the relative newness of many PGPs allows them to incorporate AHPs within their designs and to select physicians who are comfortable in such a team relationship. This may explain the differences between the Kaiser Portland experience, which after three years had nine AHPs and about 120 physicians, and the experience of the Columbia Medical Plan, where after five years there were more AHPs (nineteen) than physicians (fifteen) (Levine et al., 1976). Obviously there are many other differences between the two settings, but the opportunity to design a practice setting from the ground up has certain real advantages.

At a deeper level the question of who is in charge must be addressed. The teamwork and role definition implied in the use of AHPs is threatening to many physicians. In an FFS setting physicians are solely responsible for the style of practice, even if they form a group and share an administrative staff. We would expect them to be less likely to use AHPs in such a setting than salaried physicians working within a group that is under pressure by a health plan to increase efficiency. In fact Record and Greenlick (1975) point out that the AHPs were employees of the Kaiser Portland health plan, not the physician partnership; thus the physicians received increased leisure at zero cost, while the health plan obtained faster service for its members. It is important to note that in many cases the physician group either controls the HMO or is relatively independent of it. The HMO incentives nonetheless will be more likely to encourage such adaption in practice patterns.

Tests of these predictions must await future research. One crude set of comparative data does relate to these issues. The Gaus, Cooper, and

Hirschman (1976) study of utilization behavior by Medicaid enrollees in HMOs and FFS controls includes total ambulatory visits per person, classified by physician and nonphysician contacts. The expectation is that HMOs, particularly PGPs, will have a higher proportion of visits in which they see only nonphysicians. This is not the case. For the group practices and controls PGP enrollees had 12.1 percent of their visits administered by nonphysicians, in contrast to 10.9 percent for the FFS population, an insignificant difference. Surprisingly, the proportion of nonphysician contacts is higher in the IPAs (19.7 percent) than in their controls (15.2 percent), and both are substantially larger than the PGP proportions. In part this may reflect geographic variation.

In a separate study of enrollees in the Seattle Prepaid Health Care Project, it was found that outpatient professional costs were slightly lower for GH than for KCM-BC members. This was the result of GH's using a less costly mix of providers (e.g., AHPs, general practitioners). The average cost for a visit to the same type of provider was 22 percent higher at GH (McCaffree et al., 1976, p. III-24).*

SUMMARY

This review of evidence concerning differences in the content of ambulatory visits, practice patterns, and productivity between HMOs and other provider types underscores the need for careful data evaluation. Reports abound in health services literature concerning the emphasis on preventive services, homogeneous practice patterns, and the use of new types of allied health personnel in HMOs. (See Steinwachs et al., 1976; Lairson, Record, and James, 1974). For some these are positive changes; for others they are negative. Regardless of how one values them, it is important to examine whether or not such differences would be expected to occur, and whether in fact they appear.

In general the review of the potential effects of incentives in HMOs relative to those in FFS practices resulted in few strong predictions. In fact, predictions made with respect to one characteristic were often countered by those stemming from another characteristic. Thus even greater reliance must be placed on empirical evidence, which is unfortunately very sparse. The data with respect to the content of ambulatory visits suggest that some PGPs have high rates of laboratory and X-ray use, while others have low

---

*It should be noted that the Group Health costs are based on uniform accounting procedures, while the KCM-BC "costs" actually represent charges. One might expect this to inflate the KCM-BC figures and thus make the results all the more striking. On the other hand, KCM-BC charges for X-rays were 35 percent higher than GH costs, and KCM-BC charges for laboratory service were 87 percent higher. Thus FFS physicians might have been obtaining a disproportionate share of their profit from these ancillary services. (See Shroeder and Showstack, 1978.)

rates. When compared to national data, it is impossible to reject the hypothesis that there really are no consistent differences in the content of ambulatory visits between HMOs and non-HMOs. What is apparent is the wide variability of practice patterns, even among physicians in the same office. These variations may be attributable to differences in such factors as patients and quality, but there is no evidence to support that theory. In fact, the few available studies find no relationship.

Much the same pattern of "no significant differences" occurs in the examination of economies of scale and the use of various types of personnel. The empirical literature is split between studies that find economies of scale and those that find diseconomies. In fact, both appear to occur—the economist's traditional U-shaped cost curve. Group practice appears to result in higher physician productivity than solo practice, but the minimum costs seem to occur in the range of two to four physicians. Beyond that point physician productivity falls, and expenses per physician rise. In the textbook world of competitive economics, producers would not expand beyond the point at which their costs per unit begin to rise. Few health services researchers would argue that the medical care market is competitive, and it is certainly reasonable that, in the absence of such competition, some physicians choose to work in inefficient practice settings. Of course, what is inefficient from the point of view of the external observer may be highly desirable from the perspective of the individual physician. For instance, larger groups often try to attract physicians by emphasizing the easier life, which would include such things as longer vacations, more time to read journals, more assistants, and a business management staff. These benefits appear to occur in both FFS and prepaid groups, as might be expected.

Both the wide variations in practice patterns and the inefficiencies are related to the dominance of particular organizational and individual situations and preferences over economic incentives. This is not surprising; the power of economic predictions is directly related to the pressures exerted by market competition. Given the noncompetitive nature of the medical care market, providers are able to indulge in a wide range of idiosyncratic behavior. There is little evidence that this behavior is consistently different in HMOs, if one controls for the special effects of group practice. This is a strong statement, but it should not be misinterpreted. It does not say that there are no differences, just that they cannot be detected in the available data. How does this view square with the many claims of distinctive practice patterns in certain HMOs? The key point is that such claims stem from doubly biased sources. First, they come from organizations that are sufficiently interested in their behavior from a research perspective to undertake the analysis. FFS practices usually are concerned only with delivering medical services, and they do not maintain staff researchers. Also some PGPs, such as Ross-Loos, undertake no internal research. Another important point is that a strong bias exists in research toward emphasizing the new and different. When policy is being set one often wishes there were a *Journal of Nonsignificant Differences,* which could advise about whether a proposed change really will accomplish what it is supposed to. The studies outlined in this chapter offer some assistance. The new and different findings are that there is little difference in the productivity of HMOs.

EIGHT

Trends in Medical Care
Costs and Utilization

Previous chapters have provided ample evidence that health maintenance organization enrollees experience lower total costs for their medical care and have lower hospitalization rates than comparable groups of people. From a policy perspective, however, there is another important question that rarely is addressed: do HMO enrollees experience a slower rate of increase in costs, or is there simply a one-time reduction in levels? In the same way that previous chapters broke down total cost into utilization and cost per unit, this chapter will examine the time trends in the number of services utilized and the cost per unit of service.

Since the early 1960s total costs for HMO enrollees have grown at only a slightly lower rate than costs for those with conventional insurance coverage. As indicated before, at any point in time the HMO's comparative advantage vis-a-vis conventional providers is in lower hospitalization rates. Over a twenty-year period a number of HMOs show substantial long-term reductions in hospitalization, but there is also evidence of long-term reductions in hospitalization in non-HMOs. Some apparent reductions in HMO utilization can be explained by changes in the age-sex mix of the enrolled population. Costs per inpatient-day in HMOs largely reflect changes in the costs of inputs and do not demonstrate differential increases in efficiency over time. The falling number of hospital days per enrollee-year does, however, represent a resource saving, Physician productivity in HMOs actually decreases over time, but this too seems to reflect a national pattern.

These trends reinforce the belief that HMO cost advantages are almost entirely attributable to utilization patterns, rather than to the ability to provide specific services less expensively. Inpatient costs per day follow almost the same trend as those of all community hospitals. Data drawn from several sources suggest that utilization and cost patterns for HMO members and enrollees in conventional insurance plans have been changing in similar ways for at least the last decade. This still implies substantially lower costs for HMO members. As presently constituted, however, HMOs provide only limited evidence of a long-term solution to slowing the growth rate of medical care costs.

The first section of this chapter presents the evidence on changes over time in total costs of medical care. The second section examines the major source of HMO "savings"—hospital utilization—and the third section examines trends in ambulatory care and ancillary services. The fourth section presents the limited data concerning productivity and costs per unit of service. A final section summarizes the findings.

TOTAL COSTS OVER TIME

A major difficulty in examining total costs and utilization over time is that the population composition and the extent of insurance coverage can change as well, so it is difficult to determine the true causes of apparent changes. Holding the population group constant is thus particularly important. This section will present data drawn from two groups of government employees with dual choice options for health insurance. The relative homogeneity and stability of government employees makes them a serendipitous data source. A third source of data is available for the four-year experience of enrollees in the Seattle Prepaid Health Care Project.

California State Employees

Table 8-1 presents the changes in total costs (premium plus out-of-pocket) for a single employee group, California state employees and their families, in 1962–63 and 1970–71. These data indicate that Kaiser enrollees had the lowest total costs in both years. The cost increase data, however, indicate lower growth rates over the seven-year period for both commercial enrollees and those in the individual practice associations. Total costs for enrollees in BC-BS and Ross-Loos more than doubled. If the two conventional types of coverage, commercial indemnity and BC-BS, are combined, an 83 to 85 percent increase is demonstrated for enrollees. This brackets the 84 percent found for Kaiser enrollees.*

All of the plans provided improvements in their benefit packages, but it is difficult to compare individual changes. If one assumes that the relative share of premiums attributable to administrative costs is constant over time for each plan, however, changes in the proportion of total expenditures attributable to premiums may be used as a crude measure of changes in

---

*The 83 to 85 percent range indicates the alternative estimates that are obtained using either the 1962-63 or 1970-71 population bases as weights.

Table 8—1 Changes in Total Costs per Person for California State Employees and Their Dependents, 1962—63 and 1970—71 (Basic Only)

	Commercial Indemnity Plans	Statewide Blue Cross-Blue Shield	Prepaid Groups		
			Kaiser	Ross-Loos	IPAs
Total costs					
1962—63[a]	$104	$121	$ 93	$ 99	$118
1970—71	$176	$242	$171	$199	$218
Premium as % of total, 1962—63	55%	59%	76%	69%	65%
Premium as % of total, 1970—71	58%	66%	80%	70%	59%
Percent increase to 1970—71:					
Total costs	69%	100%	84%	101%	85%
Premium	79%	127%	92%	104%	66%
Out-of-pocket	57%	62%	59%	94%	120%
Proportion of employees and dependents in each plan*					
1962—63[b]	36.5%	40.2%	14.9%	1.7%	1.3%
1970—71	33.3%	26.0%	32.2%	0.7%	2.0%

SOURCES. Dozier et al., June 1964; Dozier et al., 1973, pp. 44, 99.

* Excludes enrollees in employee organization service benefit plans, thus percents do not sum to 100.0.

[a] No supplemental in 1962—63, p. 77, 1974. All 1970—71 data are for Basic Only.

[b] Table 4, p. 56, 1964.

Note: Revised numbers in this table have been provided by Health Benefits Division of Public Employees' Retirement System, Sacramento, Ca., March 1980.

relative coverage within each plan.* As seen in Table 8—1, this remained approximately constant for the two prepaid group plans and the indemnity enrollees.† On the other hand, almost all of the extra increase in costs for BC-BS members is attributable to their premiums, which were 127 percent higher than in the first period, while direct costs were 62 percent higher. This increase in the proportion of total expenditures attributable to the premium, which is a measure of effective coverage, suggests greater protection against the risk of out-of-pocket expenses and thus an improvement in welfare not captured in the average cost figures. (See the

*On a national basis, the proportion of national health expenditures identified as administrative ranged from 4.8 percent to 6.4 percent over the period 1962 to 1971, with little apparent pattern (Mueller and Gibson, 1976).

†The use of survey data to measure out-of-pocket costs results in a potential bias due to forgetfulness. While such a bias might be expected to be greatest for indemnity-type plans, the figures in Table 8-1 indicate few differences between commercial enrollees and BC-BS enrollees, either in the proportion of out-of-pocket expenses or in their rate of growth. In part, this reflects the relative similarity of coverage under the conventional plans.

discussion in Chapter 4.) The opposite movement is apparent for IPA enrollees; their costs were increasingly out-of-pocket, and thus they were bearing more risk over time.

These data suggest that for California state employees, HMO enrollment has not resulted in substantial reductions in the rate of increase of their total medical care costs. The smallest increases were experienced by commercial plan enrollees, while nearly the largest increases were borne by BC-BS members. The latter also may have had a broadening of their coverage and thus a potential reduction in their exposure to out-of-pocket costs. Enrollees in the IPA form of HMO had a rise in total costs comparable to that of Kaiser enrollees, but in the IPA this was coupled with an apparent reduction in relative coverage. Of the two PGPs, both of which held effective coverage nearly constant, Kaiser had increases slightly below the average, while Ross-Loos had increases at the high end of the range.

One important caveat must be taken into consideration—the population in each plan changed substantially. Kaiser more than doubled its proportion of the total enrollees, mostly at the expense of statewide BC-BS. This shift from most to least expensive is not surprising. But if the relatively high utilizers shifted to Kaiser in order to protect themselves from further financial risk, then the Kaiser performance is more impressive than Table 8–1 indicates. On the other hand, if high utilizers in BC-BS wanted to retain their physician relationships, while relatively low utilizers left BC-BS because their potential usage would not warrant the higher premiums, then the Kaiser figures overstate their control over costs. Just the opposite type of behavior might explain the relatively poor showing of Ross-Loos. That plan held total enrollment constant throughout the period, and thus probably had an aging and hence more expensive enrollment mix. As costs rose, some of the relatively lower utilizers may have switched out because they were not getting their money's worth. While it is impossible to determine from the available data whether such selective enrollment changes occurred, a later section of this chapter discusses the importance of population changes.

Federal Employees

Since 1960 federal employees have had multiple choice options among health care plans. Everyone is eligible for the nationwide plans sponsored by BC-BS and Aetna, while PGPs and IPAs are available only to those living in areas where such organizations exist. Table 8-2 presents data for the annual rate of increase in premiums and benefits per person in the various plans in existence for the entire period, 1961 to 1974. Both measures ignore changes in direct costs to the individual because of changing benefit packages. In spite of this limitation, these data are useful both because of the questions they answer and the questions they raise.

In general, federal employees enrolled in HMOs experienced slower

Table 8-2 Enrollment and Monthly Premiums in 1961 and Annual Changes (1961-1974) in Premiums and Benefits per Person under the High Option of The Federal Employees Health Benefits Program

Plan	1961		1961-1974 Average Annual Changes*	
	Enrollment	Self Only Premium	Premium per Person	Benefits per Person
Blue Cross/Blue Shield	2,466,150	$7.39	10.4%	10.6%
Aetna	1,064,275	6.76	10.5	10.7
Prepaid Group Practices				
Health Insurance Plan, NY	17,685	8.34	7.2	9.5
GHA, Washington, D.C.	23,023	9.90	8.4	9.7
Group Health-St. Paul	756	7.89	8.3	9.0
Group Health of Puget Sound	7,311	8.34	7.9	8.2
Western Clinic, Tacoma	640	8.34	8.6	9.2
Kaiser-Oregon	8,775	6.31	8.7	9.4
Kaiser-Northern California	78,628	7.71	9.9	9.6
Kaiser-Southern California	47,821	8.23	10.5	11.0
Kaiser-Hawaii	19,115	5.81	8.6	9.3
Ross-Loos	2,033	7.28	8.9	11.4
PGPs-unweighted average			8.7	9.6
PGPs-weighted average		7.91	9.5	9.6
Individual Practice Associations				
GHI, New York	14,976	7.02	6.4	7.1
North Idaho	493	9.47	8.4	7.6
Washington Physicians, Seattle	23,677	9.47	7.7	8.1
National Hospital Association, Oregon	3,670	7.74	4.5	6.9
HMSA, Hawaii	37,792	8.80	7.7	7.1
IPAs-unweighted average			6.7	7.5
IPAs-weighted average		8.62	6.9	7.6

SOURCE. Annual Reports of the U.S. Civil Service Commission, Bureau of Retirement, Insurance, and Occupational Health.

* Annual rates are computed from a regression equation of the log (premium income per person per month) or log (benefits per person per month) against the year. All coefficients are significant at well beyond the .001 level.

rates of growth in premiums and in the dollar value of benefits than did those in conventional insurance plans. While one would expect the premium and benefit trends for each plan to be almost identical, as they are for BC-BS and Aetna, in almost every case HMO enrollees had a more rapid growth in benefits than in premiums. This suggests that a decreasing share of their premiums was going to administration and overhead. While the average growth in PGP premiums was about 9.5 percent, the rate for IPAs was 6.9 percent. The initial IPA premiums, however, were substantially higher. The IPA performance also may be attributable to different policies with respect to coverage. In the previous section the California state employee data for IPAs showed the slowest rate of growth in premiums by far, but the highest growth in out-of-pocket costs. The net result was similar to that of Kaiser enrollees. If the same were true for the IPAs in the federal employee program, then the low growth rate in covered costs may be offset by a greater burden of out-of-pocket costs.

These data also point to the wide variation in experiences, even among apparently similar plans. For instance, the annual rate of premium increase for PGPs ranged from 7.2 percent to 10.5 percent, with both figures being drawn from large, well-established plans. The two California Kaiser plans, which dominate enrollment, have the highest rates of increase. Thus the weighted average of the annual increase in premiums is 9.5 percent versus 8.7 percent if each plan is weighted equally, as if each were an independent point. Depending upon the measures used, PGP enrollees experienced annual premium increases of 1 to 1.5 points lower than those in conventional plans, while IPA enrollees had a 3.6 point advantage. These translate to 10 to 35 percent lower growth rates, a potentially substantial difference. It must be pointed out that part or all of this could be caused by more rapid relative improvement (or catching up) of the benefit package in the conventional plans.

Seattle Prepaid Health Care Project

While the previous two sources are valuable because they provide data for several HMOs over substantial periods of time, both suffer from a subtle but important limitation. Major components of the cost data are based on premiums rather than actual costs. Although premiums and costs will be approximately equal for the entire HMO membership, they can vary widely for any particular enrollee group. This variance stems from the use of community rating by HMOs. This means that the Kaiser premium for California state employees is set to approximate costs not for those enrollees, but for all Kaiser members. This is not the case for conventional insurers and BC-BS, which experience rate premiums; so the BC-BS premiums for state employees, for example, reflect their actual experience.

The importance of this premium factor can be seen in Table 8-3, which presents premiums and paid-out costs for enrollees in the Seattle Prepaid Health Care Project. The GH premium was based on the GH community rate, adjusted for family composition. Changes in enrollment mix led to modest reductions in average premium for the first three years. The increase in 1974 reflected a GH-wide rate increase in spring of 1974. Because KCM-BC premiums were experience-rated, they show substantial increases each year, reflecting actual increases in costs. While over the four-year period premiums approximated costs for each plan, the rates of increase varied substantially. GH premiums rose only 8 percent, in contrast to a 21 percent increase for KCM-BC. The increases in total costs present a different story: a 57 percent increase for GH versus 24 percent for KCM-BC. The worse GH experience is attributable to a much more rapid rise in hospital costs for GH enrollees. This, in turn, may be explained by self-selection factors. (See Chapter 3.) Given the potential influence of selection on these figures and the differences between these findings and the long-term trends in HMO enrollee overall costs, which do not indicate such wide differences, it is best to treat these data merely as a cautionary note when examining premium data.

HOSPITAL UTILIZATION

The major source of savings in HMOs is in their lower hospital utilization rates. The question is: have these rates changed over time? This section reviews the evidence from three data sources, each increasingly specific. The first compares utilization for enrollees in three Kaiser plans and all BC-BS plans. Although crude, this comparison holds constant a measure of insurance coverage, unlike overall national utilization data, which reflect increasing insurance coverage among the poor and elderly. The second comparison is for federal government enrollees in conventional insurance plans (BC-BS and Aetna) versus those in PGPs and IPAs. These data are much more specific and hold constant the level of coverage. Everyone has the most comprehensive coverage offered under the plan, and all HMO enrollees also had the choice of BC-BS and Aetna. The third level of analysis foregoes comparisons and, instead, examines the factors that explain utilization changes of Kaiser Oregon enrollees over more than a quarter of a century.

Table 8−3   Premiums and Paid-Out Costs for Enrollees in the Seattle Prepaid Health Care Project

Year[a]	Premiums		Experience-Rated Costs	
	GH	KCM-BC	GH	KCM-BC[b]
1971	$176.56	$241.12	$148.08	$246.49
1972	173.07	246.57	158.23	262.17
1973	170.83	260.30	192.42	282.12
1974	191.07	290.86	232.12	306.58
48 Month Average	$177.68	$263.08	$183.96	$279.14
Increase	8.2%	20.6%	56.8%	24.4%

SOURCE.   McCaffree et al., 1976, Tables III−1(a) and (b).
[a] For year beginning February 1.
[b] Includes 3% BC hospital discount, payments under coordination of benefits, and administrative costs.

Kaiser and Blue Cross-Blue Shield Members, 1955-77

Figure 8-1 presents data for annual rates of inpatient days per 1000 enrollees for three Kaiser regions and national BC-BS for various years between 1955 and 1977. There is a general downward trend in utilization for the Kaiser enrollees. For instance, in the 1950s Kaiser Oregon had utilization rates in the 800 to 900 per 1000 range, while by the late 1960s this had fallen to about the 450 level. Kaiser Northern California lowered its rate from the 600 to the 650 per 1000 range in the late 1950s to 372 in 1977. In contrast to this general downward or stable trend, the national BC-BS hospitalization rates showed a marked upward trend from 1955 to 1965, increasing from about 950 to over 1200 days per 1000 members. Reflecting the removal of the elderly because of Medicare coverage in 1966, the BC-BS rate fell to about 900, and then remained constant from 1967 to 1970. Thereafter, it showed a rate of decline comparable to that of the Kaiser plans.* Thus, at least for the 1966-77 period, there is evidence of national changes in utilization levels for a conventionally insured population. This might partially account for the observed patterns in these HMOs. More importantly, in the last decade HMO utilization rates were not falling any less rapidly than rates for BC-BS enrollees.

Enrollees in the Federal Health Benefits Program, 1961-74

The above findings are partially corroborated by the utilization trends for people covered by the Federal Employees Health Benefits Program, as shown in Figure 8-2. For the 1961-62 to 1972 period, nonmaternity utilization by BC-BS enrollees was generally in the 900+ range, while that of the commercial (Aetna) enrollees showed a sharp upward trend in the first few years and then leveled out. Enrollees in both PGPs and IPA type plans had small but consistent reductions in utilization per 1000 enrollees until about 1969. This was followed by small increases. Between 1972 and 1973 there was a sharp reduction in utilization rates, from 950 days per 1000 to about 750, for both Aetna and BC-BS enrollees. There also was a substantial, although not as large, reduction in absolute terms for IPA and PGP enrollees. The proportionate reductions are comparable, on the order

*For instance, a regression estimate for the 1967-77 BC-BS data shown in Figure 8-1 yields $y = 942.87 \ (13.06) - 14.78T \ (1.92), R^2 = .87$, where T represents years, 1967 = 1, 1968 = 2, etc. (standard errors in parenthesis). The comparable estimate for the three Kaiser plans is $y = 503.13 \ (9.53) - 9.63T \ (1.40), R^2 = .60$. The larger absolute coefficient for the time variable in the BC-BS equation indicates a more rapid decline in hospital utilization. The relative change, however, is in the opposite direction; BC-BS shows a 1.6% decline per year, in contrast to 1.9% for the Kaiser plans. How this difference is to be interpreted is another issue. If the lower initial Kaiser rates are due to the elimination of unnecessary inpatient use, one would not expect further large reductions. But if the lower initial Kaiser use is attributable to a different patient mix, then the impact of changes in medical practice might be comparable in the two plans.

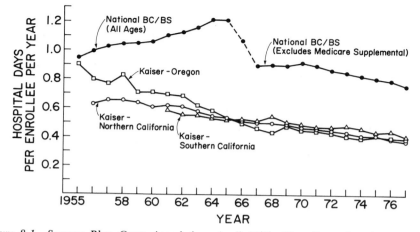

Figure 8-1 Sources: Blue Cross Association, April 1975; Blue Cross Association, 1966; Somers, 1971 (and November 1975 update); Kaiser Foundation Medical Care Program, 1967, page 24; Kaiser Foundation Health Plan Inc., 1977, 1978; Blue Cross Association, April 12, 1977; Blue Cross and Blue Shield Associations, 1978; Saward, Blank, and Greenlick, 1968, pp. 231–244; Saward, Blank, and Lamb, 1973; Marks, Hurtado, and Greenlick, 1976. *Note:* The data for Kaiser are for covered hospital days for plan members discharged within the year in question.

of 20+ percent. The substantial utilization reductions in the government-wide plans are reflected in a premium decrease between 1972 and 1973. However, premiums increased in 1973 and 1974 at about their old rate but from a lower base. It is not known what accounts for the break in the series, but it probably was caused by a systemwide change in coverage or accounting, and comparable data are not available after 1974 (Hustead, 1978). The relative advantages of HMOs remain apparent. Regression estimates on utilization rates for specific plans and groups of plans indicate statistically significant increases over time for the conventional plans (BC-BS and Aetna), essentially no change for the PGPs, and significant decreases for the two IPAs with complete data (Washington Physicians and HMSA).* These two IPAs, however, began the 1960s with very high hospitalization rates, which were later brought down to the level of the PGPs (U.S. Civil Service Commission, Annual Reports, 1961-75).

* For the three groups of plans, the regressions relating total days per 1000 to a time variable, T, and a dummy for the years 1973–74, D, are as follows:

BC/BS + Aetna	$Y =$	827	$+ 13.1T$	$- 262D$	$R^2 = .69$
		(21.4)	(3.18)	(5.55)	
PGPs	$Y =$	412	$- 2.38T$	$- 80.5D$	$R^2 = .45$
		(27.0)	(1.15)	(3.37)	
IPAs	$Y =$	521	$- 8.33T$	$- 64.6D$	$R^2 = .57$
		(19.5)	(2.30)	(1.55)	

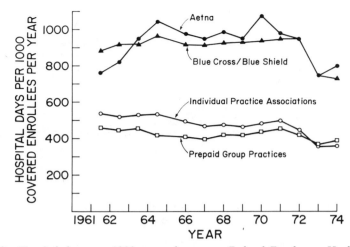

Figure 8-2 Hospital days per 1000 covered persons, Federal Employees Health Benefits Program, 1961–1974, high option, nonmaternity. *Source: U.S. Civil Service Commission Annual Report, 1961–1972.*

A Quarter-Century of Changes in Hospital Utilization in the Kaiser Oregon Plan

As one attempts to examine more detailed characteristics over time, the data become even more limited. In fact, the only reasonably complete data set is that describing the experience of the Kaiser plan in Oregon (Saward, Blank, and Greenlick, 1968; Saward, Blank, and Lamb, 1973). It must be remembered that the data in Figure 8-1 suggest that the Oregon region is atypical. Kaiser Oregon began with higher than normal (for Kaiser) utilization, and by the late 1960s had lower than average hospitalization. Thus its trends will be steeper than is likely to be the case even for other Kaiser regions, and it may be unrepresentative of other HMOs. Nonetheless, it offers important insights into some of the factors behind utilization changes.

Figure 8-3 represents data on hospital utilization by Kaiser Oregon enrollees over a twenty-seven-year period. As discussed above, there is a fairly steady downward trend in hospital days per 1000 enrollees. This reduction is attributable both to a declining admission rate, which fell from over 130 per 1000 enrollees to under 90 per 1000 and to a drop in the average length of stay, from over six to under five days. The admission rate rose steadily from 1951 to 1954 and then began a long-term decline for the next two decades. The length of stay shows a more irregular but consistent decline throughout the period, leveling off in the late 1960s and early 1970s. As can be seen by the proportionate changes, admissions and length of stay are about equally responsible for the overall changes in total hospital days.

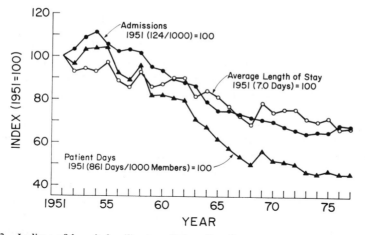

Figure 8-3   Indices of hospital utilization, Kaiser-Oregon region, 1951–1977. *Sources:* Saward, Blank, and Greenlick, 1968, pp. 235, 237; Saward, Blank, and Lamb, 1973, p. 36; Marks, Hurtado, and Greenlick, 1976, p. 11; Kaiser Foundation Health Plan Inc., 1977, 1978.

A few historical points lead to a better understanding of these data. The original health plan operated out of a 300-bed hospital located in Vancouver, Washington, about twelve miles from the major population center in Portland, Oregon. Membership grew to over 20,000 by 1953 and reached a plateau of about 23,000 from 1954 to mid-1957. In 1957 plans to build a hospital in Portland were announced, and the facility formally opened in mid-1959. When the new Bess Kaiser Hospital was opened, it had only 129 beds and was more appropriately scaled to the size of the membership. Enrollment has continued to grow since 1958. Additional outpatient facilities have been added, and a 120-bed hospital wing was added in 1966. Initially, much of this new capacity was used as an extended care facility, and the complement of regular hospital beds was slowly increased. A second hospital was added in 1976. Active efforts to reduce inpatient use also have been undertaken, such as a substantial increase in ambulatory or "do not admit" surgery since 1966. In fact, by 1974 about 35 percent of the operating room procedures were performed on patients who were not admitted to the hospital (Greenlick et al., 1978). Similarly large increases in "do not admit" surgery have also been observed in British Columbia, with a conventional FFS reimbursement system (Shah and Robinson, 1977).

In the early period the organization relied heavily on FFS utilization by nonplan members and a contract with the Veterans' Administration for treatment of VA tuberculosis patients. Even with this extra utilization, the Vancouver hospital maintained low occupancy. This meant that less pressure was placed on physicians to reduce inpatient care. The growth that began in 1958 also changed the relative importance of nongroup members in the plan. Before the expansion, nongroup members accounted for over a quarter of the total enrollees. Their proportion fell steadily until it was about one-sixth in 1971. Nongroup members are of particular interest because they are the most likely to have self-selected into the plan with the expectation of utilizing services. This situation was more likely to have influenced utilization in the early years when most nongroup members were direct enrollees; an increasing proportion of nongroup subscribers are former group members who converted when they left their employee group. Another change during this period was in the average number of persons per subscriber unit. This figure increased from 2.06 in 1950 to 2.82 in 1966; most of the increase occurred in the 1950s. This probably was due to the addition of families with children and the postwar baby boom. The change in age structure can have a major influence on hospital use averages. For instance, for the United States as a whole in 1977 children under seventeen years of age used only one-third the number of short-term hospital days that was used by the general population (U.S. National Center for Health Statistics, Series 10, no. 126, September 1978).

One clear indication of the importance of changes in the enrollee mix is given in Table 8-4. From 1965-66 to 1974 the nonobstetric discharge rate fell from 76 to 61 per 1000 enrollees and the days of hospital care from 468 to 335, substantial reductions in a ten-year period. If the age-sex specific rates for 1965-66 are weighted by the membership mix in 1974, it is apparent that one-third of the overall reduction in both discharges and days per 1000 is attributable to the changing membership mix. Although age-specific data are not available for earlier periods, the data concerning members per subscriber unit suggest that the post-1965 period was relatively stable in comparison with the pre-1965 period. Thus changes in the membership mix are likely to account for substantially more than one-third of the utilization changes in the 1951-65 period.

A Summary of the Evidence on Hospitalization

In terms of overall utilization rates, there is evidence that both PGPs and IPAs demonstrate long-term reductions in hospitalization rates relative to other insured groups. It is not entirely clear to what these trends can be attributed. For one prepaid group, Kaiser Oregon, part of the halving in the patient-day rate is accounted for by changes in the population mix. The evidence from this experience suggests that a prepaid group practice does not necessarily produce low hospitalization rates, as the present practice patterns took time to develop. Bringing the bed supply into line with the population seems to have supported those changes in practice.* (See Klarman, 1970.)

*This is not to imply that new prepaid groups must repeat that learning experience. In fact, new HMOs have produced evidence that suggests rather low hospitalization rates within a year or two of initiation. More experienced HMOs have even lower utilization rates (U.S. Health Maintenance Organization Service, 1977).

Table 8–4   Effects of Changes in Composition of Health Plan Membership on Hospital Utilization, Kaiser–Oregon Region, 1965–66 to 1977

	Excluding Obstetrics					
	Discharges/1000 Members			Days/1000 Members		
	Total	Males	Females	Total	Males	Females
(1) 1965–66 Actual rates	76	78	74	468	501	436
(2) 1965–66 Age–sex specific rates weighted by 1974 membership mix	71	71	71	424	439	410
(3) Reduction attributable to change in mix	5	7	3	44	62	26
(4) 1974 Actual rates	61	64	59	335	340	331
(5) Total reduction, line (1) − line (4)	15	14	15	133	161	105
(6) Proportion of reduction attributable to mix (3)/(5)	33%	50%	20%	33%	39%	25%

SOURCE.   Marks, Hurtado, and Greenlick, 1976, pp. 11, 25, 32, 34, 37.

AMBULATORY VISITS AND ANCILLARY SERVICES

The Kaiser Oregon region also provides data concerning trends in ambulatory visits and the use of ancillary services. Figure 8-4 presents data for doctor office visits and inpatient and outpatient laboratory and radiology services. Except for 1951-54, the doctor office visit rates are remarkable for their lack of trend. Instead, there is relatively random variation in the range of 3 to 3.5 visits per person. The use of radiology services suggests a strong time trend, resulting in a three-fold increase in twenty-five-year period. Superimposed on this is a cyclical pattern with peaks in 1955, 1957, 1962, 1966 and 1974. The use of laboratory services per 1000 members shows a similar cyclical pattern, although with a less pronounced time trend until the late 1960s. Freeborn et al. (1972) point out that much of the recent growth in laboratory use was for preventive or nondisease services, supporting the hypothesis that new members use a disproportionate share of such services. Mullooly and Freeborn (1978), however, show that new members are not more frequent users of ambulatory visits; so these data may reflect the use of laboratory and X-ray to obtain baseline data. An additional factor in the late 1960s was the removal of a 50 percent copayment for laboratory and X-ray services in some contracts (Freeborn et al., 1972).

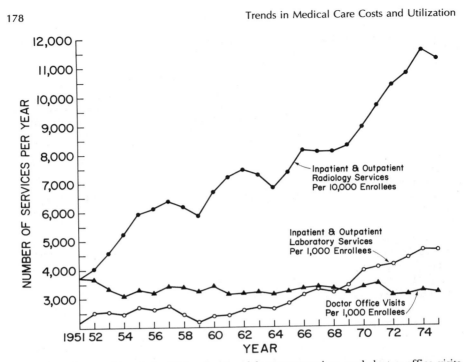

Figure 8-4 Sources: Trends in X-Ray services, laboratory services, and doctor office visits per enrollee per year, Kaiser-Oregon, 1951–1975; Saward, Blank, and Greenlick, 1968, pp. 231–244; Saward, Blank, and Lamb, 1973; Kaiser-Permanente Medical Care Program, Oregon Region, 1971–1975.

For both laboratory and X-ray services, there seems to be a long-term utilization increase that may reflect medical advances and technological change. While time-series data for these services for the general population are not available, data from the PAMC, a predominantly FFS California group practice, show roughly similar increases. (See Table 8-5.) Although the absolute levels of services differ substantially, largely reflecting different practice patterns, the periods of rise and plateau seem to parallel one another, suggesting the influence of new equipment or the coming into vogue of new tests. Data from HIP of New York indicate a 41 percent increase in laboratory tests per enrollee between 1961 and 1970 (HIP Statistical Report, 1971 *in* Birnbaum, 1972). The comparable increase for Kaiser Oregon was 62 percent.

Thus for both hospitalization and ancillary services long-run changes in the Kaiser Oregon experience appear to be the results of external changes in medical practice and technology, deliberate planning to control the availability of beds, HMO incentives, and changes in membership. Enrollment growth and mix changes may be encouraged by the HMO, for example, by offering maternity coverage to attract young couples (Hudes

Table 8−5   Laboratory Tests and X-Rays per Physician Office Visit, Palo Alto Medical Clinic and Kaiser−Oregon, 1964−75

	Laboratory Tests per Visit		X-Rays per Visit	
	PAMC	Kaiser	PAMC	Kaiser
1964	0.85	0.84	0.118	0.218
.	.	.	.	.
.	.	.	.	.
.	.	.	.	.
1968	1.07	0.96	0.122	0.244
	.	.	.	.
1970	1.61	1.16	0.146	0.264
1971	1.64	1.16	.	.
1972	1.70	1.35	0.165	0.338
	.	.	.	.
1974	2.10	1.43	.	.
1975	2.11	1.46	0.177	0.356

SOURCE.   Personal correspondence, Anne Scitovsky, May 18, 1977; for Kaiser data, see notes to Figure 8−4.

et al., 1979). They also may occur through factors not under the HMO's control, such as demographic changes in the community.

COST PER UNIT OF SERVICE

The Kaiser Oregon region data also allow an investigation of long-term trends in hospital costs and physician productivity. Figure 8-5 presents hospital cost data for Kaiser and for all short-term general and other special hospitals in Oregon. The Kaiser Oregon data have the particular advantage of having been drawn from a single, consistent source. Data that should be comparable, chosen from the annual American Hospital Association hospital guide, have been examined for all Kaiser hospitals in each state. While broad trends are similar, the AHA data exhibit much more variability, even when averaged over a large number of hospitals, and this variability seems to reflect differences in reporting, rather than true expenditures.

The costs per patient day in the Kaiser Oregon hospital began somewhat below the Oregon average, but by the end of the period they were somewhat above average. The higher cost per patient day may be a reflection of the shorter length of stay in Kaiser Oregon hospitals. There was a decline in Kaiser costs in the years surrounding the opening of the Bess Kaiser Hospital in Portland, but all Oregon hospitals exhibited a slowing in cost increases in that period. (In fact, both Kaiser and all Oregon

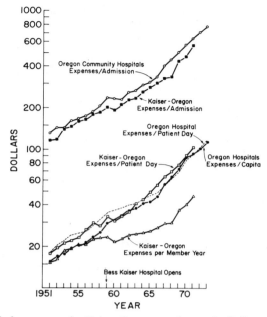

Figure 8-5 Hospital costs trends, Kaiser-Oregon region and all Oregon community hospitals. *Sources:* Worthington, 1975, Table 1; American Hospital Association, 1962, p. 414; Saward, Blank, and Lamb, 1973, p. 39; Saward, Blank, and Greenlick, 1968, pp. 231–244. *Note:* Data for Oregon hospitals refer specifically to nonfederal, short-term general, and other special hospitals.

hospital costs per admission show an absolute decline in 1960.) Of course, costs per patient day may well be an inappropriate figure for comparison because of changes in length of stay and case mix over time. This is especially true when there are major changes in utilization patterns.*

The data for expenses per admission capture the effects of differences in length of stay. In this instance the Kaiser expenses are below the Oregon average, and there appears to be a somewhat widening differential, especially in the post-1959 period. To the extent that simpler cases were treated on an outpatient basis, the cost per admission understates cost control. As discussed above, 1959 saw both the opening of the new hospital,

---

*The expenses per patient day figures do not reflect the recent American Hospital Association adjustments to account for increased outpatient use. Although outpatient visits have increased markedly in community hospitals, there is corresponding evidence of substantial increases in "do not admit" (or ambulatory) surgery at Kaiser (Greenlick et al., 1978). When it is not known precisely how these trends differ, adjusting only one series is probably worse than leaving both series unadjusted.

which may have been more efficient, and substantial membership growth, which tended to lower the utilization rate. The population mix changes resulting from the rapid growth may also have contributed to the reduction in length of stay. (The differences in length of stay may also explain why the costs per day were growing more rapidly in the Kaiser hospital in the later period if, as is usually the case, the first few days of a hospital stay are more expensive than the last few.) The clearest cost advantage for Kaiser is in the comparison of cost per member year and cost per capita; there is a much slower rate of growth for Kaiser members. The preceding discussion indicates that these overall savings are not due to major technological efficiencies in the provision of specific services, such as performing an X-ray more efficiently. Instead, they largely stem from the long-term fall in admissions per member and a shortening of the average length of stay.

One rough comparison in hospital cost trends for the 1970-76 period has been developed by the California Health Facilities Commission (Carter and Allison, 1978). Kaiser hospitals in Northern and Southern California were compared with non-Kaiser hospitals in the same regions. While average costs per case and per day were lower for Kaiser hospitals, probably reflecting differences in case mix, the trends in costs were similar. On a per admission basis, Kaiser costs in Northern California rose at an average annual rate of 14.1 percent, in contrast to 13.2 percent for non-Kaiser hospitals; while in Southern California the relative performance was reversed, 14.7 percent for Kaiser and 16.8 percent for non-Kaiser. Reflecting a slight decline in average stay for Kaiser patients, their costs per patient day rose more rapidly than for non-Kaiser hospitals—15.5 percent versus 14.0 percent in the North and 16.2 percent versus 15.2 percent in the South (Carter and Allison, 1978, pp. 25, 27).

Physician productivity can be crudely measured by the volume of doctor office visits per physician, as shown by Figure 8-6. While there is a slight downward trend in productivity over the entire period and a substantial fall in the last few years, the most remarkable thing is the wide variation from year to year. The graph of full-time-equivalent (FTE) physicians per 1000 members and doctor office visits per physician traces almost exactly inverse patterns. This follows from the basically uniform level of ambulatory visits per enrollee. The number of physicians in the group each year explains the productivity pattern. The medical group substantially expanded in 1954, probably in response to previous growth and to pressures on physicians. At that time physicians were seeing 5000 to 5500 patients per year. Membership growth stopped in 1954; so productivity fell markedly, as there were more physicians to handle the same number of enrollees. It is of interest that the doctor office visit rate shows only a small increase in the 1954-57 period, suggesting that the sharply increased supply of physicians per enrollee was not translated into more patient visits, but into productivity changes. The membership expansion that began in 1958 quickly pushed productivity up again. However, since 1960 an increase in FTE per member has led to a decline in doctor office visits per physician. Data for all Kaiser regions combined suggest similar declines in physician productivity (Palmer, 1977).

These data need to be placed in perspective in two ways. First, the substantial long-run decline in plan member hospitalization should allow Kaiser physicians to spend a larger fraction of time with ambulatory patients. This suggests that the decline in productivity per unit of office time is probably greater than appears in the graph. On the other hand, the increased substitution of ambulatory visits for inpatient care might increase the complexity of the average unit. Second, national data show a long-term (at least since 1965) reduction in the number of hours and weeks worked by physicians in general (Owens, 1976, 1978). There also is evidence of a decline in patient contacts per physician during the 1959-76 period (Wilson and Begun, 1977; Falk, 1978). This may reflect the increased supply of physicians. It would not be surprising if lightening of the work load for Kaiser physicians reflected this trend.

These cost and productivity trends strongly reinforce the belief that HMO cost advantages are almost entirely attributable to differences in utilization patterns, rather than to economies in the provision of specific

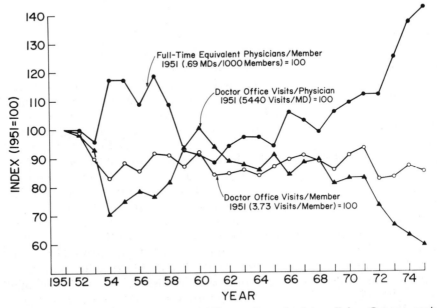

Figure 8-6 Indices of physician availability and productivity, Kaiser-Oregon region, 1951–1975. *Source:* See notes to Figure 8-4.

services (National Advisory Commission on Health Manpower, 1967). Inpatient costs per day followed almost the same path as those of all Oregon community hospitals. Similar results for more recent years are apparent for Kaiser hospitals in California. Some increased savings in the costs per admission over time were obtained by shortening the length of stay. The major relative reductions in costs per member, versus costs per capita for the population as a whole, were achieved through reductions in the admission rate. Physician productivity, as measured by doctor office visits per physician per year, has exhibited a substantial decline, but this may be little different from that experienced nationally as physicians work fewer hours per year.

SUMMARY

Comparisons of people in HMOs with those having conventional insurance yield consistent results showing lower costs and hospital utilization for HMO enrollees. This chapter has addressed the question, do HMOs also lower the growth rate of costs over time? While the answer is not as clear as one would like, the evidence points to a cautiously affirmative answer— HMOs have achieved a slightly slower growth rate. This answer must be qualified because the data are drawn from a wide variety of often noncomparable sources. What would be desirable is a complete analysis of the performance of a large number of HMOs. Such analysis would include not only the crude, aggregate statistics used here, which are available to the outsider, but also age-sex specific utilization and cost figures and the ability to trace down the reasons for various changes. The latter information, if available at all, is usually embedded within internal data systems and the personal recollections of HMO administrators.

There is only one set of data that allows direct comparisons in total costs (premium plus out-of-pocket) for people in various types of health plans. These data indicate somewhat lower growth rates for HMO members than for those with conventional coverage. Unfortunately for those who prefer unambiguous answers, there is as much variation within types of plans as there is across types. Results from the Federal Employees Health Benefits Program support the view that premium costs for HMO enrollees have been growing at a slower rate than costs for conventional coverage, but again there are important differences within groups of providers. Some of the higher rates of premium growth in conventional plans may reflect broadening coverage. Simultaneously, the individual practice associations seem to be lagging behind both PGPs and conventional insurers in depth of coverage. Trends in hospital utilization, however, indicate somewhat more control by HMOs. While utilization rates in the conventional plans tended to increase over time, those for HMOs remained flat or decreased.

This analysis also indicates that a great deal about HMOs is not explained merely by financial incentives. For instance, the early years of the Kaiser Oregon plan were marked by excess hospital capacity and a high hospitalization rate. The development of new practice patterns over time, a new hospital with more tightly constrained resources, and a change in enrollment mix seem to account for an important part of its significantly lower current hospitalization rate. In the early 1950s, when a combination of additional medical staff and slower enrollment growth produced a substantial increase in the ratio of physicians to members, there was little change in the rate of visits per member. Instead, the increased effective supply was translated into more leisure for physicians, rather than more visits for members. Over the last decade, however, there has been a nearly steady decrease in office visits per physician. Prior to this period, special efforts had been made to maintain productivity levels (Saward, 1978).

These data also make it clear that HMOs operate within the context of the much larger medical care system. For instance, their hospitals are subject to the same rate of inflation in the cost of inputs. Thus it is to be expected that costs per patient day show little difference. The Kaiser Oregon plan exhibits the same pattern of rapid increases in laboratory and X-ray usage as does an FFS clinic in California. Similarly, the rate of doctor office visits per physician shows a steady decline in HMOs, just as it does nationally. Thus long-term changes in HMO costs come not from improved productivity in providing a unit of service, or micro-efficiency, but from relative reductions in the number of services rendered. If this is achieved at no perceptible reduction in quality, there is a clear gain in overall or macro-efficiency.

NINE

Preventive Care

There has been a great deal of discussion about whether health maintenance organizations possess more incentives to provide preventive health services than do FFS practices. The usual argument is that because HMOs are responsible for all medical care required by their enrollees, they will use preventive services to reduce the need for more expensive treatment. Sometimes the argument is buttressed with data showing more inoculations, Pap smears, or annual checkups among HMO enrollees than among people with conventional insurance coverage. Counterarguments claim that HMOs have incentives to undertreat patients, and thus might skimp on preventive care (Schwartz, 1978).

This chapter presents evidence that both sides are correct. HMO enrollees do, in fact, receive more preventive services than do people with conventional coverage. This is not because HMOs discovered that an ounce of prevention is worth anything like a pound of cure. Nor is it due to a particular health maintenance philosophy. Instead, the greater number of preventive services for HMO enrollees seems merely to result from the lower prices HMO patients pay for ambulatory visits. In short, patient and provider incentives matter more than philosophy. This is not to deny the importance of beliefs. HMOs typically offer better coverage for preventive care because their founders and members believe in providing such services. However, the system most likely to maximize the number of preventive services is FFS with complete ambulatory insurance coverage.

The first section of the chapter presents a framework for discussion by outlining the theoretical arguments concerning the use of preventive services in various medical care settings. The HMO debate generally focuses on economic incentives, and these are not as clear as is generally believed. Compounding the problem are various professional and legal incentives that may also influence behavior. The second section presents the major studies of preventive use in various settings. The third section demonstrates how these often conflicting studies can be understood when examined in terms of differential ambulatory coverage, rather than HMO versus FFS incentives. It also discusses why more preventive care does not take place in HMOs. A final section summarizes the major findings and offers some policy suggestions.

A FRAMEWORK FOR DISCUSSION: THEORETICAL INCENTIVES FOR PREVENTIVE SERVICES IN VARIOUS SETTINGS

Most discussions of preventive services suffer from two problems: (1) many studies focus only on the provider or the consumer but not on both; and (2) in the various studies it is often unclear what is meant by preventive services. Thus differences are sometimes definitional rather than substantive. This section first outlines the economic incentives for the provision of preventive services. It then discusses some noneconomic factors that may be more important than the financial incentives. Finally, it outlines some of the problems with and approaches to defining preventive services.

Economic Incentives

The economic incentives of preventive services must be derived from a model that includes what economists call "a production function for health," that is, the causal relationships between preventive and therapeutic services, on the one hand, and health status on the other (Phelps, 1978). The general assumption is that preventive services and early treatment will catch a problem in its initial stages and eliminate the need for extensive curative services at a later stage. The focus of this discussion is on what is often called secondary prevention, or the screening for and early treatment of disease. Primary prevention, of which immunization is an example, refers to an action taken to forestall a disease from occurring (Fielding, 1978).

Whether one chooses a preventive or a curative strategy depends on the natural course of the disease and the costs and benefits associated with each strategy. Many diseases have a presymptomatic phase in which they can be detected by a screening program and treated early. For some diseases there is little advantage to early treatment. In such cases the symptoms will lead a patient to seek treatment that is as effective as earlier treatment would have been. For example, gonorrhea in males creates symptoms that are sufficiently clear to make screening unnecessary; while for females the symptoms are subtle, and active case-finding is preferable. The optimal choice of strategy in such cases is made from a social viewpoint, reflecting existing technologies for screening and treatment and alternative uses of resources. In other words, more "prevention" requires a reallocation of resources.

The social perspective is useful to decision-makers primarily for determining the optimal mix of preventive and curative services. In order to determine what is likely to happen, one must examine the prices and incentives faced by individual decision makers (Luft, 1976a). The market will reach the optimal allocation only under stringent conditions. One of these conditions is the requirement that prices reflect resource costs; this often is not true in the medical care system. Fees are usually set by relative value scales that include substantial distortions in the prices assigned various types of services (Schroeder and Showstack, 1978).

Even if relative fees did reflect true costs, medical insurance would continue to change the prices seen by patient and provider. The effective price changes due to insurance are the crucial aspect of discussions about different provider systems. While any particular setting will not quite match the model, there are three major combinations of ambulatory care financing. (See Chapter 1.) At one extreme is the conventional FFS system in which the patient pays the physician directly for each service. (Although most people have some health care insurance, coverage is often poor or nonexistent for ambulatory and particularly nonillness care (Andersen, Lion, and Anderson, 1976)). At the other extreme is the HMO plan that contracts to provide the enrollee with all ambulatory services for a fixed annual fee. In this case the enrollee faces no monetary price when the service is rendered, and the plan, while incurring some extra expense, receives no additional revenue. A third model involves prepayment for enrollees, usually through an insurance scheme, and payment to providers on an FFS basis by the plan, not the patient.

Applying these financing models to the preventive care question leads to a number of predictions. (See Pauly, 1970.) FFS providers will prefer to offer those services yielding the greatest net profit. For instance, in an extreme view, they may prefer to discourage preventive care if in the long run they make more from therapeutic care. Prepaid plans, on the other hand, will promote whatever costs least in the long run, be it prevention or treatment. For example, some types of screening, such as annual physical examinations for business executives, have little long-term medical benefit and would not be offered by prepaid plans, even though they are profitable in the FFS setting, where they are encouraged (Breo, 1976). On the demand side, a patient who bears the cost of care directly is less likely to request as much service as a patient for whom services are prepaid or covered by insurance. Obviously, the outcome of this theoretical discussion depends on the exact shape of the supply and demand curves. These, in turn, are to be derived from the specifics of the illness and the efficacy of preventive and therapeutic care. Data for such predictions are not available; all that can be done is to examine behavior and make inferences from these observations.

Noneconomic Factors in Preventive Services

The economic factors discussed above may be taken as tendencies, if everything else is held constant and the system is competitive, so that noneconomic behavior is difficult, if not impossible. Unfortunately for the analyst, the medical care system has many market imperfections, so other factors enter into the analysis. Perhaps of primary importance are the physician's professional training, ethics, and concern for the patient. Economists have long recognized that physicians are expected to behave in noneconomic ways and provide the best possible care (Arrow, 1963). The malpractice liability system reinforces this expectation. Furthermore, medical school training largely conditions the style of practice of most physicians. This training tends to emphasize diagnosis and treatment of disease on an inpatient basis. In contrast, screening for asymptomatic disease and providing preventive health care is often dull, and such activities offer fewer psychological rewards than does a "cure."

While the physician and organization are generally much more influential than the patient in determining what services are rendered, it is in the area of preventive care that consumer influence is greatest. Psychosocial orientations toward prevention are important factors in determining how often a patient will want a checkup or screening test (Becker et al., 1977; McKinlay and Dutton, 1974). The absence of specific symptoms makes the preventive visit more apt to be postponed, and it may therefore be more sensitive to convenience or access barriers (Dutton, 1977).

Identifying Preventive Services

Preventive care is defined by Kasl and Cobb as "any activity undertaken by a person believing himself to be healthy, for the purpose of preventing disease or detecting it in an asymptomatic stage" (1966, p. 246). Although the concept is simple, the empirical application of this definition is complex. For example, one might clearly count as preventive the annual physical examination or checkup. But how should one count a visit initiated for a sprain or other acute problem during which certain preventive procedures or diagnostic tests are undertaken? The management of chronic conditions often involves periodic return visits to the physician and retesting to determine whether the condition is stable or has worsened. Are such visits preventive? Specific procedures also raise a problem of definition. For instance, rectal and pelvic examinations usually are performed with prevention in mind, but in some cases they are in response to specific symptoms. Thus it is impossible to derive exact measures of preventive care within a particular setting, let alone across organizations. There also are biases built into data collected from different systems. For example, medical insurance often pays for treatment but not preventive visits, so there is an incentive to classify visits as follow-ups, rather than checkups.

Rather than offering a strenuous argument for what ideally should be classified as prevention, this chapter is limited to a review of previously collected data. These measures include physical examinations and checkups; immunizations; screening tests, such as Pap smears; and early prenatal care.

STUDIES OF PREVENTIVE SERVICES IN HMOS AND COMPARISON POPULATIONS

This section presents major findings concerning the use of preventive services by HMO enrollees and comparison groups with conventional insurance coverage. The studies are drawn from a comprehensive review of the literature, which was designed to include all available results. After this brief set of summaries, the next section will attempt to reconcile their conflicting findings.

Health Insurance Plan of Greater New York (HIP)

One of the first and most detailed examinations of preventive services is the comparison of HIP enrollees and the overall New York City population (Committee for the Special Research Project, 1957). These data for 1951 provide several measures indicating that HIP enrollees received more preventive services than nonenrollees. Among women who were pregnant and delivered in 1951, 84.2 percent of the HIP enrollees saw a physician in their first trimester, in contrast to 73.6 percent of the New York City sample. HIP enrollees had an average of 10.5 physician visits before delivery versus 9.3 for the New York City women. The rate of physical checkups or routine health examinations in the eight weeks preceding the interview was also higher for HIP enrollees—11.1 per 100 versus 9.7 per 100. Most of this difference is attributable to a higher rate of general checkups, 6.7 versus 5.4, rather than school, employment or insurance, or an "other and not reported" category. The content of these examinations was measured by the proportion that included each of thirteen specific components, such as temperature, pulse, urinalysis, and rectal examination. When classified by reason (school, employment, insurance versus general checkup), there were few differences in content for HIP enrollees and the New York City sample. Thus it appears that the lower cost for HIP ambulatory visits led to more preventive utilization. However, once a visit was sought, the content was similar.

Los Angeles School Children with Health Problems

Cauffman, Roemer, and Shultz (1967) investigated the medical care received by a group of Los Angeles school children who had been identified by school physicians as having dental, otological, or other medical problems. As expected, children in insured families were much more likely to have received attention for their problem (52.3 percent) than those without insurance (37.7 percent). Among those with insurance there were no significant differences in utilization by provider type—group versus individual practice or commercial versus provider-consumer insurance plan. In contrast to this lack of difference in utilization for a specific problem, 50 percent of the children enrolled in prepaid group practices reported having periodic health examinations, in contrast to 36.2 percent of those with conventional insurance and FFS practitioners (p < .05). When the social class of the child's neighborhood is held constant, this relationship disappears for the upper-class children but remains for those in lower socioeconomic neighborhoods.

Alameda County Human Biology Laboratory

Alameda County, California, was the site of two population-based surveys. In one, the focus was on the proportion of women aged twenty and over who had taken a Papanicolaou test (Breslow and Hochstim, 1964). The data in Table 9-1 exhibit a clear insurance effect and a substantially higher examination rate for native white women in Kaiser relative to those with other insurance.

The second survey focused on the proportion of men and women who had a general health maintenance examination in the last year (Breslow, 1973). The data in Table 9-2 are adjusted for age and income. In addition, parallel data concerning the proportion with dental checkups allow a test of the general propensity to obtain preventive care. (None of the insurance

Table 9−1 Percentage of Women Who Have Taken Papanicolaou Test, by Health Insurance Plan, and Race−Nativity, Alameda County, California, 1962

Insurance Status	All Women	Native White Women	All Other Women
Total	51	57	32
With Kaiser plan	70	77	51
With other health insurance plans	54	57	37
Without health insurance plans	34	43	19

SOURCE. Breslow and Hochstim, February 1964, p. 112.

Table 9−2 Percentage of Persons with Health Maintenance Examinations and Dental Checkups within Past Year, Adjusted for Age and Income Level, by Sex and Type of Health Insurance Coverage, Alameda County, California, 1965

| Type of Coverage | Men | | Women | |
	Health Maintenance Examination	Dental Checkup	Health Maintenance Examination	Dental Checkup
Kaiser	58%	50%	63%	62%
Blue Cross−Blue Shield	45	50	56	60
Other insurance	46	49	57	57
None	43	34	49	41

SOURCE. Breslow, November 7, 1973, p. 4.

plans provided significant coverage for dental examinations.) Male Kaiser enrollees had substantially higher rates for health maintenance examinations than those with other coverages, while dental checkup rates were the same for all three groups. Although female Kaiser enrollees also had higher examination rates, this was paralleled by a higher proportion with dental checkups, suggesting that they may have been more prevention oriented.

Enrollees in Southern California Health Plans

Hetherington, Hopkins, and Roemer (1975) collected data from samples of enrollees in six Southern California health plans. Information on specific preventive procedures was drawn from medical records (Table 9-3). Regardless of the measure used, the data suggest more preventive care for the prepaid group practice enrollees (Kaiser and Ross-Loos).* They consistently have the smallest proportion of families without preventive services and, with minor exceptions, the highest average number of preventive procedures per person. Hetherington, Hopkins, and Roemer also offer a summary factor analytic score per ambulatory visit. This measure is significantly higher for the PGPs than for the other plans, but the two PGPs are not significantly different from one another.

Washington, D.C., Families Using Five Health Care Systems

Utilization behavior of people using different providers was examined in great detail by Dutton (1976), using household interviews with families in two Washington, D.C. neighborhoods. She estimated multiple regression equations for several measures of utilization with a wide range of independent variables, including health problems, age, sex, race, education, family income, health insurance coverage, attitudes, and usual source of care. Preventive use was identified by: (1) the number of checkups received by the respondent; and (2) the frequency of children's checkups. Patients of solo FFS practitioners were taken as the baseline, and estimates were made of the differential use by patients in other health care systems, holding constant their personal and family characteristics. On both measures of

---

*The interpretation of these data is somewhat obscure. For instance, it is difficult to believe that only 4 percent of the families in the large commercial plan had any adult with an annual checkup (row 1, column 1). The problem seems to be in the underlying data, not the interpretation of the table. For instance, the authors note in the text that: "For children the record of the large group practice plan is the most impressive, where only 58% of the families with children 18 years and under went without annual checkups and about three out of five of these children had such an examination during the study year. In contrast, fewer than three among 20 children 18 years and younger received annual checkups under the large commercial plan" (page 155). For the large group (Kaiser), this implies that only 42 percent (100−58 percent) of the families had *any* children with a checkup, but the children in those families who did have checkups account for 59 percent of *all* children in the sample. While this is possible, it seems unlikely.

Table 9—3   Measures of Preventive Care Utilization for Enrollees in Six Southern California Health Plans, 1967—68

	Large Commercial	Small Commercial	Blue Cross	Blue Shield	Kaiser	Ross-Loos
	Proportion of Families with None					
Annual checkup, persons aged 19+	96.1	90.6	87.5	83.7	73.6	61.2
Annual checkup, persons aged 18 and under	90.6	79.5	86.9	76.0	57.8	74.6
Pap smears, adult females	80.7	63.9	66.9	60.9	55.7	54.1
Pelvic exams, adult females	76.2	66.7	69.1	59.6	58.6	57.8
Rectal exams	94.6	85.5	75.6	81.7	63.8	58.8
Immunizations	87.8	84.5	82.9	85.0	58.8	77.6
	Average Procedures Per Person					
Annual checkup, persons aged 19+	0.03	0.05	0.09	0.11	0.21	0.30
Annual checkup, persons aged 18 and under	0.14	0.18	0.38	0.38	0.59	0.30
Pap smears, adult females	0.20	0.39	0.36	0.40	0.45	0.53
Pelvic exams, adult females	0.45	0.74	0.69	0.72	0.82	0.73
Rectal exams	0.03	0.06	0.14	0.13	0.18	0.24
Immunizations	0.04	0.09	0.12	0.10	0.22	0.18
	Prevention Factor Score per Person per Ambulatory Visit					
Mean score	0.375	0.412	0.401	0.410	0.455	0.435

SOURCE.   Hetherington, Hopkins, and Roemer, 1975, pp. 155, 157.

preventive use PGP enrollees had the highest scores among the five health care systems: FFS solo, FFS group, PGP, public clinics, and hospital outpatient department/emergency rooms. There were no significant differences among utilizers of FFS solo, FFS group, and PGP on the respondents' checkup measures. For children's checkups, PGP enrollees had significantly higher utilization than solo FFS users, with users of FFS groups and public clinics in an intermediate position.

Dual Choice Enrollment of Employees in Two Midwestern Firms

All of the above studies are based on population surveys, without particular concern for whether or not people were in a dual choice situation.* This

*Perkoff, Kahn, and Haas (1976) report a much higher utilization rate of preventive services for people in the Medical Care Group of Washington University, in contrast to those in the control group (traditional insurance). Unfortunately, these data were collected in a way that led to systematic underreporting of preventive ambulatory visits in the control group, a point recognized by the authors.

comparison and the next examine dual choice situations, but as a consequence, their scope is limited. Slesinger, Tessler, and Mechanic (1976) rely on interview data from families of employees of two firms who chose either BC-BS or a prepaid group practice. (The BC-BS plan had some outpatient coverage but did not reimburse physician charges for office visits or physical examinations.) For adults, there were no significant differences in the proportion of respondents having any of the eight selected types of preventive care—general checkup, chest X-ray, tuberculin skin test, urine test, blood pressure, blood test, Pap smear (women only), and sickle cell anemia screening test (blacks only). It is of note, however, that in every instance the proportion in the prepaid plan was slightly higher. (If the two groups were identical, one would expect such an outcome to occur due to sampling in 4 per 1000 trials.)

The situation was different for children. PGP enrollees had significantly more regular checkups and tuberculin skin tests. No significant differences were found for the receipt of five specific immunizations in the preceding year. A different picture emerges if attention is paid to the proportion of children who had been fully immunized at any time against measles, polio, rubella, and mumps. Children under five showed no significant difference between plans; in fact, the PGP children had a lower rate. A significantly higher proportion of PGP children aged five to twelve were fully immunized, 53 versus 40 percent. This suggests that there may have been some self-selection among enrollees, with those more concerned about prevention joining the PGP. It may also reflect different approaches by physicians in encouraging follow-ups and booster shots.

Sault Ste. Marie, Ontario

A series of reports compare member utilization of the Group Health Centre (GHC) in Sault Ste. Marie, Ontario. Two studies refer to the 1967-68 period, when the comparison group was composed of employees who chose the indemnity insurance option. In one study the rate of checkups for GHC enrollees was 1.6 times that of the control group, while the immunization rate was 3.0 times as high (Hastings et al., 1973, p. 96). However, these data were drawn from two different sources: claims forms for the indemnity enrollees and internal records for GHC members. That this may have led to an undercounting of visits for the indemnity group is suggested by the second study, which is based on household interviews. In this instance there was little difference in the immunization status of children under five years of age enrolled in the two plans (Mott, Hastings, and Barclay, 1973, p. 187).

Five years later another household survey was undertaken, this one using a random survey of the entire population (DeFriese, 1975). In the intervening period the provincial government had inaugurated a comprehensive health insurance plan that provided identical ambulatory and inpatient coverage for everyone. The only remaining differences were in the organization of practice—group and salaried versus solo and FFS. In the 1973 survey, about half of the respondents reported using solo practitioners as their predominant source of care there, while the remainder split their allegiances between GHC and solo providers. The survey indicates that GHC member respondents (but not their spouses) were less likely never to have had a physical examination. On the other hand, solo and GHC-solo users (respondents and spouses) were more likely to have had a checkup in the last six months. If the focus is instead on whether each of six specific diagnostic procedures was performed during the respondent's last physical examination, the GHC users indicate somewhat higher scores, which are statistically significant (DeFriese, 1975, pp. 141-142).

Medicaid Beneficiaries

A key aspect of the DeFriese study outlined above is that universal provincial health insurance allowed the same coverage for GHC members and nonmembers. Perhaps the most common instance of a similar situation in the United States is when Medicaid recipients, who receive complete ambulatory coverage, have the option of joining an HMO. Two studies report on such situations. Fuller and Patera (1976) focus on an experimental group enrolled in Group Health Association in Washington, D.C. The other study is based on a survey of nine HMOs and comparison groups across the country (Gaus, Cooper, and Hirschman, 1976).

Medicaid Beneficiaries in Washington, D.C. Fuller and Patera (1976) report a larger proportion of PGP members aged six years or more receiving each of seven types of preventive services: routine physical examinations, blood pressure, urinalysis, chest X-ray or tuberculin skin test, Pap smear, and breast exam. The differences in the two groups were statistically significant for all but Pap smears and breast examinations. Fuller and Patera point out that these findings are not surprising, because the PGP encouraged everyone to have a routine physical examination at the time of enrollment. It is of interest that the type of preventive visit that is most frequently scheduled by the patient, the gynecological visit, exhibits the smallest differences.

Fuller and Patera (1976) examined the proportion of children under six years of age that had ever received each of five immunizations, as well as a routine physical examination in the last six months. A smaller proportion of the PGP children had received each of the six services, and the differences were statistically significant for three of the five immunizations.

A final measure of preventive use in this study is the pattern of prenatal care. Sixty percent of PGP mothers were seen in their first trimester, in comparison to 74 percent of the control group mothers. About the same proportion of both groups had no prenatal visit or visits only in the third trimester. Once they began seeing a doctor, 100 percent of the control group women had visits at least monthly, in contrast to only 88 percent for the PGP (p < .05). Furthermore, all of the control group mothers had a six-week follow-up after a full-term pregnancy versus 76 percent for the PGP mothers (p < .01).

Medicaid Enrollees in Nine HMOs.   Gaus, Cooper, and Hirschman (1976) collected data from Medicaid enrollees in nine HMOs and from Medicaid beneficiaries with FFS providers in the same Zip Code areas. They used several measures of preventive services, and their rather consistent findings from nine sites across the country are presented in Tables 9-4 and 9-5. They summarize their results as follows:

First, measures of maternity care—in terms of number of prenatal visits, trimester of first visit, baby check-up, and mother check-up—were used. Although statistics varied among the sites, the overall results were quite similar for HMOs and controls. About 52 percent of women with live births in the group-practice plans compared with 60 percent in the controls, had 11 or more prenatal visits. About four-fifths in both groups had their first in the first trimester, nine-tenths had baby check-ups, and somewhat more than four-fifths of the mothers had check-ups. The foundations [IPAs] and their controls showed similar relationships, as Table [9-4] indicates.

Measures of preventive care in the total population were also made and included physical exams, well-baby check-ups, and immunizations. In a 1-month period, about 6 percent of the group-practice plan enrollees had at least one preventive-care procedure and the controls had 9 percent [Table 9-5]. In no site was preventive care greater in the HMO than the control. In several sites it was significantly less. There was no difference between the foundations and their control groups.

As a proportion of all visits, preventive care represented 20 percent of visits for group-practice enrollees and 29 percent for the controls. It is possible that during visits for specific problems some preventive procedures are administered and the patients are not aware of it. If an HMO is especially preventive-care conscious, this situation may occur more often in the HMO than in fee-for-service. Nevertheless, it is doubtful that HMOs are providing more preventive care than fee-for-service. (Gaus, Cooper, and Hirschman, 1976, p. 11).

Seattle Prepaid Health Care Project

Diehr et al. (1976) describe the findings of the experimental Seattle Prepaid Health Care Project. Low-income but nonpoverty families in the Seattle Model Cities neighborhood were given the choice of enrolling in the GHCPS or a service benefit plan sponsored by the local BC-BS plans. Both options were available at no cost to the enrollees and offered comprehensive inpatient and ambulatory coverage. Table 9-6 presents their findings for various ancillary services, of which the first five immunizations are clearly preventive, while some of the other services may have been

Table 9–4 Pregnancy-Connected Services for Women with Live Births in HMOs and Control Groups, by Plan[a]

Plan	Percentage Distribution, by Number of Prenatal Visits					Percentage Distribution, by Trimester of First Prenatal Visit				Percent of Births with—	
	Total	Less than 5	5–10	11–15	16 or more	Total	1	2	3	Baby Checkup	Mother Checkup
Group practice	100	20	28	35	17	100	79	20	2	86	83
Control	100	14	27	42	18	100	78	19	3	92	85
Central Los Angeles Health Project	100	b	b	b	b	b	b	b	b	b	b
Control	100										
Consolidated Medical System	100	3	13	81	3	100	74	23	3		
Control	100	6	6	88		100	79	15	6		
Family Health Program	100	41	25	16	19	100	75	25		81	86
Control	100	19	47	32	4	100	74	21	4	96	96
Group Health Cooperative of Puget Sound	100	9	9	79	2	100	88	12		100	87
Control	100	12	2	85		100	88	8	5	90	87
Harbor Health Services	100	18	8		75	100	80	20		93	73
Control	100	5	7		88	100	77	23		93	87
Harvard Health Plan	100	21	55	24		100	79	16	5	100	83
Control	100	16	43	35	6	100	82	14	4	94	81
Health Insurance Plan of Greater New York	100	31	38	24	7	100	83	17		88	100
Control	100	23	41	20	6	100	75	23	2	84	77
Temple Health Plan	100	19	50	19	12	100	72	25	3	79	79
Control	100	14	42	34	10	100	72	26	2	93	93
Foundation and control											
Redwood	100	18	52	24	6	100	72	24	4	90	77
Control	100	14	52	14	19	100	76	24		95	74
Sacramento	100	21	41	31	7	100	100			90	80
Control	100	30	30	37	3	100	80	17	3	95	84

SOURCE. Gaus, Cooper, and Hirschman, May 1976, p. 12.

[a] Based on 1-year period. Tests of significance not completed.
[b] Data not available.

Table 9–5 Utilization of Preventive Care Services by Persons in HMOs and Control Groups, by Plan[a,c]

Plan	Percent of All Visits for Preventive Care[b]	Number of Persons per 100 Using Preventive Care Services[b]			
		Total[b]	Physical Examination	Well-Baby Checkup	Immunizations
Group practice	20	0.06	0.03	[d]	0.03
Control	29	0.09	0.04	[d]	0.04
Central Los Angeles Health Project	[e]	[e]	[e]	[e]	[e]
Consolidated Medical System	[f]19	0.06	0.02	[d]	0.04
Control	[f]29	0.09	0.02	0.01	0.06
Family Health Program	[f]16	0.04	0.01	[d]	0.02
Control	[f]37	0.10	0.03	0.02	0.06
Group Health Cooperative of Puget Sound	[f]16	0.06	0.04	[d]	0.03
Control	[f]23	0.10	0.04	[d]	0.06
Harbor Health Services	[f]12	0.04	[d]	[d]	0.03
Control	[f]26	0.07	0.02	[d]	0.04
Harvard Health Plan	29	0.06	0.05	0.01	0.02
Control	35	0.07	0.05	0.02	0.02
Health Insurance Plan of Greater New York	25	0.09	0.05	[d]	0.03
Control	28	0.10	0.06	[d]	0.04
Temple Health Plan	23	0.06	0.04	[d]	0.01
Control	25	0.08	0.06	[d]	0.02
Foundation and control:					
Redwood	25	0.09	0.03	0.01	0.05
Control	29	0.09	0.03	[d]	0.06
Sacramento	13	0.06	0.03	[d]	0.03
Control	16	0.06	0.02	0.01	0.03

SOURCE. Gaus, Cooper, and Hirschman, May 1976, p. 12.

[a] Based on 1-month period.
[b] Unduplicated total.
[c] Tests of significance not yet completed.
[d] Less than 0.005 percent.
[e] Data not available.
[f] Difference statistically significant at the 95-percent confidence level.

Preventive Care

Table 9−6   Ancillary Services by Plan in the Seattle Prepaid Health Care Project

Variable Definition	Mean		Partial Correlation[a]
	GH	KCM-BC	
Total NSLABS/person-years exposure[b,c]	3.82	2.81	
NSLABS/years exposure (per person)[b,c]	3.82	2.87	−.09
Pap smears[c]	0.21	0.13	−.10
Flu immunization[c]	0.004	0.014	.06
DPT-OPV[c]	0.37	0.14	−.20
Measles immunization[c]	0.04	0.01	−.11
Other immunization[c]	0.24	0.07	−.16
Hematology[d]	0.18	0.12	−.08
Urine[d]	0.63	0.54	−.033
CBC[d]	0.31	0.32	−.01
Battery (chemistry profiles)[d]	0.12	0.28	.08
Smears and cultures[d]	1.04	0.33	−.20
Total X-rays/total person-years exposure[c]	0.38	0.61	
Annualized X-rays (per person)[c]	0.36	0.60	.09
Chest[d]	0.18	0.27	.03
Upper extremities[d]	0.03	0.06	.03
Lower extremities[d]	0.04	0.09	.04
EKG[d]	0.04	0.12	.06

SOURCE.   Diehr et al., November 1976, page II 91.
[a] Partial correlation between provider and variable, holding AGE, SEX, RACE, AGESEX, Health Status, and FAMSIZ constant. $n = 3,804$ because of unknown values, "other" race. Correlation positive if KC higher, negative if GH higher. A value of .032 is significant with a 2-tailed .05 level test; .042 at .01 level; .053 at .001 level.
[b] Totals for labs include immunizations.
[c] $n = 5110$ for KC, 2253 for GH. All four program-years.
[d] $n = 3709$ for KC, 1503 for GH. Final nineteen program-months only.

performed either for screening or for diagnostic purposes. The GH enrollees had significantly more immunizations, with the exception of flu shots for the elderly. As indicated by the partial correlation coefficients, these results are statistically significant, even when age, sex, race, health status, and family size are held constant. These results are reversed for X-rays (including EKGs); BC-BS members had substantially more per person. Examining the results in other ways, such as tests per visit and tests controlling for length of time in the plan, does not alter these patterns.

Enrollees in Three HMOs and Rochester Blue Cross-Blue Shield

Employees in one large industrial plant in Rochester, New York, were offered a multiple choice option of retaining their conventional BC-BS coverage or choosing one of three HMOs: an IPA or one of two PGPs.

Premiums for all four options were paid by the employer. While the basic BC-BS plan did not cover preventive service, all three HMOs covered them at either no charge or a nominal $2.00 per visit. (Berki et al., 1977b). The survey identified those who had enrolled in one of the HMOs six months earlier, those who had newly enrolled in one of the HMOs, and those who remained in BC-BS. Focusing only on preventive visits of adults, the research team found that PGP enrollees were significantly more likely to have had preventive visits than BC-BS enrollees, while IPA members were slightly more likely to be users.

It was also found that PGP enrollees expressed somewhat higher levels of health concern. Using a multiple regression model that included health concern, health status, illness visits, satisfaction, convenience, cost, and plan, it was found that PGP members used significantly more preventive services, while IPA member usage was not different from that of BC-BS members. When interpreting these findings it is important to remember that all of the PGP members had joined a new, closed panel group within the preceding year. They had to establish a relationship with a new physician and were encouraged by the plan to have an initial health assessment, which would have been counted as a preventive visit (Wersinger and Roberts, 1977). Few of the IPA enrollees had such a change in provider relationship.

Federal Employees in Washington, D.C.

Meyers, Hirschfeld, and Riedel (1977) examined the ambulatory visit experience of federal employees in the Washington, D.C., area who belonged to either BC-BS or Group Health Association (GHA). BC-BS did not cover preventive examinations, while GHA provided complete coverage for such services. Substantial differences in utilization and enrollment occurred by race. Controlling for race, the research team found that a higher proportion of GHA members had at least one preventive contact (42 versus 32 percent), and the mean number of contacts per enrollee was greater (1.36 versus 0.95). In both instances the differences are significant at the 5 percent level.

Stanford University Employees

Scitovsky, Benham, and McCall (1979) examined the use of physican services by Stanford University employees who chose either Kaiser or a prepaid option offered by the PAMC. The clinic is predominantly FFS but offers a package to Stanford that requires a 25 percent copayment for all physician and outpatient ancillary services. Kaiser members had a token $1.00 copayment per visit.

Over a twelve-month period, 37 percent of clinic members and 26 percent of Kaiser members had one or more routine physical examinations. Among females aged seventeen to sixty-four, 47 percent of clinic members had a Pap smear, while only 34 percent of Kaiser women had one. After including a number of independent variables, such as age, sex, marital status, years in plan, income, other insurance coverage, satisfaction, and health status, these differences remained statistically significant. A major source of explanation, however, was the question of whether the enrollee had as a regular source of care a specific plan physician, any physician within the plan, or no regular source within the plan. This regular source of care variable accounted for much of the variation in utilization, and a much larger proportion of clinic members named a specific plan physician.

INTERPRETING THE FINDINGS

The findings of the above studies can be divided into two groups that appear to imply contradictory findings. The first group supports the hypothesis that HMO enrollees receive more preventive services of various types (Committee for the Special Research Project in HIP, 1957; Cauffman, Roemer, and Schultz, 1967; Breslow and Hochstim, 1964; Breslow, 1973; Hetherington, Hopkins, and Roemer, 1975; Dutton, 1976, Slesinger, Tessler, and Mechanic, 1976; Hastings et al., 1973; Diehr et al., 1976; Berki et al., 1977b; Meyers, Hirschfeld, and Riedel, 1977). The second group of studies suggests that there are no differences in the use of preventive services or that HMO enrollees receive even fewer services (DeFriese, 1975; Fuller and Patera, 1976; Gaus, Cooper, and Hirschman, 1976; Diehr et al., 1976; Scitovsky, Benham, and McCall, 1979).

A closer look suggests that the two groups of findings are not really in conflict. With a few exceptions, the different results can be explained by focusing not on the distinction between HMO enrollees and nonenrollees, but on whether the individuals had insurance coverage for preventive visits. (See Table 9-7.) Such coverage is almost universal with HMOs, but it is rare with traditional insurance (U.S. Congressional Budget Office, 1979). Thus those studies that involve a comparison between HMO enrollees and people with traditional insurance coverage, the first group above, are actually testing two variables: (1) an HMO health maintenance effect; and (2) differential financial coverages for preventive care. In the few instances in which the third party covers preventive visits, the second group of studies, the second (insurance) variable is held constant, and there appears to be little or no HMO health maintenance effect. In fact, those studies comparing HMO enrollees with people having full coverage for FFS providers typically have ambiguous results; the HMOs provide more preventive care of some types and less of others.

Rhetoric versus Behavior

How can one explain the apparent disparity between the rhetoric of health maintenance and the behavior discussed above? In part, the behavior does

Table 9—7   Summary of Findings of Preventive Services in HMOs and Comparison Groups (All Comparison Groups Had FFS Payment of Providers)

	Comparison Groups with FFS Payments by the Patient	Comparison Groups with No or Minimal Extra Charges for the Patient.
HMO enrollees received more preventive services than comparison group	HIP-NY (Committee for the Special Research Project)	Sault Ste. Marie, specific tests (DeFriese)
	Los Angeles School Children especially poorer ones (Cauffman, Roemer, and Schultz)	Washington Medicaid, seven services for people aged 6+ (Fuller and Patera)
	Alameda County Women and Pap Smears (Breslow and Hochstim)	Seattle Prepaid Project, immunizations (Diehr et al.)
	Alameda County, Health Maintenance Exams (Breslow)	
	Southern California Health Plans (Hetherington, Hopkins, and Roemer)	
	Washington, D.C., Families (Dutton)	
	Two Midwestern Firms (Slesinger, Tessler, and Mechanic)	
	Sault Ste. Marie (Hastings et al.)	
	Rochester employees in PGPs (Berki et al.)	
	Federal Employees (Meyers et al.)	
HMO enrollees received the same or fewer preventive services than comparison group		Sault Ste. Marie, physical exam (DeFriese)
		Washington Medicaid, children and prenatal care (Fuller and Patera)
		Medicaid Enrollees in nine HMOs (Gaus, Cooper, and Hirschman)
		Seattle Prepaid Project, X-rays (Diehr et al.)
		Stanford Employees (Scitovsky, Benham, and McCall)

support the rhetoric: HMOs, almost by definition, provide full coverage for preventive services, in contrast to the usually nonexistent coverage offered by traditional providers. But if everyone had complete coverage for preventive services, say through national health insurance, then the results probably would be like those on the right side of Table 9-7, and HMO enrollees might receive even fewer services than nonenrollees.

A partial explanation for this behavior is that financial incentives tend to encourage the provision of services in an FFS setting and discourage them in the HMO setting. There is little reason for such incentives to be any more or less pervasive, everything else being equal, for discretionary ambulatory care than for discretionary surgery. As will be discussed below, there is considerable controversy in the medical profession over the efficacy or usefulness of many preventive services. Thus HMO financial incentives to do less may well be supported by good clinical judgment.

The question about preventive services focuses on two major issues: (1) potential benefits of services relative to their costs; and (2) the extent to which physicians actually take steps to realize these potential benefits. It should be recognized that at least two types of services fall under the "preventive" heading. The first type, primary prevention, includes those services, such as immunizations, that are by nature preventive and that require no follow-up procedures.* Secondary prevention includes tests and examinations that are designed to identify diseases at an early stage. Such tests, such as mammography for breast cancer, may be highly specific. Others, such as the multiphasic or the preventive checkup, cover a wide spectrum of individual tests.

The immunization type of service rarely is challenged on cost or efficacy grounds although in some cases routine immunizations have been discontinued or rejected. For example, smallpox vaccinations have been discontinued, because the small number of people who have adverse reactions to the innoculation far exceeds the number of cases that would be prevented, even if there were a new outbreak. Vaccination for whooping cough also has been challenged recently (Northrup and Bishop, 1977; Grady and Wetterlow, 1978). Even prior to the recognition of Guillaum-Barré syndrome, the 1976-77 swine flu program faced strong public resistance, in spite of a massive public campaign.

Preventive services that involve testing an otherwise asymptomatic patient are subject to two problems, costs and follow-up. The financial costs of screening a large number of people can be substantial, especially when relatively few people have undiagnosed problems. For instance, Kaiser has undertaken several long-term trials of multiphasic screening. The results indicate that only for middle-aged men do the potential savings in earnings resulting from reduced mortality and morbidity exceed the costs of the test (Collen et al., 1973). Of course, such cost figures are subject to a wide range of interpretation. Thus, for mammograms, the low prevalence of even suspicious findings in women aged forty-eight and over implies a cost of over $2000 per true positive (Collen et al., 1970, p. 463). But Garfield, of

---

*This discussion quite consciously omits the evaluation of various preventive behaviors that the individual can adopt, such as good diet, exercise, nonsmoking, or that can be accomplished on a collective basis, such as a clean and quiet environment and workplace. It is very possible that such factors are substantially more important, at the margin, than most current medical care activities. However, the focus here is primarily on actions likely to be taken by medical providers in HMOs and elsewhere.

the same Kaiser program, argues that instead of focusing on the $2000, one should emphasize the fact that "[it] costs $4.00 each to assure 499 women that there is no evidence of breast cancer by mammography and to detect one cancer that, through early surgery, may have a better prognosis" (Garfield, 1970, p. 1087).

The controversy goes beyond just the test costs. Every test misses some people who have the disease (false negatives) and indicates disease in some people who are disease-free (false positives). The actions that are undertaken in such instances, such as false reassurance or unnecessary biopsies, also entail costs and risks.* (Hedrick, 1977). Such testing errors also can be embarrassing to the program (*Wall Street Journal* Staff Reporter, 1977). Furthermore, the test itself may entail risks. For example, mammography involves a radiation hazard. Much of the current controversy about mammography relates to the magnitude of such risks in relation to the potential benefits (Bailar, 1976). Depending upon the true prevalence rates in the population and the accuracies and risks of the test, it may be advisable not to test on purely medical-risk grounds, even if the test is available at no financial cost (Reiser, 1978). The examples here are drawn from the literature on multiphasic tests and mammography, but other tests also have been questioned. (See Sagel et al., 1974; Abrams, 1979; Foltz and Kelsey, (1978); Cochrane and Ellwood, 1969; Chamberlain, 1975; Holland, 1974; Sackett, 1975.) It is noteworthy that much of the critical examination of tests has come from the United Kingdom and Canada, where there is direct government interest in health care costs.

Even if a test is cost effective, problems can occur in its implementation. For a test to be beneficial, its results must be interpreted and appropriate action taken. Williamson, Alexander, and Miller (1967) document the difficulty in getting a medical staff to take note of abnormal test results with appropriate follow-up. Olsen, Kane, and Proctor (1976) found that previously unknown abnormalities identified by multiphasic testing prompted retesting for confirmation in only 28 percent of the cases. These abnormal findings led to treatment in only 15 percent of the cases.

These discouraging results probably are not due to financial incentives, but rather to the physician's traditional orientation toward curative care. (The clinician's negative attitude toward screening is supported by evidence that most abnormal findings are laboratory errors, variations in the definition of "normal," not clinically significant, or not treatable [Bradwell, Carmalt, and Whitehead, 1974].) This orientation does not preclude positive attitudes toward preventive care in general. Behavior just does not measure up to rhetoric. Thus 84 percent of the physicians in the Olsen, Kane, and Proctor study acknowledged a role for automated multiphasic screening in the health care system. Strikingly similar attitudes were found

---

*Of the 500 women discussed in the preceding paragraph, about one will be reassured when, in fact, she has cancer, and four women will be biopsied because they had suspicious findings later proven to be negative. (See Shapiro, 1976).

in Mechanic's survey of United States general practitioners and pedia-tricians in FFS solo practice, FFS groups, and PGPs. For the six combina-tions (two specialty types and three settings) between 76 and 86 percent of the physicians strongly or moderately approved of multiphasic health screening as part of a doctor's or clinic's practice (Mechanic, 1975, p. 201). There were no differences in approval by setting.

There also is evidence that at least some HMOs, as organizations, feel preventive services are more important than do physicians who practice in groups. HIP of New York pays its medical groups on a capitation basis with supplemental payments for meeting specific goals. Included in these incentives are payments for medical records having histories, physical examination results, and the results of three of four specific diagnostic tests. Additional payments are also made for having a high Pap smear rate (HIP, 1970, p. 22). The existence of such incentive payments suggests that the desired behavior would not always be met without special incentives. Similar findings with respect to Kaiser physicians are suggested by Wil-liams:

Judging from spontaneous comment in interviews, Permanente physicians tend to be less enthusiastic about promotional emphasis on preventive medical services "keeping people well"—than do Kaiser Health Plan representatives. Except for those doctors involved in the automated multiphasic screening program or other aspects of preventive medicine, the typical medical attitude toward disease preven-tion is one of skepticism, with the obvious exception of immunizations. The doctors not only say healthy patients "clog the system"—this could be a misperception of the primary care problem—but they question the general effectiveness of annual health examinations in reducing morbidity, mortality, and disability. They also point out that the uncovering of many abnormalities that may or may not progress to clinical disease requires follow-up observations of the patient and further stresses the demand-supply balance (Williams, 1971, p. 53).

Since then, Kaiser has formally shifted its stance on health examinations. For instance, the handbook sent to all Northern California health plan members in 1978 stated that, while many people assume that annual checkups are the most effective way of maintaining health, the "medical profession generally, does not agree" (Kaiser Foundation Health Plan, 1978, p. 13). Healthy living habits were stressed, and the following recommendations were made concerning checkups: school-age children: checkups at school entry, one before and one during adolescence; adults: two examinations between the ages of 18 and 29, three between 30 and 39, four between 40 and 49, five between 50 and 59, and annually for 60 and over; for women of child-bearing age: initial pelvic exam and annual tests until gynecologist suggests longer intervals. Of course, these recommenda-tions are qualified by the admonition that the enrollee should seek care promptly if there is any change in well-being. Similarly, Group Health

Cooperative is attempting to alter the "massive and inappropriate overexpectation on the part of the general public as to what physicians at the level of office practice can deliver, on the one hand, and the massive and inappropriate 'overkill' on the part of our physicians on the other" (Thompson, 1979, p. 71).

A final and important point in evaluating preventive services is that many consumers are less than enthusiastic about some services. Olsen, Kane, and Proctor (1976, p. 929) report that 22 percent of their sample refused a free multiphasic health examination when it was offered to them. Preventive care usually comes at a price. Table 9-8 presents the preferences expressed by California state employees for adding preventive health services to their benefit coverage for specified additional monthly cost. In general the PGP plans already covered these services. Among those people who thought they were not covered, the only clear support was for the additional coverage for Pap smears. There was overwhelming opposition to coverage for children's immunizations and well-baby care, and this opposition does not seem to come just from the childless. A breakdown of the results by plan and type of enrollment indicates that employees in the indemnity and service plans covering themselves and two or more dependents were the most strongly opposed to these benefits (Dozier et al., 1973, pp. 120-121).

SUMMARY

These findings suggest that, contrary to the rhetoric of health maintenance advocates, the greater use of preventive services by HMO enrollees appears to be attributable to their better financial coverage, not the preventive care ideology. When people have full coverage for preventive ambulatory visits, they have at least as many, if not more, services under the FFS system as in an HMO. These results are entirely in accord with data for hospitalization. HMO enrollees seem to get fewer services if everything else is held constant.

While results of this type may be theoretically sound and empirically defensible, some discussion is warranted when strongly held beliefs are questioned. It is undoubtedly true that if one is seeking a health plan that offers more preventive care, the average HMO will win hands down, when compared to the average health insurance plan. In policy discussions, however, we want to know what is likely to happen if things are changed. Adding complete ambulatory coverage to traditional insurance plans is an easy although expensive change. It is almost certain that such a change would be easier to implement politically than would enrolling the whole population in a system of HMOs. If for some reason more preventive service is the goal, then complete ambulatory coverage is likely to be the easiest policy to implement.

Table 9–8 Preferences for Adding Preventive Health Care Benefits
California State Employees, 1971

Proposed Added Benefit	Extra Monthly Premium		Percentage Distribution of Employee Preferences				
	Employee Only	Employee + 2 or More Dependents	All Employees	Add Benefit	Don't Add	Benefit Already in Plan	No Answer
Pap test	$0.06	$0.15	100.0	34.7	18.6	36.1	10.5
Immunization for minor children	0.00	0.70	100.0	19.4	50.4	15.7	14.5
Well-baby care, first year	0.00	0.34	100.0	13.8	53.0	16.9	16.3
Chest X-Ray, urinalysis, blood tests, etc. in annual physical checkup	1.12	2.51	100.0	22.8	24.7	43.5	9.0
EKG	0.45	0.75	100.0	25.7	25.3	37.9	11.0

SOURCE. Dozier et al., 1973, pp. 35, 120–124.

But it is not at all clear that more is necessarily better. Although some preventive services are probably better than none, and there is convincing evidence supporting the value of certain procedures, there is a large gray area in which the services do no harm and little good.* They are, however, almost always costly. Thus it may be expected that HMOs will begin to try to ration the use of at least certain types of services, as in the case of the attempt to replace the annual physical with the triannual physical. Whether such changes can be made at *no* health risk is unlikely. Whether the patients would prefer the extra risk in exchange for the potential savings will depend on many factors, among the first of which is some evidence of the effectiveness and costs of such procedures.

---

*Some preventive services may actually do more harm than good. The smallpox and whooping cough examples were mentioned above. Another type of harm stems from labeling individuals as having a disease (Curran, 1974).

TEN

Quality

Quality ... you know what it is, yet you don't know what it is. But that's self-contradictory. But some things *are* better than others, that is, they have more quality. But when you try to say what the quality is, apart from the things that have it, it all goes *poof!* There's nothing to talk about. But if you can't say what Quality is, how do you know what it is, or how do you know that it even exists? If no one knows what it is, then for all practical purposes it doesn't exist at all. But for all practical purposes it really *does* exist. What else are the grades based on? Why else would people pay fortunes for some things and throw others in the trash pile? Obviously some things are better than others ... but what's the "betterness"? ... So round and round you go, spinning mental wheels and nowhere finding anyplace to get traction. What the hell is Quality? What *is* it? (Pirsig, 1974, p. 178)

Evidence presented in the previous chapters provides strong support for the contention that costs and utilization are lower for HMO enrollees. Although there is some controversy over specific figures, particularly those relating to ambulatory care, few people argue with these general conclusions. The key question is, have the apparent savings been obtained at an unacceptable sacrifice of quality?

Quality is a devilishly elusive concept. People use different measures for quality determination, and while there often is some correlation among them, there also are substantial differences. Measures of quality are difficult to interpret; more is not always better, nor is it always worse. For instance, prescribing an appendectomy for every patient with abdominal pain would produce poor quality, as would a situation in which no appendectomies were performed. However, merely knowing that the optimal proportion is somewhere between 0 and 100 percent does not help us to decide whether setting A, with a 60 percent rate, is better than setting B, with a 50 percent rate.

This chapter is designed to shed light on the controversies surrounding the issue of quality of care in HMOs, particularly as they are compared to traditional providers. A number of important issues related to quality are discussed in other chapters. These include measures of utilization, access to care, preventive services, distributional equity, and consumer satisfaction.

Each is important enough to warrant a separate chapter. This chapter focuses on those factors that are traditionally thought of as medical quality. To do so, however, requires first a discussion of the difficulties inherent in the major quality measures. The remainder of the chapter contains a review of the available evidence, under the headings of structure, process, and outcome measures.

THE ELUSIVE QUALITY MEASURE: AN OVERVIEW

One way to approach quality measurement in health care is to ask what it is that people really want. In most cases the goal is the maintenance or improvement of one's health, rather than the mere consumption of medical services. Thus quality should be measured in terms of outcomes. However, as will be discussed below, there are severe drawbacks to measuring outcomes with an agreed-upon index. In addition, people are concerned with means, as well as ends. Therefore, other measures, such as structure and process, are frequently used.

Another more subtle factor may be behind the general avoidance of outcome measures—they may be unflattering. Charles Lewis (1974) recounts the efforts of Emory Codman in 1916 to measure quality on the basis of end results. This led to a survey by the predecessor organization to the American College of Surgeons of United States hospitals with 100 or more beds. Apparently, only 89 of the 692 hospitals studied met *any* reasonable standards for quality of care. The detailed findings of the survey were suppressed, and instead, various structural criteria for hospitals were established, which were to serve as the basis for accreditation.

While almost any standard would show that quality has improved in the last sixty years, there is still substantial resistance to the use of outcome measures. This is understandable in part because on an *absolute* scale the results still may not be favorable. People continue to die and suffer from diseases. Individual providers recognize that they practice within the context of both the larger medical care system and the entire social environment. Thus the provider is justified in disclaiming responsibility for patients who seek care too late or for others whose living conditions work against medical treatment. If quality must be assessed, providers probably will be more comfortable in being judged on the basis of whether what they do has been done well.

While it is not difficult to develop theoretical tests to measure whether a certain increment of medical care leads to improved outcomes, the implementation of such a test is beyond our capabilities (McAuliffe, 1979). The difficulty arises from an inability to measure health status on a sufficiently fine and accurate scale to identify small but important differences. It is possible, however, to measure outcomes for large groups of people, such as all patients treated in a hospital over the period of a year.

(See Stanford Center for Health Care Research, 1976; Shortell, Becker, and Neuhauser, 1976). But such undertakings require substantial data banks, and they do not provide conclusive explanations of why such differences in outcomes exist. Thus there is the common reliance on measures that are more generally acceptable and easier to apply.

Although there are many ways to categorize approaches to quality of care assessment, the tripartite classification of *structure, process,* and *outcome* is a simple and common one (Brook, 1973a; Donabedian, 1966, 1978b). The *structural approach* measures various characteristics of providers, such as place of medical training, number of journals received, specialty certification, and medical society membership. Similar variables can be used to evaluate institutional characteristics, such as staffing ratios, availability of specific equipment, and accreditation status. The last is usually based on a series of more detailed structural measures, many of which are related to building codes. However, accreditation is increasingly dependent on process and outcome measures.

Process measures are based upon a review of actions taken in specific cases or groups of cases. Process evaluation is generally performed by reviewing medical records, although it can be done through direct observation of medical care delivery. It is important to recognize that the former method places great weight upon the record-keeping abilities of the provider. Although a process has been carried out, if it was not recorded it is not counted. The use of records also limits the process evaluation to those items that normally are recorded, such as laboratory tests. It omits most interpersonal processes, such as provider-patient interactions, which may be far more important. The available data can be evaluated in two ways. The "implicit approach" involves ratings by a well-qualified physician of the overall quality of care. The "explicit approach" involves the development of a list of specific criteria, which are expected to be met. In some cases these lists can be very complicated, with allowance for a wide range of contingencies, such as: if A is present, then B should be prescribed (Greenfield et al., 1974). A key feature of the explicit approach is that a nonprofessional can audit charts to determine whether the criteria have been met. This results in substantial cost savings.

Outcome measures focus on the end results of medical care. They were developed in order to avoid the necessity of focusing on *how* things are done. At least three major approaches to outcome studies have been proposed. Williamson, Alexander, and Miller (1967) and Williamson et al. (1975) argue for the use of outcome measurements that may be compared to expert opinion of what the outcomes are likely to be, given (a) no treatment, (b) present treatment, and (c) adequate treatment. Under this approach, data on outcomes from a group of patients with a specific condition are compared to the acceptable levels. Brook (1973a) points out that there are a great many problems involved in implementing this type of outcome evaluation because of inadequate knowledge of the natural history of disease, a lack of training among physicians in probabilistic thinking, and the general unavailability of data, especially on long-term outcomes. An alternative approach requires the comparison of two or more settings with respect to various outcome measures, such as mortality and morbidity. Of course, the key problem in such comparisons is in assuring that the mix of patients and severity of diseases are comparable. A third approach combines outcomes and process measures by examining patient records to decide whether outcomes could have been better if the processes had been improved.

Brook (1973a) provides a discussion of the difficulties involved in collecting the necessary data and undertaking quality assessment studies. He also provides a comprehensive review of problems related to interpreting the findings. In particular, how strong is the evidence that structure and process studies really measure quality? The answer to this question depends on what is chosen as the "true" quality measure, as well as the specific studies one selects to evaluate. Although Brook (1973a) and Shortridge (1974) find some positive relationships between structure and process measures, these are neither stable nor reliable. Thus in some studies the physician's training is positively related to quality, while in others, even with the same methodology, there is no measurable relationship.

The situation with respect to the relationship between process and outcome measures is similarly disappointing. Brook has reviewed the literature and undertaken a number of studies that support the view that process and outcome may be related only tenuously (Brook, 1973b; Brook, Berg, and Schechter, 1973; Brook and Stevenson, 1970). Other investigators report similarly discouraging findings (Gordis and Markowitz, 1971; Fessel and Van Brunt, 1972). McAuliffe (1978, 1979) argues that the low correlation between process and outcome is attributable to a lack of validity on the part of the outcome studies and that more emphasis should be placed on process measures. However, some studies show positive relationships, and more importantly, there is little evidence that what is generally considered to be good medical process actually results in poorer outcomes.* (See Payne et al., 1976.) When using the various quality measures to compare plans, one must confront yet another problem: all delivery systems exhibit substantial deficiencies when evaluated against specific standards, and in general these deviations from the standards are far larger than the differences between HMOs and FFS providers.

A final question may be asked concerning the relevance of outcome measures. These measures usually are defined by clinicians and relate to items such as mortality, morbidity, and blood pressure levels. Yet little

---

*This is not to be interpreted as meaning that more is better or that some medical care does not lead to worse outcomes. In such situations the expert opinion is usually mixed, and many physicians would argue that even though the "pure technical process" was well done, the patient's condition did not warrant the procedure with its attendant risks.

effort has been made to determine patient preferences for different types of outcomes. Patients usually do not have the information to judge the technical quality of medical care, but they probably can decide, for example, whether they would prefer lower expected mortality at the cost of a restricted diet and difficult drug regimen. (See Lewis, 1974, p. 805; McNeil, Weichselbaum, and Pauker, 1978.) In fact, some studies indicate low correlations between patient evaluations and the more objective measures (Lebow, 1974, p. 333). The next chapter focuses in more detail on patient evaluations; at this point it is important to remember that outcome studies measure only selected aspects of quality.

Thus we have come full circle. While it may be possible just to *know* what good quality is, à la Pirsig, it is difficult to develop valid and reliable measures of it. Certainly, end results or outcomes are important aspects of quality. Quality also has some clear process connotations. While few people would argue that structure really is a dimension of quality, it may well be necessary in order to achieve certain types of quality. This review of the data recognizes that structure, process, and outcome measures all are far from perfect, that they may measure different things, and that better research may well reverse the conclusions.

STRUCTURAL MEASURES

Structural measures are furthest from "true quality." They are used because various researchers believe them to be causally related to quality and because the data are easy to collect. An important weakness is that they usually have been developed from a single model of medical care delivery, with little regard for changes over time. For example, specialty training may have been an indicator of high quality in 1949, when only 36 percent of active physicians were full-time specialists. Specialization was less likely to be associated with quality twenty years later, when 77 percent of active physicians were full-time specialists (Stevens, 1971, p. 181).

Problems in Interpreting Structural Measures

Given the weaknesses of structural measures, it is useful to examine them in order to determine whether certain inherent biases are likely to occur in the comparison of HMOs and conventional FFS practice. For instance, a key aspect of HMOs is that they have a formal organizational structure. This may be the medical group in a PGP or the peer review system in an IPA. The insuring role of the HMO (its fixed revenues and obligations to provide service) requires that it develop formal or informal mechanisms to review utilization. This suggests that a simple comparison of HMOs and solo FFS practitioners is likely to identify more organizational structure and peer review in the former setting. However, the potential bias implies that the comparison is not fair. If the FFS setting is expanded to include its financing mechanisms, such as Blue Cross and Blue Shield, then more structure and utilization review is likely to be found. Similarly, while the HMO may have a formal peer review structure to evaluate quality of care, informal peer review also takes place within the medical staffs of most community hospitals. Furthermore, federal legislation establishing Professional Standards Review Organizations mandates formal quality review among FFS practitioners. Of course, the vigor with which all such peer review groups search for quality is the key issue, and this is beyond the scope of a structural assessment.

The HMO organization presents a potential for greater control over practitioners, because requirements can be established for new providers, and they may be asked to leave if their performance is poor. A hospital medical staff in the FFS sector can exercise similar control in order to improve quality. Except in the rare instance of license revocation, while poor performers may be asked to leave their hospitals, their ability to practice is unaffected.

It may be argued that because PGPs are identifiable organizations seeking enrollees, they have a greater incentive to promote quality. The failings of one practitioner within a PGP can taint everyone in the organization. Such incentives are less likely to exist among solo practitioners. In fact, the presence of the group may be the key variable here. FFS groups also may attempt to maintain a high quality image, while incentives for IPAs may be less strong. (It is important to note that those situations in which public image is important are the most likely to lead to visible structural improvements that may be independent of true quality performance.)

There are other situations in which group practice may be the key variable, rather than HMO financial incentives. For instance, it is often argued that groups are more conducive to continuing professional education because of better coverage possibilities, and because physician proximity encourages more informal consultations (Graham, 1972). The sharing of patients within a group also is expected to lead to better recordkeeping. Another even less subtle factor is that many groups, prepaid and otherwise, are formed solely of specialists. Thus they will of necessity have an above-average proportion of specialists. Even if such requirements are not imposed, group practices tend to be new and thus are more likely to have younger than average physicians. This suggests that as the average level of training and specialization increases over time, groups will tend to score better on such structural measures, merely because of their age mix. If, however, a comparison is made with all practitioners of the same age, the differentials are likely to be smaller.

This discussion strongly suggests that care should be exercised in evaluating the data presented below. The meaning of the various measures is sometimes unclear, and it is difficult to determine what accounts for the observed differences. Also any data that reflect upon quality are, at the very least, sensitive. One would not expect unflattering results to be widely disseminated. Most comparative data refer to the qualifications of providers, which generally are matters of public record. These will be discussed below. Subsequent subsections address the issues of informal consultations, continuing education, and internal quality review.

Qualifications of Physicians and Hospitals

Table 10-1 presents the available data concerning the types of providers and hospitals used by various HMOs, in comparison to other groups. In general it is assumed that certified specialists are better than other specialists, who in turn are better than generalists. Similarly, voluntary hospitals are thought to be better than proprietary hospitals. The first three studies relate to HIP of New York. All show that substantially larger proportions of HIP enrollees are treated by specialists (usually board certified specialists) than is true for the general New York population or for those who have other insurance. This is not surprising, given the requirements established by HIP concerning the qualifications of physicians in its medical groups (Health Insurance Plan of Greater New York, 1970, p. 5). The quality evaluation with respect to hospitals used by HIP enrollees is substantially different. On one hand, HIP enrollees were most likely to have operations in a hospital affiliated with a medical school. On the other hand, a much larger fraction of HIP operations was performed in proprietary hospitals, and the proportion done in nonaccredited hospitals was nearly twice that of all New York City Blue Shield subscribers. The high usage of such hospitals is attributed to discrimination against HIP physicians, rather than to the surgeons' qualifications.

The fourth study compares the facilities and physicians used by Kaiser enrollees with those used by samples of union members enrolled in a major medical plan and New Jersey Blue Cross. It was found that few nonaccredited hospitals were used. The different proportions using accredited facilities of various types largely reflect the different mixes of hospital beds in each region (Columbia University, 1962a, p. 166). The qualifications of attending physicians were essentially the same for all three groups.

The Hastings study emphasizes the weaknesses of these structural measures. It points out that:

A claim often made by advocates of multidisciplinary group practice is that this form of organization facilitates the appropriate use of professional specialists and, indeed, leads to a greater degree of specialization of medical practice. In the particular setting of Sault Ste. Marie, it was quite predictable that the proportion of services rendered by specialists would be higher in the G.H.A. simply because its staff included a higher proportion of physicians with some type of formal specialist qualification, while a number of the independent practitioners (who were on

Table 10−1   Qualifications of Physicians and Accreditation Status of Hospitals Used by Various Health Plans

Percent of Families in 1952 Who Use a "Special Doctor for Children"[a]	HIP Enrollees	All New York City
For children under 1 year	89.8%	50.2%
For children 1−3 years	65.5	41.1
For children 4−6 years	42.2	36.8
For children 0−6 years	63.3	42.4

Percent of Deliveries in 1955 Attended by[b]	HIP Enrollees	All New York City	All Privately Attended New York City Births
Board certified Obstetrician/Gynecologists	72%	24%	39%
Other Obstetrician/Gynecologists	28	15	25
Other physicians (mostly general practitioners)	0	22	36
Hospital ward physicians	0	39	—

Percent of Surgical Procedures in 1958:[c]	HIP enrollees	GHI enrollees	NYC Blue Shield
In voluntary hospitals	59.7%	64.2%	73.6%
Affiliated with a medical school	(17.6)	(10.1)	(13.4)
Proprietary hospitals	38.8	33.5	25.3
Government hospitals	1.5	2.2	1.1
All accredited hospitals	63.7%	71.2%	79.4%
By board-certified surgeon	83.5%	56.6%	61.2%
Full-time surgical specialist	11.5	16.4	14.8
Part-time surgical specialist	2.3	10.2	8.5
General practitioner	2.3	14.6	11.6
Nonsurgical specialist	0.3	2.2	3.3
All others	0.1	0.0	0.5
By board-certified surgeons in accredited hospitals	56.3%	46.4%	53.7%
Board-certified surgeons in unaccredited hospitals	27.0	10.3	7.9
Other physicians in accredited hospitals	7.4	24.8	25.6
Other physicians in unaccredited hospitals	9.3	18.5	12.8

Percent of stays in 1958 in hospitals that are[d]	Kaiser	GE Major Medical	NJ Blue Cross
Affiliated with a medical school	1%	6%	2%
Others, approved for intern or residency	88	33	79
Other accredited	9	59	14
Nonaccredited	2	2	5
Percent of attending physicians for hospitalized patients who were "Recognized specialists": [d]	~44%	~44%	~44%

Qualifications of Providers Rendering Services in Sault Ste. Marie in 1967−68 to Members of Specific Plans[e]	Group Health	Indemnity
Percent in-hospital surgery by general practitioners	1%	22%
Percent in-hospital operations with anesthesia given by GPs	7	48

Qualifications of Providers Rendering Services in Sault Ste. Marie in 1967−68 to Members of Specific Plans[e]	Group Health	Indemnity
Percent obstetric care given by GPs	15	38
Percent of ambulatory visits for children aged 0−1 given by:		
Family physician	17	46
Pediatrician	76	30
Other specialist	7	24
Percent of eye refractions done by:		
Optometrists	96.8	36.7
Ophthalmologists	3.2	63.3

Percent of 16 Selected Surgical Procedures Done by a Properly Qualified Surgeon, 1968[f]	San Joaquin (FMC)	Ventura County
	54.9%	48.7%

Percent of 45 HMOs Surveyed[g]

That required board certification or eligibility	42%
With physicians having teaching responsibilities	24

Ratio of Staff Practitioners to Enrollees[h]	California Medical Group	Six Established HMOs
Family practitioners	1:3,438	1:2,300−1:8,435
General surgeons	1:8,462	1:8,056−1:17,824
Internists	1:13,750	1:2,192−1:7,510
Pediatricians	1:55,000	1:4,545−1:10,357
Obstetricians	0:110,000	1:9,000−1:14,500

Percentage of board certified specialists October 1972[i]	California Medical Group	All Calif. physicians participating in Medicaid
Full-time staff	23%	}32%
All medical staff	12	

Characteristics of Pediatricians[j]	Prepaid Group	Group	Nongroup
Full-time practice	87%	86%	96%
Member of county medical society	40	84	98
Level of postgraduate trainings:			
≤ 12 months	6	26	16
13 − 36 months	54	49	50
37+ months	40	26	34
With specialty boards	75	67	74
With membership in specialty society	50	63	71

Table 10–1 (continued)

Characteristics of General Practitioners:[j]	Prepaid Group	Group	Nongroup
Full-time practice	91%	96%	94%
Member of county medical society	35	91	97
Level of postgraduate training:			
≤ 12 months	59	71	60
13 – 36 months	34	19	21
37+ months	6	11	19
With specialty boards	4	7	1
With membership in specialty society	22	65	66

[a] Committee for the Special Research Project in the Health Insurance Plan of Greater New York, 1957, p. 66.

[b] Shapiro et al., September 1960, p. 1305.

[c] Columbia University School of Public Health and Administrative Medicine, 1962B, pp. 199, 200, 211. The data concerning the hospital in which the procedure was done exclude those cases for which the hospital was unknown. This represents 4 percent of the NYC Blue Shield cases, 1.5 percent of GHI cases, and 38 percent of HIP cases. It is not known how this exclusion affects the results.

[d] Columbia University School of Public Health and Administrative Medicine, 1962A, pp. 166, 171. Exact figures are not given for the proportion of "recognized specialists" other than "about 44 percent of each group." The term "recognized specialist" means that the physician was board certified or taught at a medical school or was a fellow of one of the professional organizations known as colleges (pp. 168–169).

[e] Hastings et al., March–April 1973, pp. 97, 100.

[f] Roemer and Gartside, November 1973, p. 812. The data are limited to procedures performed on Medicaid patients in each county. For each of the sixteen procedures, a panel of three physicians determined what type of physician should be entrusted to perform it under normal conditions.

[g] Group Health Association of America survey results reported in Consumers Union of U.S., Inc., October 1974.

[h] Moore, Jr., and Breslow, 1972. The six established HMOs and HIP, Kaiser–Portland, Kaiser–Northern California, Kaiser–Southern California, GHC Puget Sound, and GHA Washington, D.C.

[i] Gibbens, 1973, p. 14.

[j] Mechanic, March 1975, p. 193.

average several years older) had, in effect, specialized for many years without acquiring formal qualification. (1973, p. 100)

The data certainly support those expectations. It is interesting to note that specialists are not always considered to be better. The almost complete reliance on optometrists by GHA members is discussed in the context of task delegation.

Only one study is available comparing an IPA with FFS practice. Roemer and Gartside (1973) examined surgical procedures performed on MediCal (the California Medicaid program) patients who lived in two counties and who were closely matched on several variables. The qualifications of surgeons who performed particular procedures were compared with qualifications that had been designated as necessary for performing the procedure in question. Unfortunately, all procedures performed by surgical groups were eliminated, because no particular surgeon was identified in such situations. This may have produced some biases, as might the differences in availability of physicians in the two counties. However, the data suggest that appropriately qualified surgeons perform a high proportion of the surgical procedures in the San Joaquin FMC. The results are statistically significant for the totals and for seven of the sixteen procedures as well, six of which are "in favor" of the San Joaquin Foundation for Medical Care.

The Moore-Breslow (1972) and Gibbens (1973) studies both refer to the California Medical Group (CMG), the provider group used by HMO International (HMOI). HMOI is the largest of the California prepaid health plans (PHPs), and it primarily serves Medicaid enrollees. (PHPs contracted with the state to provide services to MediCal eligibles. The problems of the PHP program are discussed in Chapter 13.) The HMOI case is particularly interesting, because along with a number of other PHPs, it has been widely criticized for providing poor quality care to MediCal beneficiaries while reaping excessive profits. (See testimony in U.S. Senate, Permanent Subcommittee on Investigations, 1975.) Moore and Breslow base at least part of their indictment on the facts that HMOI hospitalization rates are only about half those of Kaiser, and that the availability of specialists is far below that of other, well established HMOs. The Gibbens report is essentially a defense of the CMG, but it does admit that the proportion of board-certified specialists is well below average.

Mechanic (1975) reports various characteristics of pediatricians and general practitioners in prepaid groups, groups in general, and nongroup practice. Major differences appear in local medical society membership, but the traditional antipathy of such organizations to groups suggests that it is a particularly poor measure of quality. Based on measures such as specialty board certification and length of postgraduate training, prepaid group pediatricians appear to be somewhat better qualified than nongroup pediatricians, while general practitioners in the two settings seem comparable. The low proportions of PGP physicians who belong to specialty societies may be a reflection of their exclusion from some county medical societies.

Table 10-2 presents data concerning the physicians used for various conditions by enrollees in the Seattle Prepaid Health Care Project. For each condition Group Health enrollees were substantially more likely to have seen a general practitioner or new health practitioner, such as a pediatric nurse practitioner. In some cases the differences are striking: only 15 percent of GH enrollees were treated for hypertension by an internist, in contrast to 45 percent of the KCM-BC enrollees. None of the upper respiratory infections in children were treated by pediatricians in GH in

Table 10-2   Distribution of Patients by Plan and Physician Specialty
Seattle Prepaid Health Care Project

| | Specialty of Physician | | | | | | | | | |
| | General Practice | | Internal Medicine | | Ob/Gyn | | Pediatrics | | Other/ Unknown | |
Illness	GH	KCM–BC	GH	KCM–BC	GH	KCM–BC	GH	KCM–BC	GH	KCM–BC
Hypertension[a]	76%	47%	15%	45%	—	—	—	—	9%	8%
Diabetes mellitus	67	48	19	39	—	—	—	—	14	13
Urinary tract infection[a]	78	52	1	22	5	18	—	—	15	8
Pediatric upper respiratory infection[b]	55	52	—	—	—	—	22	47	22[c]	1
Adult upper respiratory infection[b]	79	84	0	6	—	—	—	—	18[c]	9
Gynecological disease[b]	70	49	3	5	18	32	—	—	9	14
Otitis media	68	45	—	—	—	—	23[d]	33[d]	9	21
Pneumonia[e]			6	25						

SOURCE.   LoGerfo et al., 1976, Tables IV–2, 9, 16, 19, 23, 27, 31, and p. 30.

[a] KCM–BC patient distribution is adjusted for sampling fraction.

[b] KCM–BC and GH patient distribution is adjusted for sampling fraction.

[c] Includes new health practitioners at GH.

[d] Includes sixteen GH patients (all 23%) seen by pediatric nurse practitioners and one (3%) KCM–BC patient. The PNPs work under the supervision of a pediatrician.

[e] Only the figures for internists are given in the text. These figures refer to episodes of illness rather than patients.

219

contrast to 44 percent in KCM-BC. The standard structural interpretation of these figures would indicate lower quality in GH. Yet, as will be seen below, process measures for these patients indicate higher quality for GH.

Other Structural Measures of Quality

One potential advantage of the group practice variety of HMOs is the greater ease of informal consultations among physicians. However, Weinerman comments that "group conferences, medical audits, and informal office consultations are, in my experience, more common in the descriptive literature than in daily practice" (1968, p. 1429). Such a statement is in itself more descriptive than concrete. Guptill and Graham (1976), however, provide useful data comparing hours spent per week by physicians in nineteen Iowa multispecialty group practices with the experience of age-specialty-location matched solo practitioners. Their results, which are presented in Table 10-3, strongly suggest that group physicians spend less time per week having informal consultations than do solo practitioners. The data with respect to formal consultations are less clear, but it is difficult to make the case that groups lead to more time consulting with other physicians. Guptill and Graham speculate that the results might have been different had the question focused on the *number* of consultations.

Continuing education programs are another structural measure of quality. Many HMOs emphasize their efforts in continuing education. (See Health Insurance Plan of Greater New York, 1970; Permanente Medical Group, 1973.) An independent review group commented favorably on the strong educational orientation in the Kaiser program (National Advisory Commission on Health Manpower, 1967, pp. 203-205). Comparative data are provided by Mechanic (1975, p. 193). Over 80 percent of PGP pediatricians participated in formal course work in a twelve-month period, in contrast to 65 percent of pediatricians in any type of group and 57 percent in solo practice. For general practitioners the proportions are 77, 77, and 71 percent for the three categories. Guptill and Graham's data also support the argument that group physicians attend more continuing education programs (1976, p. 178).

A final structural measure that appears to have a particularly strong linkage to some "true measure of quality" is the existence of internal quality review procedures. Graham (1972, p. 52) argues that it is easier for groups to establish formal and informal review mechanisms. Furthermore, a central aspect of the foundation model or IPA is peer review of claims, which can be easily extended to quality review by examining provider profiles. Thus, while a penicillin injection is often appropriate, a physician who gives one to almost every patient is probably providing poor quality care. Similarly, if injections or acceptable substitutes are never given, one may also question the quality of the care provided. A 1959 national survey of group practices reported that about two-thirds had formal methods of

Table 10−3   Estimated Hours per Week Spent in Formal and Informal Consultation

Hours per Week	Formal Consultation		Informal Consultation	
	Clinic Group	Comparison	Clinic Group	Comparison
One or less	40.6%	46.5%	54.0%	46.0%
Two	14.9	6.0	12.0	8.0
Three	18.8	10.1	19.0	23.0
Four or more	25.7	37.4	15.0	23.0

SOURCE.   Guptill and Graham, February 1976, p. 176.

maintaining quality (Raup and Altenderfer, 1963, p. 90). Large FFS and prepaid groups are much more likely to use formal methods. In fact, PGPs listed an average of 4.5 formal mechanisms for maintaining quality, including medical audit and direct supervision.

Specific HMOs often emphasize their quality review procedures. For example, Kaiser reported that its medical groups had developed various forms of comprehensive quality assurance schemes (Kaiser Foundation Medical Care Program, 1974, p. 9). The National Advisory Commission commented favorably on the specific chart review procedures used by Kaiser physicians (National Advisory Commission on Health Manpower, 1967, p. 204). Hurtado described the audit procedures used in the Kaiser Oregon region. He noted that outpatient care review has been more difficult to implement than inpatient care. Furthermore, the reviews seem to depend upon the specific department in question. The Department of Medicine had maintained audits for at least six years; the Department of Pediatrics had been doing them but stopped, and the Departments of Surgery and Obstetrics and Gynecology had not done outpatient audits (Hurtado, 1973, p. 115). This suggests that, at the very least, there is substantial variation in the implementation of review processes. HIP emphasizes formal control processes to improve the quality of care provided by the various groups with which it contracts. This includes a medical control board composed of outstanding physicians from the community at large, as well as from HIP group physicians. A medical care survey team also visits the groups periodically to evaluate the quality of care they provide. (See Health Insurance Plan of Greater New York, 1970; Morehead, 1967; Logsdon, Magagna, and Varela, 1975.)

Such review mechanisms are not universally available. The GHAA survey of PGPs reported that only 32 of the 45 HMOs, or 71 percent, had a formal peer review program of any type (Consumers Union, 1974, p. 7). Another survey of 30 PGPs indicated that 18 had their own formal procedures for the review of hospital care, and 6 participated directly with hospitals. Eleven of the 13 PGPs with their own hospitals had review procedures, in contrast to 7 of 17 PGPs without hospitals. Of the 30 PGPs, 22 had instituted or were instituting ambulatory care review (*Group Health*

News, 1977). Furthermore, the availability of information does not imply that it is used effectively. Freidson and Rhea's (1963) classic study of a large prepaid group points out that medical records were not used to evaluate the technical quality of care, even though they were readily available. The implementation of quality control often relies on much more informal sources of information. More importantly, Freidson and Rhea's discussion of punishment and sanctions indicates that even when information is available and used, control is difficult to exert, except in the most extreme cases. This suggests that even when a formal peer review mechanism exists, it can be little more than a formality.

In summary, the structural data suggest that the quality of medical care is at least as good in HMOs as it is in the FFS sector. A number of large, well established HMOs have higher proportions of board-certified specialists and are more likely to use qualified surgeons. However, there are some counterexamples, and at least one California prepaid health plan has been sharply criticized for its low quality, primarily on the basis of structural measures. In some cases the absurdity of structural measures is apparent, as in a comparison of a specialist group practice with a substantially older population of FFS practitioners. Similarly, one need not look far to find special circumstances to explain the HIP situation in which over a quarter of the operations were done by board-certified specialists in unaccredited hospitals. Some potential advantages of group practice appear to be more rhetoric than reality. Informal consultations apparently occur no more frequently in group practice than elsewhere. Formal peer review mechanisms appear in many but not all HMOs, but the mere existence of formal peer review structures says little about the vigor of their implementation. The one clear advantage that groups seem to have is in providing continuing education opportunities for their physicians. Whether this is to promote quality, to serve as a fringe benefit, or both, is unknown.

Thus the structural data support the view that there is little reason to expect the quality of medical care in HMOs to be higher than it is in FFS practice. On the other hand, there is even less evidence that it is lower. HMO organizational characteristics do not appear to be used to any special advantage, although HMO physicians tend to have better formal qualifications than the average FFS physician. Thus, in at least one sense, the HMO does offer an informational advantage: a randomly chosen HMO physician is likely to be better qualified than an FFS practitioner randomly chosen from the Yellow Pages. The real question is whether such structural measures actually translate into the quality of medical care.

PROCESS MEASURES

As was suggested above, process measures are not necessarily related to improved outcomes. However, they are the criteria most often used by the medical profession to measure quality of care. Process measures have a particularly important role in any evaluation of quality, because the burden of proof rests with organizations found wanting on the basis of such indicators, requiring them to demonstrate their quality of care using alternatives, such as outcome measures.

Just as structural measures are biased in favor of certain types of delivery systems that emphasize specialty care and formal organization, process measures also have certain biases. Some of these biases tend to favor HMOs, while others work against them. For instance, most process evaluations are based on the review of medical records, and cases with incomplete or illegible records are severely downgraded. One may expect both PGPs and IPAs to have, on the average, a greater emphasis on good recordkeeping than the average solo FFS practitioner (Nesson, 1977). The frequent sharing of patients in the PGP makes a clear and comprehensive record much more important than is the case for the solo family physician who gets by on the basis of continuous treatment, memory, and some selected bits of information in a self-defined code. Having computerized medical records also makes it substantially easier to undertake quality review activities (Winickoff et al., 1977). The emphasis on claims review in the IPA may also lead to more careful record keeping. While there is evidence that good records are related to other process measures, the relationships are not demonstrated overwhelmingly (Lyons and Payne, 1974).

A second bias in most process measures is that they focus on the technical management of illness (Brook, 1973a, p. 120). Thus settings that emphasize tests, procedures, and referrals, all of which generate record entries, tend to score higher than those that emphasize long discussions between patient and provider as substitutes for medical technology. The highly structured PGP may be representative of the former and the traditional solo practitioner of the latter. On the other hand, there are powerful financial incentives for FFS practitioners to shift toward more technology (Schroeder and Showstack, 1977; Fox, 1977). HMOs have clear incentives to do less whenever possible. This, of course, may lead to lower ratings on those process measures that assume that more is better. As the measures become more sophisticated and it is recognized that too much may be as bad as too little, this will become less of a problem. (For an extensive discussion of this issue as applied to questions of malpractice, see Bovbjerg, 1975.)

It is important to keep these potential biases in mind when examining the process data. The first subsection focuses on studies of specific HMOs, while the second involves broader, less detailed comparisons. A third subsection deals with a particular subgroup of process measures, the use of prescription drugs.

Process Evaluations of Specific HMOs

One of the earliest process evaluations was undertaken in 1949 by HIP in order to produce an objective appraisal of the activities of its medical groups (Makover, 1951). Cases were chosen from each of the twenty-six medical groups and evaluated using the implicit criteria method. Individual record scores were then combined with some overall nonclinical factors, such as referral methods and efforts to promote continuity of care. The total scores allowed the categorization of the medical groups into four classes. While there is no way to compare these categories with the quality of care provided in other settings, the descriptions provided by Makover suggest that some aspects of good practice were definitely lacking in the Class IV groups.* One important finding was that while medical group distribution formed an approximate bell-curve, subscribers were much more heavily concentrated in the better quality groups. There were four groups in Class I, nine in Class II, eight in Class III, and five in Class IV. However, two-thirds of the subscribers were enrolled in Class I and II groups, one-quarter in Class III groups, and only one-fourteenth in Class IV groups.

The Makover study was only the first in a series of quality evaluations performed by HIP. For obvious reasons the detailed results of these studies have not been made public, especially those of the later audits that focused on individual physicians. HIP has also attempted to prevent the publication of reports undertaken by the New York City Health Department (Bird, 1975). Because the studies refer only to HIP practices, it is impossible to compare the quality assessments with those of other providers, even if the data were published. However, in discussing some of these audits, Morehead (1967) suggests that the distributions of HIP physicians were probably comparable to those found by Peterson in his 1953-54 study of North Carolina general practitioners. The HIP audits resulted in scores for each physician that were used to improve the quality of care. Scores between 46 and 60 were taken to indicate below-average performance, and scores below 46 represented poor quality. While Morehead does not give

---

*Makover provides the following descriptions of the characteristics of Classes I and IV:

"*Class I*—Generally speaking, some form of unit record existed in each of the medical groups in this class. The records provided information suitable for maintaining a proper continuity of care. Specialists' notes and reports of laboratory services were adequately entered and displayed in the records. The histories and reports of physical examinations were reasonably complete; in the physical examinations, rectal and pelvic examinations were frequently reported, as were routine and indicated laboratory procedures. The health examinations conformed fairly closely to the minimum standards of HIP. In most of the medical groups in this class, efforts were made to use routine screening procedures such as examinations of urine, serological testing for syphilis, and in several of the medical groups, routine x-rays of the chest. In respect to their initial complaints, the great majority of patients were handled with good judgment. Follow-up care was adequately provided and noted.

Class IV—The records of Class IV were characterized by incompleteness, lack of uniformity, and were even further removed from an adequate method of correlation than were the records of the other classes. Greater variations in the adequacy of care were characteristic of the medical groups in this class. Some patients did not receive the diagnostic services or the follow-up that were indicated by the provisional diagnoses entered in the chart. With respect to the use of laboratory services and screening procedures, the performance of medical groups in this class was inferior to that of the medical groups in the first three classes, and it was evident from the records that even certain clearly indicated procedures were sometimes completely omitted" (1951, p. 829).

the proportion of physicians in each category, she does note that most physicians with the lowest scores were subsequently dropped from the groups. Furthermore, "several years after the completion of the study, one-third of the physicians whose scores had been between 45 (sic) and 60 had ratings above 60, one-third had left the medical group of their own volition, and the remaining third were still a point of disagreement between the group and the headquarters office." (Morehead, 1967, p. 1647). Logsdon, Magagna, and Varela (1975) note that continuing process evaluations are part of the HIP quality assurance program.

Mott, Hastings, and Barclay (1973) and DeFriese (1975) offer some evidence on the quality of care provided members of the Group Health Centre in Sault Ste. Marie, Ontario. Two process measures are available: (1) completeness of the most recent physical examination; and (2) continuity of care. The GHC users scored significantly higher on the completeness measure than did users of solo practitioners, but the difference is relatively small (DeFriese, 1975, pp. 141-142). The measurement of continuity of care is considerably more problematic. For instance, of GHC members who had an ambulatory visit for an acute condition in a two-week period, only 10.4 percent used a provider other than GHC. In contrast, 22.2 percent of visits by people with indemnity coverage was to locations other than a private physician's office—usually a hospital outpatient department or a company clinic (Mott, Hastings, and Barclay, 1973, p. 178). This suggests greater continuity among GHC members. A different picture emerges if one considers the particular physician seen, as indicated in Table 10-4. It is apparent that, while GHC members are more likely to use their "usual source of care," they are much less likely to see their "usual physician," even in cases involving chronic conditions. Thus institutional continuity is greater in this PGP, but individual continuity is less. Similar findings are reported, for example, in the Seattle Prepaid Health Care Project (Richardson, Shortell, and Diehr, 1976). Starfield et al. (1977) show how changes in the medical record can improve patient problem recognition by different physicians in the same clinic. (Issues of continuity are discussed in more detail in Chapter 11.)

The study by Hetherington, Hopkins, and Roemer (1975) of enrollees in six Southern California health plans includes extensive analyses of medical records data aimed at evaluating quality. One major factor in their quality

Table 10-4　Measures of Discontinuity of Care in Ambulatory Visits

Percentage of Visits to	Acute Conditions		Chronic Conditions	
	GHC	Indemnity	GHC	Indemnity
Other than usual doctor	58.2%	27.6%	37.0%	24.5%
Doctor not visited before	47.6	18.0	35.2	18.4

SOURCE.　Mott, Hastings, and Barclay, May-June 1973, p. 179.

measure is the use of preventive services. These results were discussed in Chapter 9. In brief, they indicate that substantially more preventive care was received by enrollees in the two PGPs. They also examined rationality, verification, and continuity, which were derived from a factor analysis of a set of twenty variables.

The rationality factor includes procedural variables, such as physical examinations, histories, and diagnoses, consideration of social factors, consultations, and the use of injections and surgery. They are interpreted as representing the various steps taken by the practitioner to evaluate, diagnose, and treat a given illness. The results indicate that the average factor score per ambulatory visit is significantly higher in the PGPs than in either commercial or BC-BS plans. However, the difference is entirely attributable to the Kaiser plan. The data for Ross-Loos are no different from those of FFS practitioners. This interpretation holds for both the summary factor scores and the underlying component data. Hetherington, Hopkins, and Roemer also offer insight into the importance of physician attitudes with respect to record keeping. The rationality factor scores seem to be directly related to the importance placed on record keeping. However, no significant differences were found across plans in physician attitudes toward record keeping (Hetherington, Hopkins, and Roemer, 1975, pp. 176-177).

Hetherington, Hopkins, and Roemer use the concept of verification to describe the use of various laboratory and X-ray procedures in ambulatory care. The two group practice plans have substantially higher utilization rates for such procedures, as well as higher factor scores for this dimension. The potential bias of this type of process measure is clear, as the PGPs offer much more extensive coverage for such tests. Furthermore, the relation of tests to quality is tenuous.* The last dimension of quality examined in their study is continuity of care. This is measured by referrals to specialists and paramedical workers, as well as by follow-ups requested. The two PGPs had higher referral rates, which count against continuity, somewhat lower follow-up rates, and a larger proportion of visits to different physicians. However, the pattern in this continuity dimension is less clear than those in other dimensions, with the commercial plans being similar to the PGPs. BC-BS enrollees received substantially better scores.

Some of these findings with respect to Kaiser are supported by the implicit chart review undertaken by the National Advisory Commission on Health Manpower (1966, pp. 203-205). The review team sampled records at each clinic and hospital visited and found them to be of "high quality, complete, and thorough." Routine laboratory tests were performed almost uniformly. The one criticism noted was that "some patients come to the

---

*An interesting example of this is given when Hetherington, Hopkins, and Roemer present the verification factor scores for physicians having different qualifications within the Kaiser plan. The scores were substantially *higher* for physicians from foreign medical schools and for those who had less experience (1975, p. 186).

clinic with frequent minor illnesses over a 4 or 5-year plan period without having a comprehensive history and physical examination" (National Advisory Commission on Health Manpower, 1967, p. 205). This may reflect the relative lack of continuity of care discussed by Hetherington, Hopkins, and Roemer.

An extensive study of the quality of medical care in Hawaii allows a comparison of Kaiser Hawaii with several other types of practices (Payne et al., 1976). The study has several components: (1) an episode-of-illness study that examined the ambulatory and hospital care of a sample of hospitalized patients; (2) an office care study focusing on the management of common conditions; and (3) a continuing education project to change behavior over time. Various physician panels were set up to establish specific criteria for selected conditions. These criteria were used to analyze: (1) the appropriateness of hospital admission; (2) the appropriateness of length-of-stay; and (3) the appropriateness of specific services ordered by the physician. The last measure was converted to a physician-performance index (PPI), which is the ratio of the weighted score to the best possible score. The episode-of-illness study is based on data from all twenty-two nonfederal, short-term general hospitals in the state, and includes twenty-three diagnostic categories representing thirty-two percent of all discharges.

The results of the episode-of-illness study are summarized in Table 10-5. They indicate that the PPI was substantially higher in Kaiser (79.4) than in the overall sample (71.2). This better performance is also reflected in the proportions of appropriately admitted cases and appropriate lengths of stay. However, two key variables must be examined: hospital size and the modal, or characteristic, specialist for the particular diagnosis. When these two variables are held constant, there are no important differences between Kaiser (the PGP), FFS groups, or solo practice. As Payne et al. emphasize: "The single most critical factor in performance (appropriate use of facilities and physician performance) is care by the modal specialist, with hospital size acting as a subsidiary factor. The important effect of the prepaid multispecialty group practice appears to be almost totally that of assuring care in large hospitals by modal specialists" (1976, p. 18). This is not a trivial advantage. The proportion of patients cared for by the modal specialist in all hospitals varied markedly by provider type: 93 percent in Kaiser, 71 percent in FFS multispecialty groups, and 34 percent in solo practice.

The office care study evaluated PPIs for the treatment of eight common conditions and five types of periodic examinations. The overall weighted PPIs suggest a small advantage for Kaiser, with an average index of 44.8 versus 40.9 for FFS groups, and 39.2 for solo practitioners. (These differences are not statistically significant.) However, the pattern is not strong, and in seven of the thirteen cases, the FFS groups had higher scores than the Kaiser physicians.

The continuing education aspect of the Payne study provides a valuable

Table 10–5   Summary Data, Episode-of-Illness Study, 1968

Study Variable	Physician Performance Index[a]	Percent Appropriately Admitted[a]	Percent of Appropriate Admissions with Appropriate Length of Stay[a]	Patients with Appropriate Admissions and Lengths of Stay, as a Percentage of Total Patients Admitted[a]
All variables	71.2 (3,316)	89.9 (3,316)	82.3 (2,573)	74.5 (3,316)
Hospital size[b]				
Large	73.7 (2,560)	91.4 (2,560)	84.7 (2,019)	71.8 (2,560)
Small	63.8 (756)	85.5 (756)	76.5 (554)	66.5 (756)
Specialty				
Modal specialists	77.9 (1,851)	94.0 (1,851)	88.0 (1,497)	83.0 (1,851)
Others	64.0 (1,455)	85.4 (1,455)	75.6 (1,072)	65.3 (1,455)
Hospital size and specialty				
Modal specialists in large hospitals	78.4 (1,720)	94.7 (1,720)	89.1 (1,397)	84.7 (1,720)
Modal specialists in small hospitals	70.7 (131)	86.6 (131)	77.6 (99)	69.5 (131)
Others in large hospitals	64.6 (833)	86.0 (833)	74.8 (620)	65.4 (833)
Others in small hospitals	63.3 (622)	85.1 (622)	76.3 (452)	65.7 (622)
Practice setting				
Prepaid multispecialty group	79.4 (679)	96.9 (679)	90.3 (565)	87.8 (679)
Fee-for-service multispecialty group	74.2 (581)	93.5 (581)	85.2 (467)	79.3 (581)
Solo practice	69.5 (2,045)	88.2 (2,045)	80.6 (1,537)	71.7 (2,045)
Large hospital, modal specialists by practice setting				
Prepaid multispecialty group	80.4 (610)	97.6 (610)	90.8 (512)	88.9 (610)
Fee-for-service multispecialty group	77.7 (385)	91.6 (385)	87.8 (315)	82.1 (385)
Solo practice	78.4 (725)	94.4 (725)	89.4 (569)	85.0 (725)

Reprinted, with permission from *The Quality of Medical Care: Evaluation and Improvement*, by Beverly C. Payne, M.D. and staff, p. 14. Copyright 1976 by the Hospital Research and Educational Trust, 840 North Lake Shore Drive, Chicago, Il 60611.

[a] Number in parentheses indicates total number of cases used in determining value of variable.

[b] Large hospitals are defined as those that discharged over 4,000 cases in 1968; small hospitals are those that discharged fewer than 4,000 cases in 1968.

insight into changes in quality over time. Data were collected from hospital discharge records for patients in eight diagnostic categories in six hospitals for 1968, July-October 1970, and July-October 1971. Four of the hospitals were large general hospitals in metropolitan areas. One of these, hospital C, was the Kaiser hospital. The other two hospitals, E and F, were small community hospitals on another island. In 1970 the Hawaii Medical Service Association (Blue Shield) instituted an aggressive program of utilization review and retrospective denial of charges for excessive length of stay. Independently, continuing education seminars were held in February 1971 in hospitals A to D. While this makes the analysis of the follow-up data more difficult, it does provide a useful natural experiment.

The key findings are presented in Figure 10-1. The first part of the figure shows that in 1968 the proportion of cases with an appropriate length of stay was highest in the Kaiser hospital, and the other hospitals were clustered at a level about 15 points lower. By the latter part of 1970, the non-Kaiser hospitals were more tightly clustered, but at a level about five points *above* the Kaiser facility. A year later the pattern is even stronger, with a 12-point spread. The major change in the non-Kaiser hospitals took place between 1968 and 1970 and is probably related to the new claims review procedures by Blue Shield. The continued increase in appropriateness of stay between 1970 and 1971 may be partly attributable to the continuing education seminar, but it seems unlikely. Hospitals E and F, on another island and without the seminar, showed at least as great an improvement. On the other hand, the Kaiser hospital (C) had the seminar and continued its fall.

The second part of the figure suggests a potential explanation for this "perverse" movement by Kaiser. It started with the shortest length of stay, 10.2 days, for the eight conditions, and continued to reduce it to 8.3 days by 1971. In the same period, the other hospitals reduced their average from about 12.5 to 10.2, exactly where Kaiser had started. The Payne method of computing appropriateness allows for both overstays and understays. In 1968 the non-Kaiser hospitals had a relatively large proportion of overstays, which was eliminated by the Blue Shield crackdown. Surprisingly, Kaiser had a decrease in understays and an increase in overstays (Payne and Lyons, 1972).

The third part of Figure 10-1 suggests that the reduction in length of stay did not adversely affect the physician performance index. Kaiser continued to increase its average PPI, as did the other hospitals, with the major changes occurring between 1968 and 1970. In fact, with the exception of Kaiser, the three hospitals having a seminar experienced a decrease in their PPIs, while the two small hospitals without seminars held constant. The most reasonable interpretation of these results is that the quality of care in the Kaiser facility is about the same as that of the other large urban hospitals.

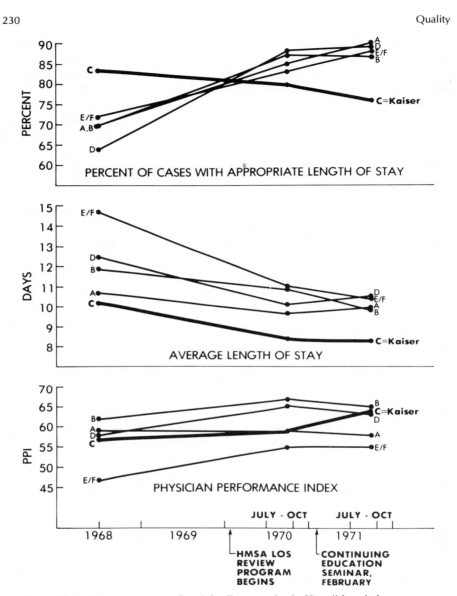

Figure 10-1   Process measures for eight diagnoses in six Hawaii hospitals.

Rhee (1976) offers a multivariate analysis of these data from the episode-of-illness study. He controls for type of hospital, physician's specialty, type of medical school, and time in practice, as well as for type of ambulatory care setting. The most important determinant of quality is type of hospital, with the Kaiser Foundation Hospital and the large urban teaching hospitals doing significantly better than the others, in both unadjusted and adjusted scores.* The Kaiser hospital actually has a higher score than the urban teaching hospitals, but the differences are small. With respect to the type of ambulatory practice, physicians in large, multispecialty groups, regardless of the method of payment, offered the best quality care using the unadjusted data (p < .001). When the other variables were taken into consideration, the differences were not significant, although large group physicians still ranked highest. There was no difference in quality between Kaiser and the large FFS multispecialty groups. Surprisingly, FFS solo practitioners ranked second, after the large multispecialty groups, and medium-sized multispecialty groups with some prepayment had the lowest ratings.†

Several quality assessment studies were performed as part of the Seattle Prepaid Health Care Project (LoGerfo et al., 1976). Studies included ambulatory treatment of various chronic and acute conditions, management of pregnancy, and justification for specific surgical procedures. The ambulatory conditions included hypertension, diabetes mellitus, urinary tract infection, upper respiratory infection, common gynecologic conditions, otitis media, and pneumonia. Patient records were drawn from GH and KCM-BC enrollee groups and evaluated with respect to specified criteria to develop a physician performance index similar to that of Payne and Lyons. A summary of these PPIs is presented in Table 10-6. In general, the process of care was similar in the two settings, but a few significant differences were found, and these all favored GH. (See also LoGerfo, Larson, and Richardson, 1978.) The major cause of these differences is the more appropriate use of the laboratory in the GH setting and the more appropriate use of antibiotics. It should be noted that this finding is contrary to what might be expected from the economic incentives—KCM-BC physicians could receive additional revenue for more testing, while GH would not. On the other hand, the proximity of the GH laboratory, as well as peer influence, may have been deciding factors.

To evaluate preventive care in the two settings, Lo Gerfo et al., examined various aspects of care before, during, and after delivery. GH mothers were slightly (but insignificantly) more likely to have had earlier prenatal visits. They were significantly more likely to be attended by an obstetrician. The labor and delivery process was generally comparable. Although a significantly higher proportion of GH deliveries were induced (23 versus 13 percent), a significantly higher proportion did not involve the use of forceps (.65 versus .31). The GH mothers were also much more likely to

---

*These findings are consistent with those of other studies that identify differences across hospitals as being much more important than differences among physicians within hospitals (Saywell et al., 1979).

†It would be very interesting to know more about these other settings, in particular the medium-sized group with a mixed FFS and prepaid practice. For instance, was there a difference in the quality of care rendered the prepaid and FFS patients by the same physicians? Unfortunately this information is not available.

Table 10−6   Seattle Prepaid Health Care Project Summary of Physician Performance Indexes for Ambulatory Care

Disease	Index	GH Score	KCM/BC Score
Hypertension	PPI-W[a]	49	46
Diabetes mellitus	PPI-W	41	36
Urinary tract infection	PPI-W	52	35*
Upper respiratory infection			
Children	PPI-W	28	25
Adults	PPI-W	31	27
Common gynecologic disease	PPI-UW[b]	62	57
Otitis Media[c]	PPI-W	29	22*
Pneumonia[d]	PPI-U[d]	50	37

SOURCE.   LoGerfo et al., 1976.

* Denotes statistical significance at p < .05 level

[a] PPI-W denotes weighted index.

[b] PPI-UW denotes unweighted index, with only highly important items chosen. There is no PPI-W for this group.

[c] Sampling frame does not allow true population estimate of PPI-W.

[d] PPI-U denotes unweighted index.

receive local anesthetics rather than epidural or caudals. Postpartum fever was noted more frequently for GH mothers, but it generally disappeared without treatment or prolonged hospital stay. Apgar scores for GH infants were significantly lower; the difference is not explained by method of analgesia or prematurity. GH nurses were solely responsible for recording the Apgar score, because it was found that, although nurses could devote more attention to the infants, physicians tended to record higher scores. Thus there is reason to suspect the differences in Apgar score are due to differences in choice of observer.

LoGerfo et al. (1976) reviewed the records of all patients having an appendectomy, cholecystectomy, hysterectomy, tonsillectomy, or adenoidectomy. In each case specific criteria were used to determine whether the procedure was necessary or justifiable. Table 10-7 presents the ratio of KCM-BC to GH procedures for all patients and for only the "necessary" procedures. A much higher proportion of GH procedures were "necessary," 18 of 23 versus 109 of 192 for KCM-BC. On the other hand, LoGerfo et al., interpret the lower rates of necessary surgery in GH as evidence of underprovision. This view is supported by the fact that all four of the appendectomies in GH involved perforated appendices, a sign of waiting too long. However, the long delays in each case occurred on the patient's part, before coming to see a physician; there was no difference between GH and KCM-BC in the time between admission and surgery. It may be that the relative newness of enrollees to GH and the lower likelihood of having a personal physician led to the delay. This conjecture is

Table 10–7   Seattle Prepaid Health Care Project Number of Elective Surgical Procedures and Proportion of "Necessary" Procedures by Provider

Number of Surgical Procedures Performed by Each Provider	KCM	GHC	Corrected Ratio of Procedures Between[a] Providers, KCM:GHC
Appendectomy	15	4	1.7:1
Cholecystectomy	24	6	1.9:1
Hysterectomy	56	4	6.3:1
Tonsillectomy and adenoidectomy	97	9	5.8:1
Total	192	23	5.0:1 (weighted)

Number of "Necessary" Procedures Performed by Each Provider	KCM	GH	Corrected Ratio of "Necessary" Procedures between Providers
Appendectomy	12	4	1.4:1
Cholecystectomy	22	6	1.7:1
Hysterectomy	44	3	6.8:1
Tonsillectomy and adenoidectomy	31	5	2.8:1
Total	109	18	3.9:1 (weighted)

SOURCE.   LoGerfo et al., 1976.

[a] Figures are corrected for patient-months of exposure based on the appropriate age and sex distribution of the patients. The corrections for KCM-BC:GH for each procedure are 2.17 for appendectomy, 2.17 for cholecystectomy, 2.22 for hysterectomy and 2.17 for tonsillectomy.

supported by the fact that for GH enrollees in general the perforation rate is 18 percent, comparable to that of other settings. While the appendectomy rate for GH is one-third lower than in the U.S. at large, the death rate from appendicitis is one-half to one-third lower (Watkins and Howell, 1977).

The underprovision interpretation is based on applying the rate of justified procedures from the KCM-BC population to the GH enrollees. There are four logical stages at which the observed differences in surgery rates can be explained: (1) the true incidence or prevalence of the disease; (2) the rate at which signs and symptoms are presented to physicians; (3) the rate at which these patients are diagnosed as having the disease; or (4) the rate at which diagnosed patients are taken to surgery. For cholecystectomies and hysterectomies, both GH and KCM-BC surgeons operated at about the same rate, once the disease was clearly identified (Step 4). (Similar analyses were not performed for the other two procedures.) LoGerfo et al. argue that interviews with the enrollees provide no evidence of significant differences in underlying disease states (Step 1). They do not distinguish between Steps 2 and 3, attributing the plan differences to more intense case finding by KCM-BC physicians. But the distinction is crucial, because if the difference occurs at Step 3, it suggests a quality problem, while if at Step 2, it may reflect either a patient access problem, self-selection into GH by people less inclined to notice, or present symptoms, or both. The appendectomy findings support the notion that the difference occurs at Step 2, the patient; and the "normal" rate of perforations for the whole GH membership suggests that if access was a problem for the new Model Cities enrollees, it is less so for the general membership.

Additional support for the notion that differences occur prior to Step 4 is provided by Koepsell, Soroko, and Riedel (1978). A different data base is used to show that federal employees in Washington, D.C., belonging to BC-BS or GHA demonstrate a similar twofold variation in admission rate. They reviewed case abstracts for patients with ten discharge diagnoses and judged the appropriateness of admission based on explicit disease-specific criteria. Two sets of criteria were used, and both gave comparable results—no statistically significant differences between plans were found with respect to the proportion of cases meeting criteria for any diagnostic category. Moreover, with the exception of tonsillectomy or adenoidectomy, the proportion of cases failing the criteria was always less than 10 percent. When these findings are juxtaposed with an admission rate in GHA half that of BC-BS, it suggests that the differences are not due merely to less stringent indications in the FFS sector.

This section has reviewed nine studies of the quality of care in five different settings over the past quarter century. While one might wish for a broader base of studies, it probably represents far more quality evaluation per enrollee than exists in the traditional FFS sector. It is difficult to derive generalizations from such data, but a few patterns stand out. The early HIP studies indicated that there was substantial quality variation within the plan, and this led the organization to undertake corrective actions to improve quality. In part, this situation was probably due to the structure of HIP, with its independent medical groups and loose central control. The other four settings are more tightly organized, and there is no evidence of wide variations. As would be expected, the Kaiser plans and GHC Sault Ste. Marie exhibit more tests and more complete examinations, but this probably is a reflection of coverage differences, rather than ideology or underlying quality. It does, however, result in higher scores on process indices. (The Seattle Prepaid Health Care Project provided equally complete coverage to enrollees in both plans, but the enrollment in the experiment represented a small fraction of the enrollment in either setting, so physician behavior probably represents standard practice, rather than specific incentives under the experiment.) The data are also consistent with the argument that the prepayment aspect of the PGPs has little to do with their superior performance, and their major strength is in assuring each patient treatment by an appropriate specialist in a large hospital. This well-developed sorting system may lead to a high level of technical quality; however, it seems to result in less continuity of care. It is also apparent that not all PGPs are alike, and much more detailed analysis of specific organizations should be undertaken.

Multisite Quality Surveys

The studies in the preceding subsection offer intensive examinations of quality in a small number of settings. Unfortunately, it is extremely difficult to suggest generalizations based upon such small samples. A few more broadly based studies offer a wider perspective for comparison, but they contain less detail.

Morehead has undertaken a number of quality-of-care evaluations of Neighborhood Health Centers (NHCs) and some other programs that deliver care to the poor. The first ranks twenty-four Office of Economic Opportunity (OEO) Neighborhood Health Centers according to a baseline audit score (Morehead, 1970). Four of the NHCs were preexisting group practices, most of which were FFS. The groups ranked 2, 5, 13, and 14 among the 24, somewhat better than average. A second report in the series presents detailed scores for components of medical, obstetrics, and pediatric care in the OEO centers and expands the sample to include medical school-affiliated outpatient departments (OPDs), health department well-baby clinics, Children's Bureau programs, and seven group practices (Morehead, Donaldson, and Seravalli, 1971). Two of the groups were established solely to serve the indigent, and all but one of the others had an ongoing program for the disadvantaged. Of the seven, two were FFS, two were prepaid, two were "prefunded," and one was supported by a combination of means. Thus the data tell us more about groups than about HMOs; nonetheless they are informative. In the overall scores, medical school outpatient departments were scored as 100; OEO centers averaged 107, and group practices 103. All three ratings were markedly better than those given twenty solo practitioners in rural FFS practice. The groups were comparable to the OPDs in the quality of care in obstetrics and pediatrics and substantially better in adult medicine. Analysis of the components of these scores lead the investigators to suggest that "there were a few indications that economy (in the group practices) may have perhaps been overemphasized on occasion at the expense of quality. Ratings were considerably lower than OEO in some areas where unit costs play a factor; for example, laboratory and X-ray studies on adult patients and hemoglobins and urinalyses on infants. One program went so far as to state they did not provide measles immunizations because of the expense of this agent" (Morehead, Donaldson, and Seravalli, 1971, p. 1304). This finding of fewer tests is the opposite of what is usually observed in HMO-FFS comparisons and may be due to the fact that most of the groups were not HMOs. However, it is more likely that the answer lies in the fact that in this case all of the comparison programs served indigent populations with outside funding sources. This again raises questions about the validity of process-based criteria, which emphasize the performance of tests and procedures.

A recent study by Thompson and Osborne (1976) focuses on pediatric care in the office practices of 166 physicians throughout the United Utates. While the sample was designed specifically to include solo, small group, and large (six and over) physician groups, no mention was made of prepayment. In brief, there were essentially no differences between small groups and solo practitioners in the frequency with which specific criteria were recorded. However, practitioners in large groups documented performance substantially more often.

In 1956 the American Medical Association sent a team to evaluate medical care in nineteen prepayment plans.* Given the orientation of organized medicine at the time, one would not have considered the AMA Commission on Medical Care Plans to have begun with a bias in favor of prepaid group practices. However, its summary conclusions on the quality of medical care were as follows:

Based upon its observations, the committee believes that the quality of medical care rendered to subscribers by the units visited and, within the scope of services offered, is comparable to the average level of care which members of the committee have observed in their years of medical practice.

The quality of medical care has improved for many low income groups now covered by these plans since a considerable number live under conditions that have made the procurement of medical care a difficult problem.

The lack of continuity in medical care, which occurs in varying degrees in conventional medical practice, is an ever-present problem in the provision of medical service through such plans. Fragmented care and lack of personal follow-up characterizes a number of representative plans observed in operation. It appears in varying degrees and takes different forms, depending upon the type and scope of medical services provided by the individual plan (American Medical Association, Commission on Medical Care Plans, 1959, p. 52).

This statement is probably still valid today.

Prescribing Patterns as Indicators of Quality

One disadvantage of most process evaluations is the great expense of either implicit or explicit chart review. This tends to limit both the number of studies done and the sample size within each study. An alternative scheme is to analyze routinely collected data, which although less detailed, may well

*Those visited included the following well-known plans: HIP; St. Louis Labor Health Institute; GHA-Washington, D.C.; Kaiser Northern and Southern California; Ross-Loos; and PAMC-Stanford, as well as a number of union and management plans.

give a good indication of broad patterns of care. One such source of data is in the prescription records for health plans that cover drugs and therefore that would be expected to have reasonably comprehensive files. A number of plans cover prescription drugs or maintain claims files, and several published reports are available on their operations (Egdahl, 1973; Brewster, Allen, and Holen, 1964; McCaffree and Newman, 1968; Greenlick and Darsky, 1968; Greenlick and Saward, 1966; Brook and Williams, 1976). Not surprisingly, most report that when drugs are covered and the out-of-pocket price falls, utilization rises. But our focus in this chapter is on differential patterns of utilization.

Johnson et al. (1976) report on a randomized experiment at Kaiser Oregon that established drug profiles for a group of patients in an attempt to alter prescribing patterns. However, no differences were found between the experimental and control groups in terms of drug volume, class of therapeutic agent, inadequate or excessive quantities, or potential drug interactions. A major defect in the study was that the experiment involved only 1.5 percent of the plan's membership and thus had limited exposure. Furthermore, no comparison with other groups is possible.

The process assessment of quality of ambulatory care in the Seattle Prepaid Health Care Project points to substantially better prescribing patterns (LoGerfo et al., 1976). For all upper respiratory infections among both children and adults, the rate of recorded antibiotic usage was about twice as high for KCM-BC patients as it was for GH patients. More importantly, the greatest difference is in upper respiratory infections likely to be viral in origin. In such cases antibiotics are inappropriate, and GH physicians prescribed them substantially less frequently than KCM-BC physicians.

A different situation is presented in the study of a Medicaid population enrolled in GHA of Washington, D.C. (Fuller and Patera, 1976; Rabin, Bush, and Fuller, 1978). Although this group exhibited an 18 percent decline in annual prescription rate after enrollment, if the number of perscriptions per ambulatory encounter is examined, the reduction is only 4 percent. Of more importance are the findings related to prescription patterns, comparing the study group with the Washington, D.C., Medicaid population. First, the drugs were classified into 90 therapeutic categories. The top ten categories in GHA account for 56 percent of all prescriptions versus 57 percent for the Medicaid population. Eight of these ten categories are the same for both groups, and the general rankings are similar. Considering only specific drugs, the top ten in GHA account for 28 percent of the prescriptions versus 27 percent in the Medicaid population. Even at this most specific level, six of the ten drugs are identical. While there are some minor differences in ranking (GHA physicians prefer Librium to Valium, in contrast to the control group), the similarities are far more striking. The fifty most prescribed drugs of each group were then compared with the AMA list of "irrational mixtures," those drugs for which "there is no rationale for mixture" or those that contain "at least one ingredient which has not been demonstrated to be efficacious for the purpose indicated on the label" (Fuller and Patera, 1976, p. T-18). Thirteen of the top fifty drugs in the GHA group were "irrational," including three of the top ten. This was in contrast to eleven of fifty in the control.

One might expect GHA to encourage the use of generic drugs, which usually are less expensive, since the organization is at risk for drug expenses. Only five of the top fifty drugs prescribed by GHA physicians were generics, in contrast to four of the top fifty in the control group. GHA members have also had the option of coverage for prescription drugs since 1960, so there is no problem of examining the experience of only a small and unusual group with the plan. In fact, the study of the plan's 1960-61 experience pointed out that only 12.2 percent of the prescriptions were for generic drugs. Subsequently GHA physicians were encouraged to prescribe generic drugs whenever possible (Brewster, Allen, and Holen, 1964, p. 405). Although there are several comparability problems, it is unlikely that the proportion of generic prescriptions in the Medicaid population ten years later substantially exceeded that percentage.*

Although the above data suggest that it may be difficult to alter physicians' prescribing patterns, there is evidence that when specific incentives are attached to behavior changes, the responses can be substantial. Brook and Williams (1976) report on injections given the New Mexico Medicaid population over a two-year period. Decisions were made about the appropriateness of certain injections in specific cases, and after an educational period, claims that did not meet the criteria were denied. The number of injections billed fell markedly after the educational efforts began. Substantial declines were found in many categories that were considered inappropriate. Some of those that did not show a response to high denial rates appear to have been used as placebos, and thus in some sense may have been appropriate parts of particular treatment plans.

These very sketchy findings concerning prescription drugs and injections lead to a number of tentative conclusions. With the exception of the Seattle study, there seems to be no evidence that HMO physicians have substantially better or worse (more or less rational) patterns of care than do other physicians. Instead all seem to reflect conventional medical practice, with a heavy emphasis on a small number of popular drugs. However, it

---

*Exact figures are not available, but one can infer some things from the available data. The most frequently prescribed generic was tetracycline, with 3.8 percent of the prescriptions. The next four were all ranked somewhere between eleven and fifty of the most common drugs. Drug number 10, Hydrodiruril, accounted for 2 percent of the prescriptions, so the four generics combined must have accounted for less than 8 percent. Thus the five most common generics could not account for more than 11.8 percent of all prescriptions, and the true figure is probably closer to 8 percent. Another 4 percent might be attributable to all prescriptions beyond the top fifty.

does seem as though practice patterns can be changed if sufficient effort and incentives are applied (West et al., 1977). This suggests that many existing HMOs have not made major attempts to alter practice patterns. As long as the data are available on claims forms, it will be at least as easy for IPAs to undertake such changes as for groups, if they choose to do so.

OUTCOME MEASURES

As was discussed above, improved outcomes are the raison d'etre for attempts to improve the quality of medical care. However, outcome studies are difficult to carry out. Furthermore most available measures, such as mortality, capture only a small part of true outcomes of care. (Consumer assessments of medical care, an important outcome measure, will be discussed in the next chapter.) Until recently, only three outcome studies were available, all performed at HIP. Now there is a reasonable sprinkling of such studies at various HMOs, and their findings round out our examination of the quality issue. The studies can be roughly categorized into three groups: (1) those that compare outcomes against preestablished criteria, usually within the same organization; (2) those that compare specific outcomes, such as mortality or blood pressure levels, in two or more settings; and (3) those that compare broader measures of outcome, such as disability days, in two or more settings.

Outcomes versus Internally Set Criteria

The key to measuring outcomes against internally established criteria is the specification of various levels of functional impairment and the description of the acceptable distribution of patients across these levels. For example, in hypertensive patients a successful therapeutic outcome might be the documented reduction of blood pressure levels to specified, age-adjusted levels within a certain period. Three studies follow this approach. However, the investigators were not enthusiastic about their findings.

Schroeder and Donaldson (1976) describe their attempts at outcome measurement and diagnostic accuracy in a sample of patients in the George Washington University Health Plan (GWUHP). Criteria were established for meeting patients' contraceptive wishes, and for treating depression and hypertension. The investigators encountered substantial problems in implementing their data collection, and the results were generally disappointing. In terms of diagnostic accuracy, while the false positive levels were acceptable, the false negatives were unacceptably high in each of the three conditions. Therapeutic outcomes were judged acceptable for contraception and unacceptable for depression and hypertension.

It is worthwhile to consider the hypertension case in more detail, because the other two reports used it for their outcome studies, and thus some rough comparisons are possible.* The GWUHP quality assurance executive board had set 25 percent as the acceptable proportion of hypertensives with blood pressures above specified levels. The observed proportion was 39 percent and thus was unacceptable. While that level is certainly higher than the goal, it does not seem out of line with findings from other settings. For instance, LoGerfo (1975) reported that 34 percent of a sample of hypertensive patients in the Seattle Prepaid Health Care Project had diastolic pressures greater than 95mm Hg. He found this result disappointing but consistent with a screening study performed elsewhere. The third study in an HMO setting offers further confirmation of poor outcomes with standard treatment. Williamson et al. (1975) found that 36 percent of the hypertensive patients in HMO International had uncontrolled blood pressures, while the acceptable standard was 5 percent. This poor outcome led to a focused program to determine the reasons for the poor outcomes and an educational effort to correct the problems. A year later, the proportion with uncontrolled blood pressure levels had fallen to 19 percent.

Although a casual reading of these three studies suggests that the quality of care in the HMOs studied was not very good, it must be remembered that the yardstick being used is what "should be," not the available alternatives. The Williamson approach can be a valuable tool for improving medical care, but it implicitly assigns the blame for failure to the organization under study. In fact, conventional medical practice may just be less effective in a real-world situation than it would be if everything went as planned. (The situation is analogous to the miles-per-gallon estimates from the Environmental Protection Agency, in contrast to what the average driver experiences.)

Specific Outcomes in Two or More Settings

Results of comparative studies are substantially easier to interpret when they focus on specific conditions and use the same methodology. The earliest studies of this type were undertaken in HIP in the 1950s, and they involve the careful analysis of prematurity and perinatal mortality rates (Shapiro, Weiner, and Densen, 1958; Shapiro et al., 1960). The experiences of HIP enrollees were compared with those of the New York City population who used private physicians. Even when the data were controlled for race and parity, prematurity and perinatal mortality rates were significantly lower for HIP enrollees. Not only are the differences statistically significant, but the magnitudes are substantial: the HIP prematurity rate was 8 percent lower, and the mortality rate was 17 percent lower.

*While most comparisons across organizations are fraught with difficulties, there is substantial evidence that blood pressure measurements are particularly unreliable. See Burch and Shewey, 1973; Varady and Maxwell, 1972; American Heart Association, 1967. Thus the comparisons discussed below should be treated with a great deal of care.

In the early 1960s New York City contracted with HIP to provide care for 13,000 recipients of welfare and Old Age Assistance (Shapiro et al., 1967). For those living at home (about 12,000), mortality data are available for both the study year and the following year and a half. After adjustments for age, sex, and country of origin, the mortality rates were essentially identical for the study year, 7.8 per 1000 for HIP versus 7.9 for the comparison group. However, in the following year and a half, there was a large and significant difference in favor of HIP, 11.7 per 1000 versus 13.3. Mortality rates for the HIP group in nursing homes were not significantly lower, 19.9 per 1000 versus 21.8 outside HIP.

A more recent study examined the perinatal death rate among Medicaid eligibles in the area served by the San Joaquin Foundation for Medical Care and in two comparison counties in California (Newport and Roemer, 1975). One of these, Ventura, had a conventional private practice delivery system and was similar to San Joaquin in terms of sociodemographic characteristics and medical resources. The other county, Contra Costa, was chosen because it had a strong county hospital outpatient department and a strong health department (Table 10-8). Perinatal death rates were then examined by county, controlling both for ethnicity and whether the birth was in a county hospital or a "mainstream" hospital (that is, one not primarily serving the poor). In all three counties, death rates in county hospitals were substantially higher than those in mainstream hospitals. As would be expected, death rates for county hospital births were comparable in the IPA and conventional practice counties, but rates for both were substantially higher than those in the county with a strong outpatient program. However, there was no difference in death rates between the two counties for births in mainstream hospitals, and both are about double those in Contra Costa, with its strong health department. These data suggest that the IPA yields care that results in outcomes no different from those in conventional private practice. However, a county with a strong maternal and child health program does have significantly lower mortality rates.

The Fuller and Patera (1976) study of Medicaid enrollees in GHA, Washington, D.C., also provides very sketchy evidence concerning pregnancy outcomes. These data are presented in Table 10-9. Mothers in the PGP had a smaller proportion of normal births, with a correspondingly higher proportion of complications, stillbirths, and abortions or miscarriages. But the sample sizes are so small that the differences are not statistically significant.*

The Payne (1976) evaluation of the quality of medical care in Hawaii includes outcome measures, in addition to its primary emphasis on process measures. Data from the conditions for which data are available by

---

*While there truly may be no difference between the two groups, it is less likely that the experience of GHA enrollees is really superior, with the observed results due solely to sampling variability.

Table 10−8   Perinatal Mortality Rates per 1000 Total Births, Three Areas in California, 1967−68 (Standardized for Ethnicity)

	Conventional Private Practice	San Joaquin Foundation for Medical Care	Strong Health Department
Births in county hospitals	39.7	38.6	24.3
Births in "mainstream" hospitals	30.1	29.6	15.5

SOURCE.   Newport and Roemer, March 1975, p. 14. Copyright © 1975 by the Blue Cross Association. All Rights Reserved. Reprinted, with permission of the Blue Cross Association, from *Inquiry*.

Table 10−9   Outcomes of Pregnancy for Two Groups of Medicaid Enrollees in Washington, D.C.

Outcome of Pregnancy	Group Health Association Enrollees		Control Sample	
	Number	Percent	Number	Percent
Normal birth	19	44.2%	19	54.3%
Birth with complications	6	14.0	4	11.4
Stillbirth	2	4.7	0	0
Abortion or miscarriage	16	37.2	12	34.3
Total	43	100.1%	35	100.0%

SOURCE.   Fuller and Patera, January 1976, p. T−36, with adjustments for those women still pregnant.

provider type are presented in Table 10-10. The small sample sizes render the differences statistically insignificant, but some patterns of interest are apparent. The FFS multispecialty group appears to have the best outcome record for chronic cholecystitis, invasive and noninvasive carcinoma of the cervix uteri (combined), and breast cancer. The two categories of cervical cancer should be combined because of the belief that early detection can shift the case mix in favor of noninvasive cases. If this is done, it is reasonable to expect that those cases still in the invasive category will have worse outcomes, on the average, but there will be fewer of them, and the overall outcome rate will be better.* With the combined categories, Kaiser patients had the worst outcomes, even though a substantially higher proportion of them had noninvasive carcinoma. The data with respect to breast cancer also raise questions about early diagnosis and treatment in

---

*This logical rather than empirical argument is based on the assumption that earlier detection shifts those cases near the border, and that those women who delay treatment will tend to continue to do so.

Table 10—10   Outcomes of Four Conditions in Three Different Practice Settings, Hawaii, 1968—70

	Kaiser	FFS Multi-specialty Group	FFS Solo
Chronic cholecystitis, number of cases	37	25	63
Poor outcomes—recurrence of pain	0.027 (1)	0.0 (0)	0.079 (5)
Death	0.027 (1)	0.0 (0)	0.015 (1)
Pain or death	0.054 (2)	0.0 (0)	0.095 (6)
Noninvasive carcinoma of the cervix uteri, number of cases	10	19	28
Hysterectomy	0.600 (6)	0.632 (12)	0.571 (16)
Cases followed up—1—2 years	1.0 (10)	0.842 (16)	0.607 (17)
Dead by end of follow-up	0.200 (2)	0.120 (2)	0.0 (0)
Invasive carcinoma of the cervix uteri, number of cases	4	13	34
Hysterectomy	0.0 (0)	0.077 (1)	0.118 (4)
Radiation therapy alone	1.0 (4)	0.846 (11)	0.647 (22)
Died in hospital	0.0 (0)	0.077 (1)	0.118 (4)
Cases discharged alive and followed up	4	6	13
Dead by end of follow-up	0.750 (3)	0.167 (1)	0.231 (4)
Invasive and noninvasive carcinoma of the cervix uteri—cases with follow-up*	14	23	34
Died in hospital or by end of follow-up	0.357 (5)	0.174 (4)	0.235 (8)
Malignant neoplasm of the breast, number of cases	26	51	106
Previous mastectomy	0.385 (10)	0.392 (20)	0.491 (52)
Mastectomy	0.846 (22)	0.765 (39)	0.698 (74)
Died in hospital	0.0 (0)	0.0 (0)	0.264 (28)
Recurrence of cancer	0.423 (11)	0.392 (20)	0.311 (33)
Died or recurrence by end of follow-up	0.423 (11)	0.392 (20)	0.575 (61)
Months from discovery to first operation:			
Less than 1	0.240 (6)	0.522 (24)	0.341 (31)
1—6	0.440 (11)	0.283 (13)	0.352 (32)
More than 6	0.320 (8)	0.196 (9)	0.308 (28)

SOURCE.   Reprinted with permission from *The Quality of Medical Care: Evaluation and Improvement*, by Beverly C. Payne, M.D. and staff, pp. 29—36. Copyright 1976 by the Hospital Research and Educational Trust, 840 North Lake Shore Drive, Chicago, IL 60611.

( ) Indicates number of cases.

* In this instance, the number of cases with follow-up equals the number of those followed up with noninvasive carcinoma, plus the number with invasive carcinoma who died in hospital, plus those with invasive carcinoma discharged alive and followed up.

Kaiser. Kaiser patients were much less likely to have their operations without delay, especially in contrast to the FFS multispecialty group patients. Nonetheless, outcomes for these two groups of patients were nearly identical. These data are difficult to interpret because of differences in the prevalence of previous mastectomies and the mastectomy rate in the various settings. Overall, the data suggest that outcomes of Kaiser patients are comparable to those of patients who saw solo practitioners, and both groups had outcomes inferior to those experienced by patients of the FFS multispecialty group.

Dutton and Silber (1979) used a tracer methodology to assess health outcomes for children, using six types of delivery settings in Washington, D.C. Their data are based on linked household surveys, clinical examinations, and interviews with physicians identified as "the child's usual source of care." The tracers include iron-deficiency anemia, acute ear infections, chronic ear problems, residual hearing loss, and vision disorders. Various sociodemographic and family characteristics were held constant, using multiple regression techniques, and the residual impact of the delivery system was then assessed. Children using solo practitioners demonstrated higher than expected prevalences, while those using the prepaid group practice and hospital outpatient departments had lower than expected prevalences. Alternative estimates suggest that these findings are rather robust. While the better outcomes in the PGP were expected, the authors cannot explain the good results of the outpatient department.

Nearly twenty years after the original HIP perinatal mortality studies, Williams (1979) examined perinatal deaths in 504 California hospitals using linked birth-death records. He first computed an expected death rate for each hospital, based on each newborn's birth weight, race, sex, and plurality. This expected death rate was used to compute an indirectly standardized perinatal mortality ratio (ISPMR). In simple correlations, ISPMR was negatively, but not significantly, associated with Kaiser hospitals. That is, Kaiser hospitals had somewhat lower than expected death rates. After controlling for number of births, proportion of Spanish surname mothers, percentage of Cesarean sections, and for-profit ownership, in multiple regression analysis, outcomes in Kaiser hospitals were no different from those in other hospitals.

A final set of outcome data is available from the Seattle Prepaid Health Care Project (Shortell et al., 1977). The outcome data are limited to 106 patients with demonstrated hypertension. Outcomes were the last recorded blood pressure levels after an average treatment period of sixteen months. The average age-adjusted levels in the GHC group were higher, indicating a poorer outcome. Shortell et al. examine these differential outcomes in a multivariate "causal analysis" that holds constant factors such as education, number of health conditions, family size, professional qualifications, and a physician performance index. The GHC patients had poorer outcomes, in spite of the fact that their physicians had higher performance ratings on process measures. These anomalous findings may be explained by the initially higher blood pressure levels among the GHC patients. Although Shortell argues that this should not matter, given the available drugs, it is useful to consider the difficulties described by Engelland, Alderman, and Powell (1979) in the treatment of hypertension in an ambulatory setting.

To a substantial degree, it would be preferable to rest most of our evaluation of quality on specific outcome studies. Unfortunately, the quality of these studies leaves much to be desired. With few exceptions, the samples are far too small to allow firm conclusions based on any but the largest of differences. Much smaller differences than can be measured with these studies are of substantial policy importance. Aside from problems of sample size, there is often evidence that the populations in the various groups differ with respect to clinically significant variables, such as previous mastectomy or initial blood pressure levels. Thus more refined analysis is necessary in order to separate the influence of provider type on outcome. However, data interpretation has changed markedly in just a few years. For a long time, the only studies available were the original HIP studies. In reviewing the evidence available in 1969, Donabedian noted that it describes "circumstances in which life itself is shown to be related to the precise way in which the provision of medical care is organized. Should these findings prove to be more generally true, their implications would be shattering" (1969, p. 24). Donabedian's evaluation of the importance of the findings is appropriate; however, the studies that have become available since his review have not supported a generalization of the HIP results. Instead, they suggest that the outcomes of HMO enrollees are not much better than those of people in conventional practice settings and may even be worse. The safest interpretation of the data is that there no longer is solid evidence that HMO enrollees have better outcomes, and that this crucial issue requires more carefully designed research.

Broad, Nonspecific Outcome Measures

The last two sets of outcome measures are more global than the others; instead of focusing on specific outcomes of a disease or process, they compare other measures of overall health status or the malpractice experience of HMOs. The ideal comprehensive measure of health status would be weighted to include individual preferences over various states of health and prognoses. (See Chen, Bush, and Patrick, 1975.) But the available data use much cruder indices, such as disability days or work-loss days. A crucial problem in all quality measures, which is especially important in a broadly defined index, is whether the observed differences could be attributable to selection among enrollees. Thus, if healthier people choose to join HMOs, their outcomes will appear to be better, even if there is truly no HMO effect. Until carefully designed studies that eliminate this bias are undertaken, we must interpret the data with caution and attempt to place them in context.

Robertson (1971) examined the experience of Midwestern school teachers, who were members of either a prepaid group practice or a BC-BS health plan. His outcome measure was the number of work-loss days in the study year. After standardizing for age, both men and women in the PGP have fewer work-loss days—3.88 versus 4.01 and 5.93 versus 6.41, for men and women respectively. While both findings are in the same direction, neither difference approaches statistical significance (t values are .48 and 1.07 for men and women). These somewhat lower rates of work loss are in contrast to markedly higher outpatient physician contacts for PGP enrollees, even after adjustments for BC-BS deductibles, radiology, and routine, asymptomatic physical examinations (Robertson, 1972, p. 73). Thus these data are consistent with the conjecture that PGPs provide more services that ultimately lead to a reduction in work loss. Similar findings are reported for Bell Telephone employees enrolled in Kaiser-Colorado (Mitchell and Dunn, 1978). While matched enrollees in BC-BS experienced substantial increases in disability rates and frequency of absences, those joining Kaiser had a constant disability rate and a reduction in absences. Although these differences are not statistically significant, the before-after design controls for the self-selection problem.

Comparable results can be derived from the Sault Ste. Marie study of Mott, Hastings, and Barclay (1973). (See Table 10-11.) Group Health enrollees reported fewer acute and chronic conditions than those covered by indemnity insurance. The number of restricted activity and disability days per acute condition is also somewhat lower for Group Health members. This is in contrast to a slightly higher ratio of ambulatory visits per acute condition. It should be noted that acute conditions are included in this type of survey only when they involve either restricted activity or medical attention. Different results were obtained when questions were asked about thirteen specific symptom or condition complexes. In this case

Table 10–11 Measures of Health Status among Steelworker Families in Sault Ste. Marie, Ontario, 1967–68

	Group Health	Indemnification Insurance
Illness measures in preceding two weeks		
Incidence of acute conditions per 100 persons per year	132	156
Days of restricted activity, acute conditions	625	783
Days of bed–disability, acute conditions	309	400
Average restricted activity days per condition	4.73	5.02
Average bed disability days per condition	2.34	2.56
Ambulatory visits per acute condition	1.12	1.07
Chronic conditions—restricted activity days per 100 persons per year	509	531
Bed disability days	171	202
Prevalence of 13 symptom/condition complexes in past year—conditions per 1000	329.3	289.7

SOURCE. Mott, Hastings, and Barclay, May–June 1973.

GHA members reported substantially more problems. These data suggest that GHA members are at least as concerned about their health as those covered by indemnity insurance; nonetheless, they tend to have fewer problems that disrupt their lives or require medical attention.

A final set of data concerning disability days can be derived from the Gaus, Cooper, and Hirschman (1976) study of Medicaid recipients in HMOs and control groups. Their data, as well as some adjusted figures, are presented in Table 10-12. The findings in the first half of the table support their conclusions that there are essentially no differences in disability days (either bed days or activity loss days) between HMO enrollees and their controls. Of thirty-six comparison pairs, only two differences are statistically significant; this is about what would occur by chance. More importantly, in eighteen pairs HMO enrollees had more illness, and in sixteen pairs the reverse situation was found. The data suggest a different story if one examines measures of length of illness (that is, the number of bed days per person reporting bed days). In this instance only three pairs of HMO enrollees had longer illnesses, and in two of these the differences were minor. This suggests that the HMO enrollees were as likely to have health problems resulting in activity limitation, but they were able to resume normal activities sooner. Gaus, Cooper, and Hirschman also present data concerning the health status and chronic conditions of the various groups a year before the survey. There are few differences of note and none that would explain the length of illness results. Thus these data are consistent with those of the other studies in suggesting that HMO enrollees experience somewhat better outcomes as measured by disability days or disability days per illness episode.

A different overall measure of quality is the malpractice experience of HMOs. To some extent, this measure may be a reflection of consumer satisfaction rather than true outcomes, but it is often perceived as a quality measure. Curran and Moseley (1975) report on a survey of twelve PGPs. Officials of four organizations thought their experience was better than that in neighboring areas, and the remainder thought their incidence of claims and suits was comparable to the community average. Specific figures, however, were available only for GHCPS for 1972. Aetna Insurance covers 80 percent of physicians in the state of Washington and in 1972 paid $1.45 for every $1.00 in premiums; for GHC it paid only $.89 for each $1.00. For all twelve HMOs in 1972, there was one claim for every 11,400 persons, in contrast to the 1970 national experience of one for every 16,700 persons. Several factors bias this comparison, so that a direct comparison is impossible. Some HMOs have used binding arbitration as an alternative to the courts. Ross-Loos has used such a system for thirty years and has had only five cases go to arbitration over this period. Kaiser has converted to arbitration for all its members, and it reports that in jury trials, its record was about the same as the national average for all medical providers (Kaiser Foundation Health Plan, 1979).

Table 10–12 Disability Days in One Month for Persons in HMOs and Control Groups, by Type of Disability Day and Plan[a]

Plan	Percent of population with disability days[b]			Number of disability days per 100 persons			Lengths of Illness[b]		
	Total[c]	Bed-Days	Activity loss days	Total	Bed-Days	Activity Loss Days	Disability Days per Person with Disability	Bed-Days per Person with Bed-Days	Activity Loss Days per Episode
Group practice	18	13	11	133	58	75	7.4	4.5	6.8
Control	17	12	11	142	62	80	8.4	5.2	7.3
Central Los Angeles Health Project	NA	NA	NA	NA	NA	NA	NA	NA	NA
Control									
Consolidated Medical System	22	15	16	165	63	102[d]	7.5	4.2	6.4
Control	17	12	12	141	53	88[d]	8.3	4.4	7.3
Family Health Program	16	13	10	127	61	66	7.9	4.7	6.6
Control	13	8	9	130	52	78	10.0	6.5	8.7
Group Health Cooperative of Puget Sound	27	19	19	189	71	118	7.0	3.7	6.2
Control	24	15	18	187	64	123	7.8	4.3	6.8
Harbor Health Services	18	14	11	123	55	68	6.8	3.9	6.2
Control	15	10	11	111	38	73	7.4	3.8	6.6
Harvard Health Plan	9	6	4	64	35[d]	29	7.1	5.8	7.3
Control	11	8	5	84	45[d]	39	7.6	5.6	7.8
Health Insurance Plan of Greater New York	21	16	13	192	88	104	9.1	5.5	8.0
Control	24	20	10	231	124	107	9.6	6.2	10.7
Temple Health Plan	10	7	7	70	30	40	7.0	4.3	5.7
Control	16	12	10	112	60	52	7.0	5.0	5.2
Foundation and control									
Redwood	21	11	17	183	48	135	8.7	4.4	7.9
Control	20	11	15	205	59	146	10.3	5.4	9.7
Sacramento	24	15	17	184	61	123	7.7	4.1	7.2
Control	20	11	15	166	46	120	8.3	4.2	8.0

SOURCE. Derived from Gaus, Cooper, and Hirschman, May 1976, p. 11.
[a] Based on 1-month period
[b] Tests of significance not yet completed.
[c] Unduplicated total.
[d] Differences statistically significant at the 95% confidence level.
NA Data not available.

SUMMARY

Substantial interest in health maintenance organizations arises from the lower medical care costs experienced by HMO enrollees. If everything else were the same—quality, consumer and provider satisfaction, and distributional equity—then a pro-HMO policy clearly would be desirable. However, everything else is not the same. More importantly, we know relatively little about the differences. The performance dimension of greatest importance in medical care is quality. One might go so far as to say that a pro-HMO policy would never get off the ground if the quality of care in HMOs were found to be inferior, even if they outperformed conventional practice models in every other dimension. Thus it is particularly unfortunate that the quality of care area is so underdeveloped.

Quality assessment measures can be grouped under the headings of structure, process, and outcome. Each is a more or less crude approximation of what is implicitly understood by most people as "quality." The three broad measures are roughly related to each other, and each has important drawbacks and biases. However, they represent the state of the art and must be at the core of present discussions about quality.

Structural measures are furthest removed from true quality, but they are the most visible indices. The available structural data generally support the contention that HMOs are at least as good as the conventional system. They tend to have higher proportions of more educated physicians and are more likely to use accredited hospitals. However, there are a number of important exceptions: some HMOs have not been able to get ready access to the better hospitals; others apparently have chosen not to emphasize specialists and accredited, nonprofit facilities. Clearly, there is nothing in the HMO's direct financial incentives to promote structural quality, other than the fact that, as a visible organization, such obvious factors may be important in attracting enrollees. Among the other structural measures, many have to do with particular organizational types and often seem to be more rhetoric than reality. For instance, there is little evidence that group practice leads to more informal consultations among physicians. Internal quality review mechanisms are present in many HMOs, but their effectiveness is unclear. And while groups have the advantage of proximity, the claims review function of IPAs leads to the automatic development of practice profiles. Groups do seem to encourage more time for continuing education, but there is little evidence that such programs make a difference, and they may be just a fringe benefit.

Process measures are primarily designed to evaluate the technical quality of the medical care provided. Thus they often are biased in favor of organizations that keep good records and offer more technical, recordable services. HMOs have financial incentives to do less, but their coverage tends to induce patients to demand more. Practice patterns also vary among providers of different training and practice locations. Thus structural and process factors combine to suggest that the average HMO offers care that is comparable or superior to the average FFS practitioner, but not better than that of the better non-HMO settings. HMOs tend to get higher scores than conventional practitioners on process measures that are sensitive to laboratory tests and procedures, but when all patients have the same coverage, the differential disappears or reverses. Large group practices seem to have a quality advantage over small groups and solo practitioners. (This may well be due to the type of physicians who join groups, rather than to a "groupness" factor.) Thus large PGPs exhibit higher quality relative to the average FFS provider, but not relative to large FFS groups. Prescribing patterns are not inherently altered by HMOs at risk for drugs but can be changed if sufficient incentives are used, regardless of the "at-risk" situation. Similarly, conventional FFS providers may account for a large number of inappropriate hospital days, but aggressive claims-review procedures can alter those patterns substantially.

One hopes for outcome measures in quality evaluation, but the available studies focus either on narrowly defined mortality-morbidity measures or on broad outcomes, such as disability days. While population-based measures are desirable, they are difficult to develop and face almost insurmountable problems of controlling for underlying population differences. Clinical outcome studies of people already receiving care ignore potential differences across systems concerning those who enter the medical care setting. The early HIP studies showed importantly lower prematurity and mortality rates for HMO enrollees. Subsequent studies offer no such conclusive evidence in any direction. In general, the data suggest that HMO outcomes are not very different from those of conventional practice. In some cases, such as when a county health department really makes an effort, outcomes can be substantially improved, but this improvement is not limited to particular financing systems. The one apparent advantage that HMOs seem to have is in shorter illness episodes. But it is difficult to see *how* this happens.

In brief, the quality question remains unresolved, but the issue is clearer. The specific financial incentives of HMOs seem to have little direct effect on quality. The importance of this finding depends upon one's expectations. One who expected HMOs to provide substantially better care would be disappointed. But one who expected HMOs to skimp on quality in order to cut costs would find little evidence to support that contention. The organization of practice in an HMO setting appears to confer an advantage, because HMOs can select their practitioners. Thus, if an organization decides to improve the quality of care, it can select better physicians and better hospitals. An organization can be identified as providing better or worse than average care, thus conferring a substantial amount of information to potential consumers. Finally, it is apparent that considerable variation in quality exists among HMOs, and it is likely that even more variation is present among conventional practices. To obtain more specific answers to the quality issue, we must generate more specific questions and better tools.

ELEVEN

Consumer Satisfaction

Consumer satisfaction is perhaps the most important dimension of HMO performance. Regardless of the advantages of HMOs in terms of costs, quality of care, or outcomes, they must be able to attract and retain members. Even if a political decision were made to enroll people in HMOs, the presence of substantial dissatisfaction would soon lead to a reversal of that policy. (The California Medi-Cal Prepaid Health Plan experiment is an example of such a fiasco.) Thus HMO policy must include a real concern for consumer satisfaction.

Agreeing that something is important does not guarantee a common definition of its component parts. There is no generally accepted framework for evaluating satisfaction, and the few that do exist serve only as discussion outlines rather than as tools of analysis. In part, the difficulty arises because there are two approaches to the measurement of satisfaction. The first focuses on how people feel about various aspects of medical care, such as access, information transfer, quality, and humaneness. Each is considered as a separate dimension, and no effort is made to combine them. This approach directs attention to those HMO features that are particularly liked or disliked by consumers and thus encourages changes in the appropriate directions. The second approach focuses on behavioral correlates of satisfaction, such as out-of-plan use and disenrollment. It asks the basic question: when are people unhappy enough to do something? Both the feeling and behavioral aspects of satisfaction have obvious implications for the future of HMOs.

This chapter is divided into three major sections. The first outlines issues related to measuring consumer satisfaction. These include the lack of an agreed-upon conceptual framework, problems of data sources and biases, interpreting differences, and the influence of enrollment and choice when evaluating HMOs. A comprehensive review of both aspects of satisfaction follows these introductory sections. The first includes sections on subjective and objective measures of satisfaction with access, financial coverage, continuity of care, information transfer, humaneness, quality, and overall satisfaction. The second includes the two behavioral correlates: out-of-plan utilization and disenrollment. A final section offers a brief summary.

MEASURING CONSUMER SATISFACTION

The measurement of satisfaction is perhaps the most written about and least understood dimension of HMO performance. There are several reasons for this: the lack of a clear conceptual framework, the types of data available, differences in interpreting empirical findings, and special problems related to the HMO environment. Removing the existing confusion is beyond the scope of this work, but it is important to discuss the issues, as well as their influence on the evaluation of HMO performance.

Conceptual Framework

The current status of the "satisfaction literature" can be contrasted with that of the "quality literature." The latter draws upon rather widely accepted distinctions among structure, process, and outcome measures. Some researchers modify Donabedian's (1968) framework, but it is usually easy to see how the various studies relate to one another. Furthermore, it is generally recognized that structure, process, and outcome are three relatively independent measures of quality, and there is no single overall index (Brook, 1973a). The field of patient or consumer satisfaction is much less advanced. There is no generally accepted conceptual framework. Instead, almost every study uses slightly or markedly different questions, even for the same concepts. (See the extensive reviews by Ware, Snyder, and Wright, 1976; Lebow, 1974; Rivkin and Bush, 1974.)

More important than differences in the wording of questions, which substantially affects responses, are the differences in the methods of examining the data. Five major approaches have been taken: (1) using questions that relate only to some overall (consumer-defined) measure of satisfaction; (2) using open-ended interviews to allow the respondent to elaborate on specific aspects; (3) using specific questions about more than one aspect of care, such as waiting time, physicians' attitudes, and so on; (4) constructing indices based on multiple measures of satisfaction, sometimes with an empirical basis, often with arbitrary combinations; (5) constructing test instruments based on theory, empirical evidence, and accepted social science procedures. Some important efforts in this last direction are Zyzanski, Hulka, and Cassell (1974); Ware and Snyder (1975); and Ware, Wright, and Snyder (1975). An important component of these studies is in determining the reliability of the scales when used repeatedly and their validity in actually measuring what they claim to measure.

The work of Ware and associates is the most comprehensive to date and includes extensive reliability and validity tests (Ware, Wright, and Snyder, 1975). Their construct involves ten separate components of patient satisfaction: accessibility and convenience, availability of resources, continuity of care, efficacy and outcomes of care, finances, humaneness, information-gathering, information-giving, pleasantness of surroundings, and quality and competence. This construct serves as a framework for the review of HMO performance that follows.

One important caveat must be recognized. All consumer satisfaction studies have been performed by researchers or evaluators, rather than consumers (Kelman, 1976; Hessler and Walters, 1975). (However, since most researchers consume some medical care, the situation is not quite the same as one in which middle-class whites are put in the position of assessing the quality of life in the ghetto.) Problems may arise because the wrong questions were asked or because consumers give different weight to their feelings when making decisions than when answering questionnaires. As will be discussed below, some of these issues may be checked by observing consumer behavior.

Data Sources

Satisfaction studies must rely upon interviews and self-reporting, except when behavioral measures, such as disenrollment, are used. Interviews introduce the biases of selective memory and the tendency to respond positively (Ware, 1978). This leads to anomalies, such as people believing that there is a health-care crisis in America, while being satisfied with their own medical care (Andersen, Kravits, and Anderson, 1971). High levels of satisfaction with one's own provider occur in almost all studies (Lebow, 1974). While this may be explained by self-selection of provider, cognitive dissonance, or other factors, it does have important implications for HMO evaluations, particularly for PGPs (Condie and Lyon, 1975). If it is difficult to admit negative feelings about one's own physician but easy to find fault with more anonymous groups of physicians, then there may be a bias toward more negative comments about PGP physicians. The whole is likely to be seen as worse than the sum of its parts, but few people are asked comparable collective questions about independent FFS providers. There is evidence to support the conjecture that PGP consumers base their opinions on undifferentiated reports of other patients and physicians in the HMO (Freidson, 1961, p. 161).

A second important factor involves consumer knowledgeability and level of expectations. HMO enrollees seem to know more about their plans and are more likely to have opinions on almost every issue (Anderson and Sheatsley, 1959, p. 59; Columbia University, 1962a; Dozier et al., 1973, p. 104). This difference, which is probably due to the conscious choice made by HMO enrollees, suggests a difference in the quality of the responses made by consumers in different plans. The evaluations of traditional providers by consumers with the same level of interest and involvement as the HMO members might be much more critical. This issue is particularly important because few questionnaires identify standards for consumers to use in order to evaluate their providers.

When Is a Difference a Difference?

"A difference, to be a difference, must make a difference" (attributed to Gertrude Stein). In consumer satisfaction, as in other areas, one should distinguish between statistically significant and practically important differences. A more important issue is that attitude differences may not matter. For instance, we might find that members of Plan A are substantially less satisfied than members of Plan B on nine out of ten dimensions, with the reverse being true on the tenth measure. However, depending upon the relative importance of the ten factors, they may still prefer Plan A. As will be seen, this is often the case with HMOs that offer a substantial financial advantage at the cost of other amenities. For some people cost is the most important factor. Once in the plan, however, costs are not visible, and other factors, such as waiting-time and courtesy, become more important. Thus the different situations of HMO and non-HMO enrollees may bias the types of responses received in interviews.

The Role of Enrollment and Choice

HMO studies are peculiar because almost all enrollees are there by choice. While the comparison group may be drawn from people who had the opportunity to join an HMO but chose to stay in the traditional system, their choice is apt to have been passive. The first plan that people are enrolled in seems to dominate, and the newcomer, be it HMO or insurance, is at a substantial disadvantage (Yedidia, 1959). Ignorance about such things as availability of choices is surprising. For example, in one study, even after making an original choice and then receiving announcements on two open enrollment periods, one-third of the BC-BS enrollees could not recall having made a choice (Bashshur and Metzer, 1967, p. 25). Not only are HMO enrollees a self-selected population, but they are generally more informed and more active. This suggests that when dissatisfied, they may try to exercise their voice option and make their complaints known (Hirschman, 1970). Even if the situations in an HMO and the FFS system were objectively identical, there may well be more complaints in the HMO.

The dual choice option in HMOs has the advantage of offering a behavioral measure of dissatisfaction. The discussion of Hirschman's exit-voice-loyalty analysis in Chapter 3 suggests that HMO enrollees may prefer to complain, hoping for improvement, rather than exiting. This behavior is unlikely to continue forever. If the HMO does not improve, they will eventually leave. An unresponsive HMO cannot count on replacing dissatisfied members, because personal recommendations have a critical influence on enrollment (Moustafa, Hopkins, and Klein, 1971, p. 39; Galiher and Costa, 1975). Thus enrollment and disenrollment patterns offer a good indication of overall consumer satisfaction.

In summary, consumer satisfaction data are subject to many problems that become all the more troublesome when evaluating HMOs. Interview-based data are subject to several types of bias, many of which work against HMOs. It is also difficult to determine the relative importance of various observed differences in satisfaction. Given these problems, most of the data in this chapter are drawn from studies that offer direct comparisons of

HMO enrollees and those in other provider systems. This will hold constant the methodology and questions used in each study. Occasionally comparisons must be made across studies, and such results need to be interpreted with care.

MEASURES OF CONSUMER SATISFACTION

The general framework for the remainder of this chapter is drawn from Ware and Snyder. The major sections address access, continuity of care, finances, humaneness, information transfer, quality and competence, overall satisfaction, and then behavioral correlates, such as enrollment and out-of-plan use.

Access to Care

Of the various aspects of consumer satisfaction, simple economic analysis predicts that in HMOs finances will be seen as the most favorable factor and access the least favorable. The reasoning is fairly straightforward, considering the two main variables for rationing demand—money and time. Since the development of the "new consumer economics" by Becker (1965) and Lancaster (1966), economists have begun to include measures of time, as well as money, in the analysis of demand for medical care (Acton, 1975, 1976; Newhouse and Phelps, 1976). So it is not unusual to expect that when the HMO's full-ambulatory coverage eliminates money prices, time rationing becomes more important. This view is further supported by the conjecture that the low ratios of physicians and beds per population in HMOs is not a reflection of decreased need, but instead evidence that supply is used to *constrain* demand (Reinhardt, 1973). The argument follows that HMOs make access more difficult than it is in the FFS sector in order to limit the number of services rendered.

A comprehensive review of the comparative studies on access by enrollees in HMOs and the FFS system provides only partial support for the above argument, because as usual, other factors are not held constant. (The various findings are outlined in Table 11-1, and these results are summarized in Table 11-2.) The most striking finding is that there seem to be about as many instances in which access is the same or better in HMOs as when it is worse. Closer examination reveals some patterns and explanations for these results.

Two readily available indicators of access are the time that one must wait for an appointment and the waiting time in a doctor's office. Both can be evaluated as reported times (days, hours) or in terms of perceived satisfaction. There is almost unanimous agreement that HMO enrollees wait less in the office, once they have an appointment, and are more satisfied with this aspect of access than are users of the FFS system. This seems to be balanced by having to wait longer to obtain an appointment, although there are a

Table 11−1 Comparative Studies of Access in HMOs and Fee-for-Service Settings

Anderson and Sheatsley, 1959, p. 63

Union members with dual choice between HIP and GHI. Data are drawn from household interviews in 1957.

	HIP			GHI		
	True	Not True	Don't Know	True	Not True	Don't Know
Proportion agreeing with the following:						
They make you wait entirely too long when you try to see them in their office.	20%	60%	20%	12%	60%	22%
You usually have trouble getting them to come to your home when you need them.	18	40	42	10	59	31

Freidson, 1961, pp. 67, 252

Questionnaires were sent to members of the HIP Montefiore group. They were asked to check which of a series of complaints about HIP and non-HIP physicians they agreed with most.

	HIP	non-HIP practice
Waiting for the doctor even when I have an appointment	35%	43%
Feeling that the doctor's rushing me in and out of the office	29	24
Can't get housecalls	6	24
Other: physical and temporal inaccessibility of HIP	7	NA

Dozier et al., 1973, p. 106

California state employees have the choice of a large number of plans including Kaiser, Ross-Loos, Family Health Program, Foundations, statewide BC-BS, or statewide indemnity. These data are drawn from a 1971 questionnaire mailed to a sample of employees. The responses are limited to those with some medical care in the preceding year. The original responses were on a 4-point scale from "very satisfied" to "very unsatisfied."

	Kaiser	Ross-Loos/FHP	IPAs	BC-BS	Indemnity
Time to get appointment with doctor					
Satisfied	53.4	77.0	88.4	87.0	87.3
Not satisfied	43.2	19.2	7.1	5.1	3.9
No answer	3.4	3.8	4.5	7.9	8.8
Waiting time in doctor's office or clinic					
Satisfied	68.2	80.8	78.3	76.3	75.1
Not satisfied	28.9	15.6	16.6	15.6	16.1
No answer	2.9	3.6	5.1	8.1	8.8

Table 11−1 (continued)

Availability of emergency care					
Satisfied	77.7	75.0	79.4	76.9	75.3
Not satisfied	11.9	10.7	7.8	6.2	7.5
No answer	10.4	14.3	12.8	16.9	17.2
Number of different doctors to see or places to go to obtain medical care					
Satisfied	81.2	81.1	85.1	80.0	80.1
Not satisfied	15.4	13.2	6.2	6.8	4.6
No answer	3.4	5.7	8.7	13.2	15.3

Gibbens, 1973, p. 12

Medicaid enrollees in each of three groups: California Medical Systems, another "plan,"and FFS beneficiaries. Response rates were 31%, 34%, and 53%, respectively.

	CMS	Plan X	FFS
Can get an appointment when wanted?	86%	78%	86%
Wait to see a doctor?			
20 minutes or less	36	43	36
40 minutes	35	36	29
60 minutes or more	29	21	36

Condie and Lyon, 1975

Interviews with a sample of HMO enrollees in Salt Lake City and FFS patients in same neighborhoods. The 1972 interview was ten months after the HMO began. The survey was repeated two years later with new samples.

	HMO Enrollees		FFS	
	1972	1974	1972	1974
Perception of ease in getting an appointment				
Very easy	29.5%	39.6%	38.5%	41.3%
Quite easy	42.9	41.8	44.4	38.0
Somewhat difficult	15.4	13.7	11.2	15.2
Very difficult	12.2	4.9	5.9	5.5

p=.00004

p=.95

p=.0001

p=.99

DeFriese, 1975, p. 143

All persons in Sault St. Marie, Ontario, covered by national health insurance. Some are primarily users−members of the Group Health Center; others use solo practitioners. Data

Table 11−1 (continued)

are from a population based sample using Osgood style semantic differential, with 5 as the most positive score.

	GHC	Solo	p value
Parking convenience	4.2245	3.4646	<.0001
Waiting time to see doctor	3.2544	2.8257	<.0001
Lab services convenience	4.8214	3.8997	<.0001
X-ray convenience	4.7169	3.9791	<.0001
Difficulty of telephoning for doctor appointment	4.5101	4.3580	<.01
Ease of telephoning to talk to doctor	3.0618	3.6891	<.0001
Visitation by doctor in hospital	4.7896	4.7122	n.s.

Tessler and Mechanic, 1975a, p. 108

Employees of two Midwestern firms with dual choice between a PGP and BC-BS. Interviews were held in 1973, after one to two years of enrollment in the PGP.

	Prepaid Group	Blue Cross	p values
Reported time to get to doctor (in minutes)	26.86	15.57	.001
Reports it is inconvenient to get to a doctor	1.68	1.22	.001
Reported number of days wait to get an appointment (except in emergencies)	10.30	8.31	.025
Reports difficulty in getting appointments	1.36	1.19	.001
Reported waiting time at doctor's office (in minutes)	26.86	37.81	.001
Reports that waiting time at doctor's office is too long	1.31	1.46	.01

Ashcraft et al., 1976, Table 3

Interviews with employees of one firm in Rochester, New York, who had multiple choice among two PGPs, an IPA, and BC-BS. These data are from those people who had been enrolled for 18 months. Satisfaction is scored as 5 (extremely satisfied) to 1 (extremely dissatisfied).

	PGPs	IPAs	BC-BS
Mean scores for:			
Physical convenience	4.53	4.65	4.77
Waiting time for appointment	3.78	4.55	4.45
Waiting time in office	4.16	4.48	4.19
Freedom to call about problems	4.50	4.64	4.51
Patient-physician contact time	4.64	4.50	4.75

Table 11−1 (continued)

Fuller and Patera, 1976, Tables 28−31, 43, 44

Medicaid enrollees in Group Health Association, Washington, D.C., and an age-sex matched control group of Medicaid beneficiaries. Interviews in 1972, one year after enrollment.

	PGP enrollees	Controls
Transport time from home to doctor's office		
Less than 10 minutes	9%	13%
10−19 minutes	35	28
20−29	29	36
30+ minutes	27	22
Method of transportation		
Walk	7%	20%
Drive	9	8
Taxi or bus	69	47
other	13	23

Gaus, Cooper, and Hirschman, 1976, p. 13

Interviews were conducted with about 500 Medicaid families enrolled in each of ten HMOs and matched control groups living in the same ZIP code areas.

	7 PGPs and Controls					2 IPAs and Controls				
	PGP mean	Control mean	#PGP vs Controls			IPA mean	Control mean	#IPA vs Controls		
			a <	b 0	c >			a <	b 0	c >
Episodes with disability days:										
Percent of episodes with physician contact	60%	60%	4	2	1	58%	59%	1	0	1
Average time to contact physician (in hours)	6	13	5	0	2	13	11	1	0	1
Average time from appointment to visit (in days)	11	10	4	0	3	11	11	1	0	1
Average waiting time in office (in minutes)	32	32	4	0	3	24	25	1	0	1
General physician accessibility to persons attempting to call:										
Weekday: percent successful	77%	87%	5	0	2	87%	86%	1	0	1
Weekday: average time (in hours)	4	5	2	1	4	7	5	0	0	2
Weekend or night:										
percent successful	74%	80%	4	0	3	93%	84%	0	0	2
average time (in hours)	2	2	4	2	1	1.5	1	0	1	1

a = HMO < Control
b = HMO = Control
c = HMO > Control

Hetherington, Hopkins, and Roemer, 1975

Mail questionnaires were sent to samples of enrollees in six different health insurance plans in Los Angeles County.

	Kaiser	Ross-Loos	Open Market Plans
Feelings about clinic procedures (p. 260)			
Very satisfied	30%		
Satisfied	38		
Dissatisfied	17		
Very dissatisfied	15 (20% if recent illness, p. 263)		
Availability of physicians (p. 261)			
Dissatisfied	10%	7%	6%
Highly satisfied		"same picture"	
Satisfaction associated with office waiting periods (p. 267)	no complaint		present in 3/4 plans

Number of days before being able to see doctor if no regular appointments

	PGP enrollees	Controls
Within 2 days	58%	51%
3−7 days	28	28
More than a week	12	19
Waiting time in doctor's office		
Less than 10 minutes	56%	10%
10−19 minutes	29	19
20−30 minutes	9	35
Over 30 minutes	5	35
Things liked or disliked about delivery system		
Proportion mentioning convenience	66%	13%
Proportion mentioning inconvenience	15	14

Richardson, Shortell, and Diehr, 1976, pp. v.5−6

Low-income residents of Model Cities area in Seattle were given the option of enrolling in Group Health Cooperative or a Blue Cross type plan at no cost.

	GHC	KCM-BC	p value
Ease of transportation			
Hard	5%	5%	
Moderate	34	40	
Easy	60	55	<.001
Appointment waiting time			
Mean number of days	6.7	3.0	<.001

Office waiting time			
Less than 1/2 hour	79%	65%	
1/2 to 1 hour	17	25	
More than 1 hour	3	10	(not reported)
Visits without appointment as a percent of all inperson visits	20%	16%	<.001
Mean number of convenience reasons citied for not seeking care			
Resurvey I	0.32	0.30	n.s.
Resurvey III	0.36	0.30	p<.03
Mean scores on direct access barriers (inconvenient office hours, did not know doctor, not able to get appointment soon enough, could not find doctor who would accept person)			
Resurvey I	7.0	7.0	n.s.
Resurvey II	6.9	4.3	p<.001
Responses to illness episode (p. v.43)			
Illness perceived as less serious:			
percent seeking care same day	30%	27%	n.s.
percent going to usual MD or place	73	82	p<.001
percent making appointment	60	76	p<.001
mean wait in days	1.8	1.7	n.s.
Illness perceived as serious and urgent:			
percent seeking care same day	47%	56%	p<.05
percent going to usual MD or place	72	65	p<.10
percent making appointment	54	59	n.s.
mean wait in days	1.8	1.6	n.s.
Expressed reasons for dissatisfaction with illness episode: percent citing office waiting time (p. v.52)	4%	24%	p<.001
Proportion of families with dissatisfactions reporting: (p. v.56)			
Felt unnecessarily rushed	9%	1%	p<.001
Appointment waiting time	16	7	p<.05
Office waiting time	13	8	n.s.
Hulka-cost-convenience scores: (pp. v.62−63)			
Overall sample	0.08	0.12	p<.05
Those satisfied in baseline survey	0.12	0.15	
Those not satisfied in baseline survey	0.01	0.04	

Table 11−1 (continued)

Salkever et al., 1976, Table 7

Low income residents in East Baltimore, interviews in 1974.

	Usual Source of Care		
	East Baltimore Medical Plan (PGP)	Johns Hopkins Hospital	Other
Percentage of persons reporting duration of children's visit to regular source as two hours or more:			
EBMP registrants and enrollees	28.4%	38.3%	—
Housing projects near EBMP	—	67.5	45.7%
Adult visits			
EBMP registrants and enrollees	33.4	67.6	—
Housing projects near EBMP	—	76.9	48.2

number of important exceptions to this generalization. Three studies (Gaus, Cooper, and Hirschman, 1976; Fuller and Patera, 1976; and Gibbens, 1973) that reported such exceptions are based on Medicaid enrollees who may have only limited access to the FFS system.

The explanation for the differences in appointment and office waits lies in different scheduling patterns. PGPs attempt to keep their physicians fully occupied and thus maintain full-time appointment schedules. Separate access routes are offered for people with urgent or semiurgent problems to see physicians serving on a short appointment basis. The solo practitioner maintains a more flexible schedule, squeezing in urgent patient visits and perhaps consistently overbooking. This leads to longer waiting times once the patient arrives (Tessler and Mechanic, 1975; Richardson, Shortell, and Diehr, 1976). The FFS provider has an incentive to overbook, provided that does not discourage too many patients, because there are always some patients who cancel or arrive late. If there is no one in the waiting room, the physician will be idle, and this implies no income (Fetter and Thompson, 1966). To some extent this is offset by the physician's fear of losing patients if waiting times become excessive. In the prepaid setting, occasional idle time does not reduce revenue, and it may allow the physician to catch up with other work. This is not to imply that PGPs are unconcerned about "no-shows." (See Hurtado, Greenlick, and Colombo, 1973.)

For other measures of access there are fewer studies, and the available evidence is more evenly divided between better and worse performance by HMOs. These measures include telephone access to physicians, home visits,

Table 11–2 Summary of Findings on Access in HMOs and Fee-for-Service Providers

	HMOs better or same	HMOs worse
Time to get appointment measured perceived	Gaus, Cooper, Hirschman Fuller and Patera Gibbens DeFriese Condie and Lyon (1974) Dozier (IPAs)	Tessler and Mechanic Richardson, Shortell, Diehr Dozier (PGPs) Condie and Lyon (1972) Tessler and Mechanic Ashcraft Richardson, Shortell, Diehr
Waiting time in office measured	Salkever et al. Gibbens Gaus, Cooper, Hirschman Tessler and Mechanic Fuller and Patera Richardson, Shortell, Diehr	

perceived	Richardson, Shortell, Diehr
	Freidson
	Dozier (Ross-Loos, IPA)
	DeFriese
	Hetherington, Hopkins,
	  Roemer
	Tessler and Mechanic
	Ashcraft (PGP = BC, but IPA
	  best)
		Anderson and Sheatsley
		Dozier (Kaiser)

Telephone access to
physician
	Gaus, Cooper, Hirschman
	(IPA)
	Ashcraft (PGP = BC, but IPA
	  best)
		DeFriese
		Gaus, Cooper, Hirschman
		  (PGPs)

Home visits	Freidson (HIP)	Anderson and Sheatsley (HIP)
General convenience	Fuller and Patera	Richardson, Shortell, Diehr
Time allocated for appointment with physician	Freidson Ashcraft	Richardson, Shortell, Diehr
Physical access	Dozier (IPA) DeFriese Richardson, Shortell, Diehr	Fuller and Patera Dozier (KP, R-L worse) Tessler and Mechanic Ashcraft (PGP worst, then IPA, BC)
Emergency care		Dozier (KP, R-L somewhat worse)
Availability of MD	Richardson, Shortell, Diehr	Hetherington, Hopkins, Roemer
Episodes of contact	Gaus, Cooper, Hirschman	

SOURCES. See Table 11–1.

general convenience, physical access, emergency care, availability of physicians, illness episodes with physician contact, and time allocated with physicians. Generalization is impossible beyond the statement that the individual situation of each plan seems to dominate any universal effects. For example, PGPs are often thought to be physically less accessible, because they are centralized. However, in some cases members live very close to their HMO; this results in short travel times (Richardson et al., 1977). DeFriese (1975) reports on a situation in which all the solo practitioners practiced in a single medical office building that did not include laboratory and X-ray services, thus making them less convenient than a PGP that was also located in a single building but with complete ancillary services (DeFriese, 1975). There seems to be a consistent difference in the performances of IPAs and PGPs. The former are generally more comparable to FFS practice, as would be expected, because IPA enrollees usually comprise only a small fraction of each practitioner's patients, and the practitioner is paid on an FFS basis by the organization.

In addition to these comparative studies, there are a great many single-setting studies. Most report on surveys of various groups of Kaiser enrollees in different regions (Pope, Greenlick, and Freeborn, 1972; Williams, 1971; Marshall, 1971; Kaiser Foundation Medical Care Program, 1974; Health/PAC, 1973; Saward and Greenlick, 1972; Columbia University, 1962a; Pope, 1978). These generally support the view that waiting time for appointments is a major source of complaint, and that time in the office is less of a problem. A third type of data can be drawn from evaluations by self-selected consumers. Although these are often dissatisfied customers, they offer vivid descriptive material that is consistent with the statistical results (D'Onofrio and Mullen, 1977; Martin, 1976).

Overall, among the access measures, PGPs enjoy a clear advantage in shorter office waiting times. To a large extent this seems to be balanced by waiting longer to obtain an appointment. How one compares these two access measures is a personal issue, but broad differences may occur. Koutsopoulos, Meyer, and Henley (1977) suggest that people can be categorized by the access issues most important to them. They found that those primarily concerned with waiting time had higher incomes, scheduled appointments further in advance, and had fewer visits, even though they were more likely to identify a special health problem. Those concerned about costs were older, had less income, and were less likely to be employed full-time. The PGP pattern is clearly best for people with nonurgent needs, such as checkups and routine visits for chronic conditions. This is particularly true if they value their time highly. People with semiurgent acute problems are more likely to prefer FFS practitioners and the guarantee of eventually seeing their own physician. The other access measures are probably of secondary importance; they seem more dependent upon the specific organizations in question, and demonstrate no consistent patterns.

Financial Coverage

The major selling point of HMOs is that they offer covered services with little or no direct charge. Thus it is not surprising that there is almost universally greater satisifaction with HMO coverage than with other plans. (See Table 11-3.) Moreover, people are sensitive to specific variations in coverage. The much greater dissatisfaction of Blue Cross members relative to Aetna enrollees in the Gerst, Rogson, and Hetherington study is probably due to real coverage differences. Aetna offered partial coverage for routine physicals, eye examinations, dental care, and TB treatment, while BC-BS offered none (1969, p. 51). Similar variations explain some differences in the results presented by Hetherington, Hopkins, and Roemer (1975, pp. 52-59). The large proportion of highly satisfied people in the large commercial plan reflected an atypical group that had commercial insurance for hospitalization and complete medical coverage through a small group practice. The relative dissatisfaction with Ross-Loos reflects their more limited benefit package.

Some of the strangest results are reported by Richardson, Shortell, and Diehr (1976). Even though they had complete coverage, a substantial fraction of enrollees in the FFS option received bills or found providers reluctant to accept their cards. The low scores on the Hulka cost-convenience scale (.08−.12) relative to results on the other two scales (.21−.29) raises questions about the validity of the scales. Although their reliability has been tested on several occasions (Hulka et al., 1970, 1971; Zyzanski, Hulka, and Cassel, 1974), it is not clear whether these scales measure satisfaction with one's own care or concern about the medical system in general.* Both the generality of the questions (for example, "A doctor's main interest is in making as much money as he can." "In an emergency you can always find a doctor." "Most doctors are willing to treat patients with low incomes.") and the objectively good situation in the Model Cities project belie the low score on the scale.

The consistently positive evaluations of financial coverage given by HMO members are underscored by single provider studies. More importantly, this is generally the area liked best by HMO members (Pope, Greenlick, and Freeborn, 1972; Health/PAC, 1973; Martin, 1976; Columbia University, 1962a; Pope, 1978). The problems related to evaluating various dimensions of satisfaction will be discussed further in a later section that outlines conditions in which HMOs fare considerably worse. It is worthwhile to note, however, that the simple model of time prices replacing money prices as a rationing device is only partly valid. While money costs are uniformly lower for HMO enrollees, access measures are sometimes better and sometimes worse. Differences seem to occur, instead, at the more subtle levels of human interaction. The next three sections deal with

*I am indebted to Jinnet Fowles for pointing this out to me.

Table 11–3   Comparative Studies of Satisfaction with Financial Coverage

Federal Employees in Los Angeles, 1966
(Gerst, Rogson, and Hetherington, 1969)

	PGP (Kaiser)	Commercial (Aetna)	Provider Sponsored (Blue Cross- Blue Shield)
Percent satisfied with financial coverage	86.8%	80.7%	60.4%
Percent not satisfied with financial coverage	13.2	19.3	39.6
		(p = .01)	

Enrollees in Six Southern California Health Plans, 1968
(Hetherington, Hopkins, and Roemer, 1975, p. 239)

	Kaiser	Ross- Loos	Blue Cross	Blue Shield	Large Commercial	Small Commercial
Opinion of financial coverage:						
highly satisfied = 1	46.3%	15.9%	19.1%	5.7%	23.6%	1.7%
2	24.8	17.9	10.3	19.8	17.1	14.5
.	.	.	.	.	.	.
.	.	.	.	.	.	.
.	.	.	.	.	.	.
8	1.8	2.1	4.9	2.5	2.5	7.1
highly dis- satisfied = 9	2.9	4.5	20.0	5.6	9.5	6.6

$$\chi^2_{40} = 671 \ (p < .001)$$

California State Employees, 1971
(Dozier et al., 1973, p. 108)
(These data are limited to people with some medical care in the preceding year.)

	Kaiser	Ross-Loos/ FHP	IPAs	BC-BS	Indemnity
What you paid for medical care received:					
Satisfied	84.1	80.9	73.0	66.1	67.0
Not satisfied	10.1	13.6	22.4	24.8	23.2
No answer	5.8	5.5	4.6	9.1	9.8

Low-Income Residents of Model Cities Area in Seattle
(Richardson, Shortell, and Diehr, 1976, pp. v.56–62)

	GHC	KCM-BC	
Proportion of families with a dissatisfaction reporting:			
Getting bills	.06	.31	p < .001
Reluctance to accept cards	.05	.15	p < .01
Score on Hulka Cost/Convenience scale	.08	.12	p < .05

Table 11−3 (continued)

Households in Windsor, Ontario in 1954
(Darsky, Sinai, and Axelrod, 1958, pp. 135−137)

	WMS	Other Insurance
Are you generally satisfied with current insurance?		
Satisfied	84.4%	52.5%
Pro-con	10.5	15.6
Not satisfied	2.4	15.6
Don't know, no answer	2.7	16.4

various aspects of this patient-provider relationship: continuity of care, information transfer, and humaneness.

Continuity of Care

Continuity of care is generally considered to be a basic component of good medical care and has often been linked to both consumer and provider satisfaction. (See the literature review by Becker, Drachman, and Kirscht, 1974.) It may also lead to better quality care (Steinwachs and Yaffe, 1978; Starfield et al., 1976). Although continuity may not be the most important factor for consumers (Lewis, 1971), it is a desirable feature after basic access needs have been met.

What is continuity? Does it mean obtaining care from one place or from one physician? Obviously, the distinction is important for the evaluation of group practices. On one hand, seeing the same physician allows the development of the greatest personal rapport (Becker, Drachman, and Kirscht, 1974). Information in patient records is often not recognized by primary practitioners, but recognition is better when the patient returns to the same physician (Starfield et al., 1976). On the other hand, while a solo physician may be the best source of continuity, if he or she is not available or a referral is necessary, then a group of physicians sharing records may be preferred.

Measuring continuity is another matter. The most objective means is to track patients when they have illness episodes and see where they go for care (Shortell, 1976). This clearly identifies discontinuities, but it does not necessarily distinguish between referrals and emergencies, nor does it determine which individuals have no continuous provider. Thus a second, more subjective, measure is whether a person has a "personal physician."

Only three studies directly compare continuity of care between HMO consumers and those in conventional systems. Condie and Lyon (1975) compare a group of HMO enrollees with people living in the same area. Regrettably, they do not control for socioeconomic variables or insurance coverage. In their 1972 survey 50.7 percent of the HMO enrollees always saw the same physician, in contrast to 56.6 percent of the FFS users. The differences between provider types in terms of the distribution across "always," "usually," "seldom," and "never" was not statistically significant. In 1974 the HMO enrollees were somewhat less likely to have continuity, and the FFS users were more likely to see the same physician. Although this resulted in statistical significance, most of the effect is the result of an unexplained improvement in continuity among the FFS users. In both years, about half of each group was *not* bothered by seeing different physicians.

Richardson, Shortell, and Diehr provide the best comparative data, using population-based samples of dual choice enrollees in Group Health Cooperative (GH) and a Blue Shield-type plan (KCM-BC). Overall, slightly more of the GH enrollees, 89 percent versus 87 percent, reported a usual source of care. Among those reporting a usual source under KCM-BC, 87 percent mentioned a particular physician and 7 percent a hospital emergency room. Among GH enrollees with a usual source, only 71 percent mentioned a particular physician, but another 18 percent identified the Group Health clinic, and 8 percent mentioned the GH emergency room (Richardson, Shortell, and Diehr, 1976, p. V-5). This suggests at least a lessened attachment to a particular physician, if not less continuity among GH enrollees. A more subtle analysis is reproduced in Table 11-4, which identifies the source of care for a particular illness episode. When the problem was perceived as "not very serious" or "urgent," the KCM-BC enrollees had a clear advantage in continuity. Not only did many more receive care from their usual physician, but only two-thirds as many went to *neither* their usual physician nor to their usual facility. For more serious conditions the situation shifts. More of the KCM-BC enrollees still saw their usual physician (more usually have an

Table 11−4   Source of Care for Illness Episodes Reported by Seattle Prepaid Health Care Project Enrollees in Group Health Cooperative (GH) and a Fee-for-Service Reimbursement Plan (KCM-BC)

| | Perceived Seriousness and Plan | | | |
| | Less Serious | | Serious | |
	GH	KCM-BC	GH	KCM-BC
Source of care				
Usual M.D. and place	43	71	40	50
Usual M.D. only	01	02	02	05
Usual place only	29	09	31	10
Neither	27	18	28	35
Total	100	100	101	100
N	(237)	(534)	(184)	(431)
Significance level	p < .001		p < .001	

SOURCE.   Richardson, Shortell, and Diehr, November 1976, p. V−43.

identified physician), but substantially more sought care away from their usual provider or place. Thus GH enrollees with serious problems have more continuity through their medical records.

Scitovsky, Benham, and McCall's (1979) study of Stanford enrollees in Kaiser and the Palo Alto Medical Clinic exhibits substantial differences in the regular source of care. A somewhat larger proportion of Kaiser members reported having an outside physician or no regular source (7 percent versus 3 percent). However, 51 percent of the Kaiser members identified "the plan," with no specific physician, as their regular source. Only 10 percent of the Clinic members gave a similar response. This may be a reflection of the more recent enrollment of Kaiser members, but it is more likely due to the essentially FFS nature of the Clinic and the strong incentives Clinic physicians have for maintaining a close physician-patient relationship.

In addition to these comparative studies, a number of single-setting studies examine the extent to which PGP enrollees feel that they have a personal physician. For instance, 65 percent of the Labor Health Institute (LHI) members who had used LHI physicians considered their LHI doctor to be their family physician. This may be contrasted to the 60 percent of that sample who reported having a family doctor before becoming eligible for LHI (Simon and Rubushka, 1956, p. 719). Seventy-five percent of HIP enrollees in one study had a regular doctor before joining HIP, and 39 percent still considered the former doctor their regular one (Anderson and Sheatsley, 1959, p. 53).

These findings are difficult to interpret, because there are few clear standards for comparison. Even among people consistently in the FFS sector, the family doctor is far from universal. In fact there is evidence that many people prefer to doctor-shop or change providers without referrals (Kasteler et al., 1976). Evaluating the HMO enrollee's experience is subject to bias, because joining usually entails changing physicians, and establishing new ties takes time. Thus the lower rate of identification with specific physicians may be a function of newness, not of the plan itself. This is a particular problem in PGPs, because the limited choice of physicians is more certain to disrupt continuity. Anderson and Sheatsley's study showed that 13 percent of the GHI enrollees who had a regular physician before joining either had none or a different one after joining GHI (1959, p. 53). This is surprising, because GHI is between an IPA and a Blue Shield plan in terms of choice of physician. A very large number of New York City physicians are participating members. Furthermore, seeing a non-GHI physician simply means that the patient may find that GHI will not guarantee full coverage of the physician's fee.

In summary, it appears that there is less continuity of care among PGP members, particularly if this is measured by the identification of a single physician. However, a group may provide better continuity in terms of record transfer when specialists are required or urgent treatment is needed. Comparative studies are particularly vulnerable on the issue of continuity. As is discussed elsewhere, one major reason people give for not joining a PGP is an existing close tie to a physician. Thus those who enroll in the PGP are initially much less likely to have had a close relationship with a physician. In fact, they may not value continuity very highly. A better test of the continuity question would be to interview people who moved to an area at the same time, and chose either an FFS or PGP plan. Then, controlling for the extent of their physician ties prior to moving, it would be possible to see whether there are differences between plans in the development of physician ties in the new setting. One should then compare objective measures of continuity, such as revisits to the same physician, with the patient's satisfaction with continuity of care.

Information Transfer

Two crucial activities in ambulatory medical care are the physician's obtaining information from the patient and the patient, in return, getting back information about his or her condition. The importance of the first is recognized in the key role given the history and reporting of symptoms in physical diagnosis. (There is evidence, however, that modern clinicians now rely much more heavily on tests than on careful histories and that a return to simpler techniques often would be advantageous.) (See Fox, 1977; Sox, Sox, and Skeff, 1979; Marton, Rudd, and Sox, 1979; Marton, 1979.) This may be even more of a problem in tightly scheduled group practices than in solo practitioners' offices.* The second information transfer, from the physician to the patient, is less well recognized by the profession, but is equally important in terms of patient compliance and satisfaction and in overall outcome (Korsch, Gozzi, and Francis, 1968; Francis, Korsch, and Morris, 1969; Waitzkin and Stoeckle, 1976; Vuori, 1972). Thus information transfer is vital for good clinical practice, and it is a factor that patients consider when they compare delivery systems.

Table 11-5 presents comparative data from various settings. In every instance, the PGP enrollees are less satisfied with the physician's willingness to listen and to explain. Two studies (Anderson and Sheatsley, 1959; Tessler and Mechanic, 1975) asked about both aspects. In both cases there

---

*Whether more histories or tests make economic, rather than clinical, sense, is another issue. In a prepaid setting, the organization gains no additional revenue for extra laboratory tests, while it does incur additional costs. But physician time is very expensive, and it may be more economical to substitute tests for doctors. FFS practitioners, on the other hand, do not charge by the minute, so they too have an incentive to reduce patient contact time and substitute tests, especially when the latter are highly profitable (Blanchard, 1975). A counterincentive is that one of the key things offered by the FFS practitioner is personalized service and a willingness to spend time with the patient, as demonstrated in this chapter. A substantial shift in this behavior would probably remove their major comparative advantage vis-à-vis HMOs.

Table 11−5   Comparative Studies of Satisfaction with Information Transfer

Union Members with Dual Choice of HIP or GHI, 1958
(Anderson and Sheatsley, 1959, p. 63)

	HIP			GHI		
	True	Not True	Don't Know	True	Not True	Don't Know
Proportion agreeing with the following:						
They don't give you a chance to explain exactly what your trouble is	16%	65%	19%	6%	69%	25%
They don't tell you enough about your condition; they don't explain just what the trouble is	26	51	23	9	67	24

California State Employees, 1971
(Dozier et al., 1973, p. 108) (These data are limited to those with some medical care in the preceding year.)

	Kaiser	Ross-Loos FHP	IPAs	BC-BS	Indemnity
Information given on what was wrong:					
Satisfied	78.9%	85.2%	89.2%	84.0%	84.1%
Not satisfied	17.4	9.9	7.2	6.6	6.6
No answer	3.7	4.9	3.6	9.4	9.3

Residents of Sault Ste. Marie, Ontario, 1973
(DeFriese, 1975, p. 144)

	GHC	Solo	p
Secretiveness of MD regarding hospitalization	4.5106	4.5369	n.s.

Employees of Two Midwestern Firms with Dual Choice, 1973
(Tessler and Mechanic, 1975, pp. 99, 100)

	PGP	BC	p
Among those receiving services in the past year, the percentage very satisfied with:			
The amount of information given to you about your health	64%	81%	<.001
The doctor's willingness to listen when you tell him about your health	78	86	<.05
Among those with children under 12 who received services in the past year, the percentage very satisfied with:			
The amount of information given you about your child's health	73%	84%	<.001
The doctor's willingness to listen when you tell him about your child's health	77	87	<.05

Table 11−5 (continued)

Low Income Residents of Seattle Model Cities Area
(Richardson, Shortell, and Diehr, 1976, p. V.56)

	GHCPS	KCM-BC	p
Proportion of families with dissatisfactions reporting:			
Illness not made clear—resurvey I	.05	.03	n.s.
II	.11	.02	<.05
III	.06	.01	n.s.

seemed to be even more dissatisfaction with the PGP physicians' willingness to explain than with their willingness to listen. This, in combination with the generally good ratings on quality of care in PGPs, suggests that enough time is allocated to get the crucial clinical information from the patients, but perhaps not enough to allow the expression of feelings and concerns.* Furthermore, PGP patients felt that their physicians often did not spend enough time explaining things.

Some apparent differences may result from particular organizations, rather than inherent HMO characteristics. For instance, the Dozier et al. study (1973) compares Kaiser, Ross-Loos/Family Health Plan, IPAs, and conventional plans. While Kaiser enrollees were found to be less likely to be satisfied and much more likely to be dissatisfied, the results for other HMO enrollees were different. The Ross-Loos/FHP enrollees, in two smaller group practices, were nearly as satisfied as those with conventional coverage, once one adjusts for differences in the proportion answering. As would be expected, IPA enrollees, who essentially see FFS practitioners, respond almost exactly like people with traditional coverage.

Overall, the evidence strongly supports the view that PGP enrollees are less happy with doctor-patient communication. There is more dissatisfaction with the amount of information given the patient than with the physician's willingness to listen. This is consistent with the general view that PGP physicians have less time and are not as warm toward their patients. The one available study shows no difference in satisfaction between IPA enrollees and those with conventional coverage.

Humaneness

The doctor-patient interaction involves much more than just information transfer. The importance of bedside manner is well known and extends

---

*Neither study directly offers any quality measures, so this statement is based on inference from other studies. (See Chapter 10.) The Anderson-Sheatsley data are from HIP, which performed well during that period, as demonstrated in other studies.

beyond the hospital; most patients respond positively to physicians who seem warm and show a personal interest in them. The quality of personal interaction with others in the medical setting also influences patient satisfaction. Sensitive nurses and receptionists may well make a greater impact than physicians. All of these may be considered under the heading of humaneness.

Table 11-6 presents the results of patient feelings about humaneness in comparative settings. The eight studies are reasonably consistent with respect to evaluation of the doctor-patient relationship. In every case PGP enrollees were less satisfied than those in other plans. In the Dozier et al. report (1973), IPA members were about as satisfied with the courtesy and consideration shown by their physicians as were the BC-BS or indemnity patients. The same report showed substantially more dissatisfaction among Kaiser enrollees and an intermediate level for Ross-Loos/FHP members.

Other items in the table concern the staff. In cases such as "personalized service," the issue is very general, while in others it is very specific. The Ashcraft et al. (1976) comparison of PGP and IPA enrollees showed higher scores for personalized service among the latter. The Medicaid beneficiaries in the Fuller and Patera (1976) study mentioned both personal and impersonal service at GHA.

Many studies include specific questions about nurses and other ancillary personnel. These results are mixed, with some PGPs doing as well or better than FFS providers. This is somewhat surprising, because one would expect the PGPs to be more bureaucratic and impersonal in their ancillary services, but perhaps to have similar doctor-patient interactions. Instead, the reverse seems to be true. The following explanation is consistent with these and other data. As was discussed earlier, the PGPs tend to schedule appointments more carefully and reduce waiting time, but this is often at the expense of continuity with one physician. Seeing the same physician is probably a critical factor in developing a close rapport and a sense of personalized care. The more rigid scheduling does two other things: it reduces the amount of time the physician can spend on patient interaction, and it results in shorter waiting times. The latter may lead to less interaction with "other personnel" and also less anger directed toward them because of long waits. Thus increased scheduling may result in shorter waiting times and better staff interaction, at the expense of close relationships with one's physician and good information transfer.

Quality

Various measures of the quality of care in HMOs are presented in Chapter 10. All of these are from the perspective of professionals evaluating the structure, process, or outcomes of treatment. Patients have their own

Table 11−6 Comparative Studies of Satisfaction with Humaneness

Union Members with Dual Choice of HIP or GHI, 1958
(Anderson and Sheatsley, 1959, p. 63)

	HIP			GHI		
	True	Not True	Don't Know	True	Not True	Don't Know
Proportion agreeing with the following:						
The people who make appointments for them are not very considerate	12%	62%	26%	6%	63%	31%
They don't take enough personal interest in you	25	52	23	7	70	23

California State Employees, 1971
(Dozier et al., 1973, p. 109)

	Kaiser	Ross-Loos FHP	IPAs	BC-BS	Indemnity
Courtesy and consideration shown by nurses:					
Satisfied	88.7%	91.4%	88.7%	88.2%	86.6%
Not satisfied	8.2	5.0	5.5	2.5	3.5
No answer	3.1	3.6	5.8	9.3	9.9
Courtesy and consideration shown by doctors:					
Satisfied	87.0%	92.4%	93.3%	89.4%	89.8%
Not satisfied	9.8	4.0	2.6	1.7	1.8
No answer	3.2	3.6	4.1	8.9	8.4

Sample of Los Angeles Medicaid Enrollees
(Gibbens, 1973, p. 12)

	CMS	Plan X	Fee for Service
Staff pleasant?	91%	90%	94%
Doctor really interested in your health?	81	79	91

Residents of Sault Ste. Marie, Ontario, 1973
(DeFriese, 1975, p. 144)

	GHC	Solo	p
Receptionist's courtesy	4.6942	4.7147	n.s.
Receptionist's helpfulness	4.7179	4.6726	n.s.
Lab service courtesy	4.8151	4.6265	<.001
X-ray courtesy	4.8717	4.6605	<.001
Pleasantness of telephone for doctor appointment	4.6378	4.6200	n.s.
Pleasantness of telephoning to talk with doctor	4.1450	4.3977	<.05
In general, pleasantness	4.7332	4.7279	n.s.
In general, impersonality	4.1948	4.3831	<.05

274

Table 11–6 (continued)

Employees of Two Midwestern Firms with Dual Choice, 1973
(Tessler and Mechanic, 1975, p. 99)

	PGP	BC	p
Among those receiving services in the past year, the percentage very satisfied with:			
The doctor's concern about your health	70%	85%	<.001
The doctor's warmth and personal interest	67	83	<.001
The doctor's friendliness	79	89	<.001
Friendliness of nurses, receptionists, etc.	81	84	n.s.

(Nearly identical results are reported for satisfaction with children's care.)

Washington, D.C., Medicaid Beneficiaries
(Fuller and Patera, 1976, pp. T–44–45)

	PGP enrollees	Controls
Things liked or disliked about delivery system		
Proportion mentioning personalized service	31%	1%
Proportion mentioning impersonal service	12	4

Employees of One Rochester, NY firm, with Quadruple Choice
(Ashcraft et al., 1976)

	PGPs	FMC
Satisfaction with personalized care	4.34	4.69

Low Income Residents of Seattle Model Cities Area
(Richardson, Shortell, and Diehr, 1976, pp. V.56, 59, 62)

	GHCPS	KCM-BC	p
Proportion of families with dissatisfaction mentioning:			
Health professional's attitude	.32	.19	<.01
Receptionist's attitude poor	.01	.05	n.s.
Proportion of all families reporting they:			
Had been made to feel they were bothering the doctor or nurse	.14	.07	
Felt doctor or nurse thought they were not capable of understanding much	.12	.07	
Felt doctor or nurse did not particularly respect respondent's opinions	.13	.08	
Wondered why they had bothered to see doctor or nurse	.20	.13	
Hulka scale of personal qualities	.24	.29	<.01

perceptions of quality, which may or may not coincide with those of the professionals. But to the extent that quality is in the mind of the beholder, consumer satisfaction with quality is a crucial measure of performance.

The question arises: if there is so much controversy in the professional literature about what quality means, how can patients evaluate it? Perhaps a more relevant question is: what are patients really evaluating when they talk about quality? Direct answers to these questions are not available, but some studies with several questions offer some hints. Table 11-7 presents the findings of comparative studies of patient evaluations of quality. As was the case with professional evaluations, the results are mixed, although there is a greater tendency for patients to be negative about HMOs.

One aspect of quality is that the physician does what the patient wants. Patients often decide what is wrong with them, develop a treatment plan, and then go to a physician for confirmation and access to prescription drugs and other therapy (Freidson, 1960). If they do not get what they want from one physician, they continue to change physicians until they are satisfied. (For a clear illustration of this with respect to surgery, see McCarthy and Finkel, 1978.) While this type of behavior can be undertaken easily in an IPA, it is more difficult in a PGP setting. Some specific complaints about quality reflect these issues. For instance, complaints about unwillingness to get opinions from other doctors in HIP (Anderson and Sheatsley, 1959) and disagreements with diagnoses in GHCPS (Richardson, Shortell, and Diehr, 1976).

A second aspect of perceived quality is the availability and use of technology. While their evaluations of HIP and other physicians were comparable, HIP members felt that the quality of care in HIP was better. Freidson suggests that this was due to their evaluation of technical facilities (1961, p. 63). DeFriese (1975) found that GHC enrollees gave higher scores for laboratory and X-ray competence than did patients of solo practitioners. But these issues seem to be plan-specific. In Tessler and Mechanic's study (1975) the PGP enrollees were less satisfied with the adequacy of the office and equipment.

Two studies involve PGPs and IPAs. In the Dozier report, after correcting for people with no opinion, the IPA scored at the top, along with BC-BS and indemnity carriers. Kaiser and Ross-Loos/FHP enrollees were less satisfied with quality. Ashcraft et al. found that enrollees with PGP or IPA coverage evaluated their quality of care about equally.

Overall, consumer evaluation of HMO quality is mixed and perhaps somewhat more negative than evaluations of FFS practices. This may reflect differences in what is being evaluated. The consumer may respond to a gestalt and be more sensitive to whether the organization meets his or her perceived needs and expectations. Not all of these expectations are congruent with professionally defined quality standards. Each type of evaluation is probably valid for different purposes.

Table 11-7 Comparative Studies of Satisfaction with Physician's Quality or Competence

HMO Enrollees in Salt Lake City and FFS Patients in Same Neighborhoods
(Condie and Lyon, 1975)

	HMO Enrollees		FFS	
	1972	1974	1972	1974
Perception of own medical care compared with other residents:				
Much better	24.9%	20.7%	14.0%	15.4%
Somewhat better	25.1	26.4	21.1	25.1
About the same	44.9	48.4	59.2	54.7
Somewhat worse	4.5	3.8	4.5	4.6
Much worse	0.6	0.7	1.2	0.2

$p=.07$

$p=.00002$

$p=.33$ $p=.16$

Interviews with Employees of One Firm in Rochester, NY with Multiple Choice among Two PGPs, an IPA and BC-BS
(Ashcraft et al., 1976, Table 8)

	PGPs	IPAs
Mean score on 5-point scale for quality of care	4.73	4.77

Low-Income Residents of Model Cities Area in Seattle
(Richardson, Shortell, and Diehr, 1976, V−A14, p. V−52)

	GHC	KCM-BC	
Proportions of individuals reporting one or more dissatisfactions with treatments received:			
Survey I	.16	.11	
Survey II	.12	.07	
Survey III	.18	.07	
Reasons for dissatisfaction:			
Disagree with doctor's diagnosis	.54	.49	
Doctor was ineffective	.44	.33	
Office waiting time	.04	.24	$p < .01$
Diagnosis not made clear	.10	.09	
Hulka professional competence scores	.21	.24	$p < .02$

Employees of Two Firms with Dual Choice Between a PGP and BC-BS
(Tessler and Mechanic, 1975, p. 99)

	Prepaid Group	Blue Cross	p value
Percentage very satisfied with:			
Quality of medical care received	77%	88%	$p < .001$
Doctor's training and technical competence	78	93	$p < .001$
Adequacy of office facilities and equipment	84	93	$p < .001$

(Nearly identical results are reported for satisfaction with children's care.)

Table 11-7 (continued)

Persons in Sault Ste. Marie, Ontario, covered by National Health Insurance. Some are primarily users-members of the Group Health Center, others use solo practitioners.
(DeFriese, 1975, p. 144)

Score on Osgood style semantic differential with 5 as the most positive score:

	GHC	Solo	p value
Lab service competence	4.8120	4.6711	p < .01
X-ray competence	4.8800	4.7121	p = .0001
In general, competence	4.7513	4.7500	n.s.

Members of the HIP Montefiore Group
(Freidson, 1961, pp. 62−63)

	HIP	Non-HIP practice
"Did you or your wife or husband ever have a doctor who seemed to be incompetent?		
Yes, a HIP doctor	10%	
Yes, a non-HIP doctor		10%
"Does it seem to you that on the whole HIP doctors are better doctors than the ones you had before joining HIP?"		
Yes, HIP doctors are better	13	
No, non-HIP doctors are better		10
"Do you think that on the whole you've gotten better medical care from the Montefiore Medical Group than you got from the non-HIP doctors before you belonged to HIP?"		
Yes, HIP is better	45%	—
No, non-HIP is better	—	13%
(eliminating those with no regular doctor prior to joining HIP)		
Yes, HIP is better	43	—
No, non-HIP is better	—	16

Union Members with Dual Choice Between HIP and GHI
(Anderson and Sheatsley, 1959, p. 63)

	HIP			GHI		
	True	Not True	Don't Know	True	Not True	Don't Know
They don't like to get other doctors' opinions about your condition	11%	36%	53%	9%	49%	42%

California State Employees
(Dozier et al., 1973, p. 106)
These data are limited to people with some medical care in the preceding year.

	Kaiser	Ross-Loos/ FHP	IPAs	BC-BS	Indemnity
Quality of medical care:					
Satisfied	87.8%	87.3%	95.1%	88.5%	88.5%
Not satisfied	8.6	7.6	2.4	3.0	3.1
No answer	3.6	5.1	2.5	8.5	8.4

Overall Satisfaction

General questions concerning the overall satisfaction level among enrollees are difficult to evaluate, because respondents can interpret them in varying ways. Such overall measures are, however, useful summary indicators and may well represent the enrollee's own evaluation of how the plan does on various submeasures, as well as of the relative importance assigned each aspect.

Table 11-8 presents the findings of the comparative studies of overall satisfaction measures. While the results are mixed, HMOs tend to score somewhat worse than the conventional settings. There are few patterns in these data. Two studies include IPAs. In one, the enrollees are more satisfied, and in the other they are less satisfied. Among the PGPs there are slightly more studies in which they score lower than conventional providers, but the results vary with the exact measure chosen. For instance, more GHA members than FFS enrollees are very satisfied, and more are very dissatisfied (Fuller and Patera, 1976). In contrast, among Ross-Loos enrollees, fewer are very satisfied, and more are very dissatisfied (Hetherington, Hopkins, and Roemer, 1975). Sometimes the overall evaluations are consistent with generally positive or negative feelings about specific aspects of the settings (Richardson, Shortell, and Diehr, 1976; Anderson and Sheatsley, 1959). In other cases the whole is not simply the sum of its parts (DeFriese, 1975).

In two cases data are presented as mean values on a Hulka scale, and the PGPs scored significantly lower in both (DeFriese, 1975; Richardson, Shortell, and Diehr, 1976). In both studies, samples were drawn from geographically circumscribed areas with complete dual choice available to enrollees at no additional cost. This situation of equal cost and convenience is nearly unique among the available studies and in practice. Yet, despite the absence of economic incentives, these people chose to remain members of their HMOs. This was true even though they demonstrated lower satisfaction levels. This raises several alternative explanations. One is general inertia in the face of deteriorating conditions. A second is that they truly prefer certain aspects of the HMO and chose to stay and exercise the voice option in the hope that they could remedy the situation (Hirschman, 1970). A third explanation is that the Hulka scores are not good predictors of choice of plan. The next section pursues this point by reviewing the evidence on behavioral measures, such as outside utilization and disenrollment.

As an introduction to using behavioral correlates as overall measures of satisfaction, it may be helpful to examine first the relative importance of various expressed measures of satisfaction (Aday, Andersen, and Anderson, 1977) Table 11-9 presents the proportion of people in a national survey who were dissatisfied with various aspects of care. Cost and waiting time were far at the top of the list. It must be remembered, however, that while waiting time for HMO enrollees may be only somewhat better, their

Table 11–8   Comparative Studies of Overall Satisfaction

Medicaid Enrollees in Washington, D.C.
(Fuller and Patera, 1976, Table 45)

	PGP Enrollees	Controls
Satisfaction with overall care:		
Very satisfied	39%	20%
Satisfied	50	76
Dissatisfied	9	3
Very dissatisfied	1	0
Don't know or no data	1	1

Low-Income Residents of Model Cities Area in Seattle
(Richardson, Shortell, and Diehr, 1976)

	GHC	KCM-BC	
Percent citing at least one dissatisfaction			
Survey I	35%	27%	
Survey II	33	20	
Survey III	26	15	
Hulka overall score	.18	.22	$p < .01$

Enrollees in Six Health Insurance Plans in Los Angeles County
(Hetherington, Hopkins, and Roemer, 1975, p. 255)

Opinion of medical care:	Kaiser	Ross-Loos	Large comm.	Small comm.	Blue Cross	Blue Shield
highly satisfied	27.3	13.4	26.4	17.2	31.7	12.5
	17.8	16.1	21.8	25.4	14.5	30.2
	32.7	32.1	6.4	21.5	3.7	3.7
	7.3	12.4	7.1	4.7	8.3	8.4
	14.8	18.8	20.7	17.7	20.1	18.6
	2.3	8.4	4.8	8.5	2.0	8.1
	1.3	2.3	1.5	1.4	2.5	10.1
	0.5	3.0	5.3	1.1	2.2	2.4
highly dissatisfied	2.6	2.1	5.7	6.4	11.8	2.7

Households in Windsor, Ontario in 1954
(Darsky, Sinai, and Axelrod, 1958, p. 122)

	WMS	Others	None
"Are you generally satisfied with your regular doctor?"			
Very satisfied or satisfied	95.0%	98.0%	94.7%
Pro-con	1.3	2.0	1.7
Not too satisfied, dissatisfied	2.1	0	1.0
Don't know, not ascertained	1.0	0	1.7

Residents of Sault Ste. Marie, Ontario, covered by National Health Insurance
(DeFriese, 1975, p. 143)

	GHC	Solo	p value
Overall Hulka scale	5.6596	5.7221	p=.04

Table 11—8 (continued)

Union Members with Dual Choice of HIP or GHI, 1958
(Anderson and Sheatsley, 1959, p. 61)

	HIP	GHI
Taking everything into consideration, would you say you are:		
Entirely satisfied	47%	55%
Fairly well satisfied	32	35
Dissatisfied	12	3
Don't know	9	7

(The above data are for respondents. Very similar results are presented for married persons' spouses.)

California State Employees and Annuitants Enrolled in Various Plans in 1963
(Dozier et al., 1968, p. 60)

	PGPs	IPAs	BC-BS	Indemnity
For those with some ambulatory care in January—March 1963:				
How do you feel about the care received?				
Satisfied	86.6%	91.9%	90.7%	89.9%
Not entirely satisfied	11.0	6.5	7.7	7.8
Dissatisfied	2.5	1.8	1.7	2.5
For those with some hospital care in July 1962—March 1963:				
How do you feel about the care received?				
Satisfied	89.0%	92.7%	87.7%	86.3%
Not entirely satisfied	8.2	6.1	9.1	12.0
Dissatisfied	3.0	1.2	3.3	1.9

Blue Collar Workers Enrolled in Three Different, Geographically Distinct Plans
(Columbia University, 1962a, pp. 54, 88, 118)

	Kaiser	BC-BS	Indemnity
"How do you feel about _____ ?"			
Very well satisfied	56%	45%	33%
Fairly well satisfied	36	47	50
Not satisfied	7	8	16
No opinion	(5)	(8)	(20)

---

financial coverage for ambulatory visits is substantially better than that of most people with conventional insurance. Since cost is no longer an issue for HMO enrollees unless they choose to leave the plan, differences in satisfaction will be based on other factors. Pope (1978) uses multiple regression techniques to determine those factors that (a) are associated with higher levels of satisfaction or (b) discriminate between current and former subscribers. Having a regular doctor and perceived health status were significantly related to higher satisfaction and continuing membership.

Table 11−9   Percentage of Respondents Dissatisfied with Various Aspects of Their Most Recent Physician Visit, United States, 1976

Aspects of Care[a]	Percent Dissatisfied[b]
Cost: The out-of-pocket cost of the medical care received[c]	37 (1.1)
Office waiting time: The amount of time you had to wait to see a doctor, once there	28 (0.8)
Information: The information provided about what was wrong with you or what was being done for you	18 (0.7)
Getting to care:	
The cost of getting to the doctor's office	13 (0.6)
The amount of time it took you to get to the doctor's office	12 (0.6)
Quality of care: The quality of care you felt was provided at that visit	13 (0.6)
Doctor courtesy: The courtesy and consideration shown you by the doctors	8 (0.5)
Nurse courtesy: The courtesy and consideration shown you by the nurse or nurses there[d]	7 (0.5)

SOURCE.   Aday, Andersen and Anderson, November-December 1977, p. 513.
[a] Listed in order of percentage dissatisfied, from largest to smallest percentages.
[b] Includes those moderately, slightly, or not at all satisfied.
[c] Respondents who reported no out-of-pocket cost for the visit were not asked this question.
[d] Respondents who had no contact with a nurse were not asked this question.

Shortell et al. (1977) use a multiequation, causal model to evaluate various dimensions of performance and satisfaction among enrollees in the Seattle Prepaid Health Care Project. In order to include clinical measures, their analysis is limited to enrollees with hypertension. While satisfaction was higher among KCM-BC enrollees, there was no specific provider effect after controlling for other variables. Smaller family size, ease of access, and continuity of care were all positively related to satisfaction, as were physician qualification, the Payne PPI index, and blood pressure control. Williams et al. (1978) obtained similar results for diabetic patients in the two plans. The only major difference was a significantly *negative* effect of professional qualifications on patient satisfaction. Separate regressions for KCM-BC and for GH enrollees suggest different patterns of satisfaction among the two groups. Sex, continuity of care, and physician qualifications were important for KCM-BC enrollees but not for those in GH. Education and adjusted blood pressure were important for those in GH but not for those in KCM-BC. Only access and family size were significant for both groups. In general, physician and system factors were much more important in the KCM-BC regressions, while patient factors dominated the GH regressions. This suggests that, while differences occur across providers within PGP, they are much smaller than the variation across physicians in conventional practice.

BEHAVIORAL CORRELATES OF CONSUMER SATISFACTION

Some people can be unduly influenced by interviewing techniques so that their responses to questions about satisfaction do not represent true feelings. In such cases one may rely on behavior—giving people a chance to "vote with their feet." The very nature of HMOs makes it relatively easy to examine two behavioral correlates of satisfaction: out-of-plan utilization and enrollment-disenrollment decisions. But behavioral measures must be used with caution, because their meanings are often illusory. Despite these shortcomings, these data are valuable adjuncts to the questionnaire responses.

Out-of-Plan-Utilization

It seems logical that an "important indicator of consumer satisfaction might be the extent to which subscribers to prepaid group practice plans continue to use services outside the plans in preference to the corresponding services available to them within the plans" (Donabedian, 1969, p. 9). In fact, there is substantial evidence of a negative correlation between utilization and expressed satisfaction (Freidson, 1961, p. 119; Bashshur, Metzner, and Worden, 1967, p. 1998; Pope, Greenlick, and Freeborn, 1972, pp. 8-12; Hetherington, Hopkins, and Roemer, 1975, p. 271; Kasteler et al., 1976; Ashcraft et al., 1976; Franklin and McLemore, 1970a,b; Scitovsky, 1979). The reasons for this negative correlation are less clear. One explanation is that people try the HMO's services, dislike them, and then choose outside care at substantial extra cost. Another is that some people have never had much experience with the plan, and therefore, are less positive about it because of ignorance. (It is important that almost all of the satisfaction measures in the preceding sections showed only small minorities of dissatisfied members.) However, no studies were found that combine the effects of experience, satisfaction, and outside use.

Some of this controversy can be avoided if types and levels of outside utilization are distinguished. Three distinct types of outside utilization occur: (1) services not covered by the benefit package (for example, chiropractors); (2) services covered by and paid for by the plan, even though provided out-of-plan (for example, referrals, emergency, or out-of-area); and (3) services covered by the plan and not paid for because the enrollee chose to use an outside provider. Only Scitovsky (1979) and Pope, Greenlick, and Freeborn (1972) make these distinctions. It seems perfectly reasonable for an HMO member to be very satisfied and occasionally use the third type of outside services. (Use of the other two types of services hardly seems relevant to measures of satisfaction.) Such outside use may include returning to a previously used specialist, urgent care not considered a true emergency by the plan, a second opinion, or services covered by other health care insurance. Careful examination of the reasons given in the available studies show that each of these is important for some people. Other people, however, almost never obtain medical care through the HMO. If they do have dual choice and yet pay for their care out-of-pocket, then such behavior is difficult to understand, unless they are just waiting for the next open enrollment period in order to switch plans.

Aside from these conceptual issues, the data concerning out-of-plan use, while seemingly objective, are really a hodgepodge of confusing, ill-defined figures. Table 11-10 provides capsules of the various studies, and Table 11-11 summarizes the key results. Aside from the definition of an outside service, there are three major definitional problems: the time period covered, the unit of observation, and whether one measured outside users or services. Some studies use a defined time window, such as the previous year, but others refer to outside utilization at any time during one's membership. The probability of occasional outside use is an increasing function of time, not because one grows to dislike the HMO, but because of increased opportunity. Although Freidson (1961, p. 121) proposes the first explanation, his data support the second. As can be seen in Table 11-12, the proportion of people who regularly use outside services remains constant at 10 to 11 percent per year. Thus the longer the period, the higher the proportion of outside users and the more likely it is that they are occasional, rather than regular outside users.

Similar problems occur with the unit of observation. There will always be at least as large or a larger proportion of families than individuals with some outside use, just because of the increased chances for an event to occur. Compounding this is the frequent situation of differential coverage of family members, so that the apparent outside use of a spouse may really be inside a different plan.

The third problem arises from confusion about the unit of measurement, users, or services. For instance, the Freidson study shows that 46 percent of the sample had used outside services at some time and Health/PAC (1973) reports that 55 percent of the Kaiser members responding to a questionnaire had used outside services during their membership. But only 10 percent of each sample were frequent or regular outside users. Measuring the proportion of services obtained through outside sources is more meaningful. The data in Table 11-11 tend to cluster in the 7 to 14 percent range. (There are two notable exceptions at 0.5 percent and 66 percent from Medicaid studies, which are suggestive of data problems.) These figures indicate that outside use does not substantially alter the utilization picture, but they say little about satisfaction. Reasons given for outside use vary widely and certainly reflect some

Table 11−10   Use of Services Outside the Plan

Simon and Rabushka, 1956, pp. 720−721

During the study year, 65 percent of the individuals received one or more services through the Labor Health Institute. (Not all families have coverage for dependents.) Of the 199 families, 36 percent reported that they used LHI for all their medical and dental care, 48 percent reported some outside use, 10 percent reported no illness but would have used LHI, 6 percent reported no illness, but would have gone elsewhere. The 95 families reporting outside utilization accounted for 780 such services, or 23 percent of all services received by the total sample. The outside users averaged 5.95 outside services per person, in contrast to 7.42 services of all types for all people in the sample.

Darsky, Sinai, and Axelrod, 1958, p. 128

Enrollees in Windsor Medical Services received a higher proportion of their medical services from other than their regular physician, 29 percent versus 20 percent for people with conventional insurance coverage. This is consistent with more complaints by physicians of WMS patients about "doctor shopping."

Freidson, 1961, pp. 112−134

Among HIP members of the Montefiore group, 12 percent reported having had an operation or delivery by a non-HIP doctor at their own expense at some time while being in the plan. Of these, 2 percent were for emergencies or noncovered services, such as cosmetic surgery. These figures exclude outside use covered by BC-BS and use reimbursed by HIP. Of the outside use, 75 percent was by the wife, 41 percent involved childbirth, and 26 percent "female surgery." In 61 percent of the instances, a prior physician was used. When examining medical services (that is, nonsurgical, nonmaternity), 10 percent reported regular outside use, 36 percent had occasionally used outside services, but relied mostly on HIP, and 54 percent had never used non-HIP services. The regular outside users remained a constant 10−11 percent regardless of time enrolled, while the proportion with an occasional use increased with length of enrollment, from 21 percent with ≤ 2 years to 41 percent for those in HIP 4+ years.

Columbia University, 1962a, pp. 108−113

Among the Northern California Kaiser enrollees in 1958, only 8 percent of all hospitalizations were out-of-plan. Some of these were for excluded conditions, some were to return to previously used hospitals, and a few were by patients with indemnity coverage in addition to Kaiser. Excluding visits to industrial physicians, 14 percent of office and home visits were out-of-plan. One third of the families reported some out-of-plan use. Wives had nearly twice the out-of-plan use as men. (However, men had somewhat better Kaiser coverage.) Out-of-plan physician and hospital costs averaged $30.19 per Kaiser family.

Bashshur, Metzner, and Worden, 1967, p. 1998

A sample of auto workers who were members of CHA in Detroit reported that over a three-year period 36 percent of the families had some outside utilization.

Smillie, 1972, p. 290

A survey of northern California Kaiser members in 1971 indicated the following: 98 percent of families had used some Kaiser services, 49 percent within the last month. Within the preceding two years, 54 percent of the families used ten or more Kaiser services, while 35 percent had gone to non-Kaiser sources. Of the outside users, one-third had only one visit and another third had two-three visits. (Thus only 12 percent of the families had more than three outside visits.) Of all outside visits, 22 percent were for emergencies and were reimbursed by Kaiser, 8 percent were job related and treated through worker's compensation, and 16 percent were to chiropractors, podiatrists, and others not on Kaiser staff.

Pope, Freeborn, and Greenlick, 1972

Interviews with a random sample of Kaiser-Portland members, who had been continuously enrolled for 1969−70, indicate that 8 percent reported outside utilization in the previous year. These were for covered services available at K-P (6.4%), covered but not available (1.6%), not covered but available (.07%), and not covered and not available (.22%).

Health/PAC, 1973

A mail survey of 10,000 members of the Carpenter's Union with Kaiser coverage in Northern California resulted in a 24 percent response rate. Within this sample, 55 percent reported using some non-Kaiser services since becoming members, and 78 percent of them had to pay for those services. Of the outside users, 19 percent are frequent users, 32 percent had used them several times, and 49 percent only once or twice. A substantial fraction reported using a chiropractor or other services not offered by Kaiser.

Hester and Sussman, 1974, pp. 428−429

Substantial out-of-plan usage of ambulatory services was found for Medicaid enrollees in HIP. HIP reported an average of 2.0 visits per enrollee in 1973, while the Department of Social Services reported 1.3 visits to voluntary hospital clinics, 0.7 visits to municipal clinics, and 1.8 visits to private physicians, for a total of 3.8 visits per enrollee.

Hetherington, Hopkins, and Roemer, 1975, p. 94

Based on data from medical records, among Kaiser enrollees, 10.5 percent of all physician visits were out-of-plan, while for the Ross-Loos enrollees, the figure was 6.9 percent. Data from the same survey for hospitalizations by type of plan are offered in Roemer et al., 1972, p. 39. Only 7.2 percent of hospitalizations by group practice members were not covered, in contrast to 26.0 percent of BC-BS members and 29.1 percent of hospitalizations by people with commercial carrier coverage.

Fuller and Patera, 1976, pp. 74−77

The Medicaid enrollees in GHA reported 64 out-of-plan services relative to a total of 11,578 services in the year, or .5 percent. (However, Fuller and Patera note that their data probably underestimate the true value.) Most of these services were for prescription drugs when the PGP pharmacy was closed. Others were for services not covered by the plan's package or that enrollees thought were not covered. Some, however, were for doctor visits and even hospital and nursing home admissions in order to use the services of a previous family doctor.

Ashcraft et al., 1978

Of 83 PGP enrollees, 14, or 17 percent, of the families used some outside services. Those who used outside services had somewhat more visits per person and spent somewhat more out-of-pocket, but the differences were not significant.

Richardson et al., 1976, pp. I−33−34

Low-income people in the Seattle Model Cities area were enrolled in Group Health Cooperative under a dual choice arrangement. At the end of the first year, 19 percent of GHC enrollees reported at least one outside contact with a non-GHC doctor's office, emergency room, or clinic, or telephone consultation with a non-GHC physician. At the next survey, 18 months later, 16 percent reported outside contacts and the comparable figure for the final survey, at the end of 48 months, was 18 percent. These outside visits accounted for 10 to 11 percent of all visits in each period. Reasons for outside use are not given, nor is there any discussion of multiple coverage. However, among the KCM-BC enrollees (the other option), 10 percent of the enrollees had claims under coordinated benefits, representing 15 percent of all services. About half of this coverage was with KCM and half with other third parties.

Scitovsky, McCall, and Benham, 1979

Stanford University employees enrolled in Kaiser and the Palo Alto Medical Clinic were interviewed to determine their use of outside covered and noncovered services during the twelve months ending June 1974. Data are reported both for uncovered and covered services, but only the latter are of interest for this chapter. For covered physician and paramedic services, 20.3 percent of Kaiser enrollees used at least one service, in contrast to 15.8 percent of Clinic enrollees. The average number of services per enrollee was .62 and .50, respectively. A substantial fraction of outside covered services was provided free of charge by public clinics, through professional courtesy, by an employer health facility, or were covered by other insurance. Excluding such services reduces the proportion of out-of-plan users to 11.5 percent and 9.1 percent for Kaiser and the Clinic, respectively, and the mean number of visits falls to .36 and .31. For both all-covered services and "nonfree" services, about half of the out-of-plan users in each plan used only one such service, and 10 to 11 percent in each had six or more visits.

Greenfield et al., 1978

Claims records of Medicare beneficiaries enrolled in HIP were examined to determine the financial impact of out-of-plan use. Because Medicare legislation requires reimbursement regardless of source, out-of-plan use is reimbursible, subject to deductible and coinsurance provisions. Multiple visits may be included on a single form, so visit rates cannot be computed. During 1972, 31.3 percent of the HIP Medicare enrollees were reimbursed for out-of-plan services. Of this group 78.3 percent also used HIP services, and 21.7 percent used only nonplan services. Out-of-plan use was associated with hospitalization and more illness in general.

Table 11–11   Measures of Outside Utilization by HMO Members

	Period	Unit	Percent Outside Users	Percent of Services
LHI (Simon and Rabushka, 1956)	1 Year	Family	57%	23%
WMS (Darsky, Sinai, Axelrod, 1958)	1 Year	Individual		29% (use of nonregular doctor vs. 20% for non-WMS)
HIP-Montefiore (Freidson, 1961)	Membership	Individual	12% (operations/deliveries) 46% (medical)	10% regular outside users 36% occasional
Kaiser (Columbia Univ., 1962a)	1 Year 1 Year	Family Family	33%	8% hospitalization 14% office and home visits
CHA (Bashshur, Metzner, and Worden, 1967)	3 Years	Family	36%	
Kaiser-Northern Cal. (Smillie, 1972)	2 Years	Family	35%	12% only one visit 12% only 2–3 visits
Kaiser-Portland (Pope, Greenlick, Freeborn, 1972)	1 Year	Individual	8%	
Kaiser-N. Cal. (Health/PAC, 1973)	Membership	Individual	55%	10% frequent 18% several times 27% once or twice
HIP-Medicaid (Hester and Sussman, 1974)	1 Year	Individual claims		66% of ambulatory visits
Kaiser-S. Cal. (Hetherington, Hopkins, Roemer, 1975)	1 Year	Individual		10.5% of physician visits
Ross-Loos (Hetherington, Hopkins, Roemer, 1975)	1 Year	Individual		6.9% of physician visits
Kaiser and Ross-Loos (Roemer et al., 1972)	1 Year	Individual		7.2% of hospitalizations vs. 26–29% for BC-BS-commercial
GHA-Medicaid (Fuller and Patera, 1976)	1 Year	Individual		0.5% of all services
GVGHA/RHN (Ashcraft et al., 1978)	6 months	Family	17%	
GHCPS (Richardson et al., 1976)	12–18 months	Individual	16–19%	10–11%
Stanford Employees (Scitovsky, McCall, and Benham, 1979)				
Kaiser	1 Year	Individual	12% (20%)	29% (14% only once)
Palo Alto Medical Clinic	1 Year	Individual	9% (16%)	30% (15% only once)

SOURCE.   See Table 11–10.

Table 11-12   Period of Patient Enrollment in HIP and Use of Outside Services*

	Two years or less	Between two and four years	More than four years
Regular use of outside services	11%	11%	10%
Occasional use of outside services	21	36	41
Never used outside services	68	53	49
N	(133)	(81)	(418)

$\chi^2 = 18.13, p < .01$

SOURCE.   Freidson, 1961, p. 121.
* At any time during membership.

dissatisfaction with the quality, responsiveness, or range of services offered.

Once the data on outside utilization are corrected for methodological differences, they reflect a reasonably consistent pattern. About 5 to 10 percent of PGP members are regular outside users, while a comparable proportion of different people each year use an occasional service outside the plan. Overall, outside use accounts for 7 to 14 percent of all services received by PGP members. If outside use represents dissatisfaction, which it does to some degree, its extent is comparable to the proportion of members reporting substantial dissatisfaction in interviews. The question is why such people stay when there are alternative health insurance plans under a dual choice option.

Disenrollment Behavior

The dual choice arrangements available to most HMO members offer what may be the best single objective measure of overall satisfaction. Enrollees typically have the periodic option of changing plans, and one would expect them to exercise that option in order to find the plan they like the best. Several assumptions must be made when interpreting these data. First, they only measure people's preferences among the available alternatives. None of the options may be deemed satisfactory. Second, behavior often falls far short of the predictions of rational models. In particular, there appears to be a great deal of inertia, so that once in a plan, people stay unless something drastic happens. Inertia is most important in the short run, when a plan is trying to enroll new members and increase its market share. Over time, however, one can expect a plan to lose membership if it is consistently disliked by its enrollees. The potential for switching is not symmetrical between HMOs and conventional insurance plans. Most HMO members have had experience with traditional practice, so they have one or more alternatives clearly in mind. The same is not true of people with conventional coverage. HMOs, particularly PGPs, offer different and often unfamiliar styles of practice. For instance, about 16 percent of California state employees have switched plans at some point in time. The proportion ranges from 10 percent among those with conventional coverage to 22 to 25 percent for those in HMOs (Dozier et al., 1973).

When focusing on enrollee choice and turnover, it is crucial to distinguish voluntary from involuntary changes. The most important source of involuntary change is employment instability. If someone with HMO coverage switches jobs and the HMO is not offered by the new employer, then the worker is likely to disenroll. Pope (1978) examined the reasons given by people who left Kaiser Portland. Only 8 percent mentioned dissatisfaction and 5 percent cost, in contrast to 40 percent who could no longer obtain it through their employer and 28 percent who moved out of the area. (This is one reason for the mandatory dual choice option in the HMO legislation.) Turnover for all reasons combined can be high, on the order of 10 to 13 percent of all members per year (Densen, Deardorff, and Balamuth, 1958; Weiss and Greenlick, 1970, p. 458). For selected subgroups, such as thirty-five fifty-four-year-old members with two or more years in the plan, Kaiser reports annual turnover rates of 2.1 to 6.2 percent over a seven-year period, with an average of 3.5 percent (Cutler et al., 1973, pp. 198, 204).

Tables 11-13 and 11-14 present the summary data concerning choice during open enrollment periods. In most cases the exit rate, or proportion of enrollees who leave, is small, but there are a number of important exceptions. For instance, while Kaiser had a low exit rate among California state and UCLA employees in 1971, Ross-Loos lost enrollees at an above average rate. The low turnover rate among state employees enrolled in Kaiser should be contrasted to their greater dissatisfaction about various aspects of medical care reported in previous sections. People in the Seattle Model Cities Project were also more dissatisfied with the HMO option than with Blue Cross. In this case the dissatisfaction was translated into a much higher disenrollment rate, albeit one not very different from those in other studies.

The Ashcraft study (1978) is based on a small number of employees in a single Rochester, New York, firm with quadruple choice. These data are particularly interesting because they clearly demonstrate the impact of premium differences. In the first period the employer paid the full cost of Blue Cross or GVGHA coverage, while Rochester Health Network enrollees paid an extra $5.02 and those in Health Watch an extra $8.42 per month. Beginning in the fall 1974 open season the employer paid the full cost of all plans, resulting in a huge shift from BC-BS to Health Watch, an IPA that included most BC-BS physicians but offered more extensive coverage. Health Watch experienced very high utilization rates, and by fall

Table 11 – 13   Studies of Disenrollment from HMOs

Densen, Deardorff, and Balamuth, 1958

In the first four years of HIP there was an average dropout rate of about 9 percent, but this ranged from about 10 percent for those in the first enrollment year to 7 percent for those in their fourth year. These results, however, are largely reflective of the experience of New York City employees, who were the major source of HIP enrollment in its early years. Some of its other accounts showed much greater turnover rates, largely due to employment instability.

Moustafa, Hopkins, and Klein, 1971, pp. 32 – 41

This study examines employees of the University of California at Los Angeles who first enrolled in a health plan or changed plans in November 1967. There were 312 new enrollees and 157 changers, representing 5.8 percent and 2.9 percent of total eligible employees, respectively. (These figures differ from those reported on page 34 because they exclude people with no coverage through UCLA.) Questionnaires were returned by 160 new enrollees and 111 changers. Whereas Kaiser had 25.9 percent of the total market (UCLA employees in health plans), it attracted 34.2 percent of the new enrollees. On the other hand, Ross-Loos, with 4.9 percent of the market, attracted only 1.9 percent of the new enrollees. Kaiser was the source of 20.2 percent of the changers and attracted 42.1 percent of them. Its change rate was 2.2 percent of current enrollees in contrast to 2.9 percent overall. People who left Kaiser or Ross-Loos tended to cite unhappiness with services (73%) as their reason, rather than premiums, coverage, or advice of friends. In contrast, among Kaiser joiners, only 12 percent cited unhappiness with services under old plans, while 68 percent complained about not enough coverage.

Dozier et al., 1973, Annual Financial Reports of Public Employees Retirement System, Board of Administration for 1970 – 71, 1971 – 72, 1972 – 73.

HMOs substantially increased their market share among California state employees during the 1963 – 73 period. The percent of active enrollees in various years is as follows:

	1962 – 63	1970 – 71	1971 – 72	1972 – 73
Statewide service	44.9%	33.8%	31.0%	29.9%
Indemnity	36.1	30.8	29.3	28.6
Group practice	17.7	33.5	37.5	39.0
IPA	1.3	1.7	2.2	2.5
	100.0	100.0	100.0	100.0

An open enrollment period was held in February-March 1971 and about 5.5 percent changed plans. The exit rate for each plan was as follows: Statewide service, 8.5 percent; Indemnity, 6.0 percent; Kaiser, 2.4 percent; Ross-Loos/FHP, 10.3 percent; IPA, 7.7 percent. In 1971 about 16 percent of enrollees reported having switched plans at some time. HMO members were much more likely to have switched to their plans rather than being enrolled since the beginning of their state coverage. The proportion for each type is: Statewide service, 10.7 percent; Indemnity, 9.6 percent; Kaiser, 24.9 percent; Ross-Loos/FHP, 24.1 percent; IPA

21.7 percent. Overall, for those who changed either at the last period or at any time, about 20 percent were dissatisfied with medical care under the old plan. By far the most common reasons for change were that the new plan cost less or offered more benefits.

Kaiser Foundation Medical Care Program, 1974, p. 10

Surveys of members in Northern California, Southern California, Hawaii, Ohio, and Colorado were conducted from 1970 to 1973 by an independent survey organization. In answer to the question, "If you were given a choice right now, would you be likely to renew with the Kaiser Plan?" a "yes" answer was given 86 to 90 percent of the time.

Weiss and Greenlick, 1970, p. 458

Data are drawn from a 5 percent sample of Kaiser-Portland enrollees. A total of 2025 families and 5832 individuals were members at some time during 1967. The following figures give an indication of attrition: January 1, 1967—1640 families and 4597 individuals. By December 31, 1967, 1425 families and 4010 individuals remained. This implies a dropout rate for all reasons of about 13 percent within the year.

Cutler et al., 1973, pp. 198, 204

Two samples of Kaiser members were drawn to conduct an evaluation of multiphasic health testing. The member pool was 35 to 54 years old at entry and all had been Kaiser members for at least two years. The latter requirement was designed to reduce the dropout rate from the sample because "previous experience indicated members were less likely to leave the Health Plan after they had been members for two years." In the seven years of the study, the annual dropout rate for both the study and control groups ranged from 2.1 percent to 6.2 percent per year with an average of 3.5 percent.

Tessler and Mechanic, 1975, pp. 98, 110

Data are presented for the salaried employees of one firm who first had an HMO option in June 1971. At the 1972 reenrollment period only five of the 200 did not reenroll (2.5% dropout), and in the following year, only two left (1%). During this period, less than 1 percent of the Blue Cross participants chose to switch. Only half of those who said they would switch in Tessler and Mechanic's survey actually did so.

Fuller and Patera, 1976, pp. 87−93, T−48

During this period of July 1971 through February 1974 a total of 1056 persons were enrolled in the PGP. All had Medicaid eligibility redetermination waived for the duration of their enrollment, up to three years. They could, however, disenroll at any time and return to the Medicaid rolls. During the 32-month period, 175 individuals in 77 families disenrolled, a dropout rate of about 7 percent per year of exposure. Of the 175 people, the reasons for termination were ascertained for 157. Involuntary reasons, such as death, moving, incarceration, and admittance to a foster home accounted for all but 62 of these. This implies a voluntary dropout rate of 2.5 percent. Most of the voluntary dropouts expressed dissatisfaction with the

Table 11—13 (continued)

plan. Furthermore, the voluntary dropouts were more likely than the rest of the enrollees to be in families that were categorically indigent and thus automatically eligible for Medicaid. Thus the guarantee of eligibility for study participants probably served as a strong incentive for some people to stay enrolled.

Diehr et al., 1976, pp. II—204—206; Richardson et al., 1976, pp. I—110—111

Given the option of complete coverage under both the GHC and KCM-BC plans at no cost, about a quarter to a third of enrollees chose GHC. This varied at times and was somewhat responsive to encouragement in one direction or the other by outreach workers.

During the life of the Seattle Prepaid Health Care Project, there were nearly seven times as many transfers from GHC to KCM-BC as from KCM-BC to GHC, 329 versus 49. The population base in KCM-BC, however, was about twice as large, so the propensity to transfer was nearly fourteen times as high.

Ashcraft et al., 1978, Figure 2

Between April 1974 and Fall 1975 there were substantial shifts among plans. These data are shown below.

	April 1, 1974 Enrollment	Left	Joined	Stayed	Fall 1974 Enrollment	Left	Joined	Stayed	Fall 1975 Enrollment
Rochester Health Network	8	3	7	5	12	1	9	11	20
GVGHA	59	20	45	39	84	11	14	73	87
Health Watch	64	4	130	60	190	177	13	0	13

The massive disenrollment from Health Watch accompanied a substantial increase in premiums. Comparisons of disenrollees and continuing enrollees in the two PGPs suggest that those who disenrolled were more dissatisfied and found a greater difference between expectations and experience. The few continuing enrollees in Health Watch were relatively high utilizers for whom the $25 differential was worthwhile.

Wollstadt, Shapiro, and Bice, 1978

Medicaid beneficiaries in East Baltimore have the option of joining an HMO or the East Baltimore Medical Plan, or obtaining care from other providers. If enrolled, they would not be covered for out-of-plan services except in emergencies. Medicaid beneficiaries could disenroll at any time. During the 23-month study period (November 1971 to September 1973), 3138 individuals enrolled and 814 (25 percent) voluntarily disenrolled and another 636 (20 percent) lost eligibility. While the mandatory disenrollment rate was fairly constant over the period, voluntary disenrollment peaked 3.6 months after the plan opened. Those who voluntarily disenrolled had fewer in-plan services and much higher out-of-plan use than those who were continuously enrolled. Moreover, most of this difference is attributable to a much higher proportion among the voluntary disenrollers of people who used no plan services.

Table 11–14   Summary of Findings on Enrollee Choice in Open Enrollment Periods

	Exit Rate	Market Share[a]	Share of Changers Into
UCLA Employees, November 1971 (Moustafa, Hopkins, Klein, 1971)			
Kaiser	2.2%	25.9%	42.1%
Ross-Loos	4.7	4.9	0
University average	2.9	100.0	—
California State Employees, February-March 1971 (Dozier et al., 1973)			
Statewide service	8.5%	34.0%	
Indemnity	6.0	31.0	
Kaiser	2.4	32.0	
Ross-Loos/FHP	10.3	1.0	
IPAs	7.7	2.0	
Midwestern Company, Salaried Employees (Tessler and Mechanic, 1975)			
PGP: June 1972 open season, after 1 year	2.5%		
June 1973 open season, after 2 years	1.0		
Blue Cross	1.0		
Medicaid Enrollees in GHA (Fuller and Patera, 1976)			
Total annual dropout rate	7.0%		
Voluntary dropout rate	2.5		
Low-Income Enrollees in Seattle Model Cities Project (Diehr et al., 1976)			
Group Health Cooperative of Puget Sound	6.5%	31%	13%
KCM-Blue Cross	0.4	69	87
Employees of One Rochester, New York, Company (Ashcraft et al., 1978)			
Fall 1974 open season			
Rochester Health Network-GVGHA (PGPs)	34%	9%	~3%
Health Watch (IPA)	6	13	97
Blue Cross-Blue Shield	41	79	0.2
Fall 1975 open season			
Rochester Health Network-GVGHA (PGPs)	13	10	10
Health Watch (IPA)	93	41	0
Blue Cross-Blue Shield	NA	49	90

[a] Market share prior to switching.

1975, while the employer continued to pay the full premium for the other three plans, a $25 per month surcharge was made for Health Watch. As might be expected, almost everyone left.

These findings suggest that all aspects of consumer satisfaction do not count equally in determining behavior. In general, HMOs get the highest marks for their financial coverage, but they are often less well rated in terms of the other measures of consumer satisfaction. These enrollment data suggest that better coverage at a reasonable premium is often enough to maintain and attract members, even though they may complain about other aspects of the plan. Of course, financial coverage is not the only attraction. The Seattle Prepaid Health Care Project offered identical coverage at no cost to enrollees. Nearly a third chose Group Health Cooperative, and even though they were substantially less satisfied, they switched plans at a moderate rate of 6.5 percent per year. It should be remembered, however, that the identical, cost-free coverage was part of an experiment; actual costs of GHC members were substantially below those of the KCM-BC members. Any long-term version would require a premium differential, perhaps leading to shifts like those in the Ashcraft study.

Additional indications of consumer satisfaction are the long-term changes in enrollment patterns among people with dual choice options. (See Table 11-15.) The long-term perspective eliminates problems of year-to-year shifts in relative premiums and coverage. It also allows time for employees to gain first-hand experience or to talk to those who have, and thereby develop a more informed opinion of the plans. In almost every instance, the HMOs substantially increased their market share. The two major exceptions were Ross-Loos, which had not been trying to expand, and the two Honolulu HMOs, which together dominated the market as early as 1964 and could expect little further growth. These market-share data are the most convincing evidence that, despite consumer dissatisfaction with certain aspects of HMO performance, HMOs are preferred by a substantial and increasing fraction of the eligible population. It is also clear that no one type of plan—PGP, IPA, or conventional insurance—is preferred by everyone. (The dynamics of plan growth and organizational diversity are discussed in Chapter 14.)

In summary, the behavioral measures reveal that a small fraction of HMO members consistently use outside services, and a small group disenroll when given the option. They may, in fact, be the same people. Those who are dissatisfied enough to reject an HMO's services consistently should logically change plans as soon as possible. There may also be some people who use other providers for certain types of care and yet retain HMO coverage for other needs. For example, in some dual choice instances premiums for conventional insurance coverage may be substantially more expensive than for an HMO. At the University of California in 1979, Kaiser was free while Blue Cross coverage cost a single employee $209 a year. A relatively healthy individual might choose Kaiser with the intention of using FFS physicians for all ambulatory care and still save money. The record of long-term growth in the share of given enrollee groups implies that the levels of dissatisfaction are relatively unimportant. Among every cohort of new enrollees, there is a relatively small proportion who find that they do not like the HMO. These people become high outside users and eventually leave. Over time, additional people become dissatisfied for one reason or another and leave. These disenrollers,

Table 11−15   HMO Market Share Among Federal Employees in Selected Regions, 1964−73 and California State Employees, 1963 to 1971−72

	Market Share	
	1964	1973
Federal employees		
New York City		
Health Insurance Plan (PGP)	6.10%	13.10%
Group Health Insurance (IPA)	4.74	12.26
Seattle, Washington		
Group Health Cooperative (PGP)	19.35	32.73
Washington Physicians Service (IPA)	11.31	14.17
Honolulu, Hawaii		
Kaiser (PGP)	27.12	27.75
Hawaii Medical Service Association (IPA)	55.85	61.88
Los Angeles, California		
Ross-Loos (PGP)	1.43	1.27
Kaiser (PGP)[a]	a	30.02
	29.30	41.45
Washington, D.C.		
Group Health Association (PGP)	4.61	8.00
Denver, Colorado		
Kaiser (PGP) (began enrollment in 1970)	1.73	10.16
Boston, Massachusetts		
Harvard Community Health Plan (PGP) (began		
enrollment in 1971)	2.01	3.94
	1963	1971−72
California State employees		
Kaiser (PGP)	15.4%	32.4%
Ross-Loos and FHP (PGPs)	1.7	0.7
Individual Practice Associations (IPAs)	1.2	1.8

SOURCES.   ICF Inc., 1976; U.S. Civil Service Commission, *Annual Report of Federal Civilian Employment in the United States by Geographic Area,* December 31, 1973; Dozier et al., June 1964, p. 56; Dozier et al., 1973, p. 44.

[a] Kaiser began operations in the San Diego area in 1966. The bottom figures are based on federal employment in the Los Angeles, Riverside, and Anaheim SMSAs, while the top figures include San Diego.

however, are more than offset by people leaving conventional plans for HMO coverage.

SUMMARY

This review of the evidence concerning consumer satisfaction with HMOs, particularly PGPs, has resulted in two sets of apparently conflicting results. PGP members are often somewhat dissatisfied about various aspects of the medical care they receive. Some even turn their feelings into action and use outside services or disenroll. Yet enrollment trends within the same employment groups demonstrate that HMOs have tended to increase their share of the market. A more careful examination of the situation can reconcile these findings as well as other results.

The key to understanding satisfaction measures is to remember that people do not live in a world that has the simplicity of the researcher's categories. Instead, their environment requires them to make decisions, alter behavior, and reevaluate their new situation. The data clearly indicate that HMOs have tended to increase their market share within enrollee groups. Given the dual choice setting, those people who joined obviously felt that the HMO was the best option available. In making that decision, they weighed various factors—financial coverage, premiums, perceived quality, access, and the like. Some who join disenroll after gaining experience with the plan. Others remain members but use outside providers for some services. Most see the plan as their major or only source of medical care. In making these decisions, consumers use their own weights to evaluate the various characteristics of each alternative. One can assume that people with lower incomes might be more concerned than wealthy people about financial aspects. Similarly, busy people who expect to have few urgent problems are less likely to be concerned about the long time required to get an appointment in a PGP. They may be more concerned about waiting time in the office. The result of all these decisions in a dual choice setting is a substantial degree of self-selection. This is especially true for people who join an HMO because of the conscious choice that is required. Many people stay in conventional plans through inertia and ignorance of options.

Once people make a decision and join a new plan, their perception changes. People deal with parts of a situation and focus on those aspects that are most irritating (Simon, 1957). Thus, having joined an HMO to avoid the financial burden of conventional plans, they can consider the problems of information transfer, humaneness, or continuity of provider. There is little doubt that PGPs tend to score lower in these areas than do FFS providers. Yet the behavior of enrollees suggests that other features counterbalance these irritants. In many cases the financial advantages explain the behavior. The data suggest that relatively small premium differences can attract people despite negative attitudes about many aspects of the medical care delivery. But the Seattle Prepaid Health Project data strongly suggest that financial differences explain only part of the story. Enrollees in that experiment had identical coverage in both systems and paid nothing. Despite lower satisfaction among GH members on almost every dimension, a third of the sample chose the PGP, and disenrollment rates were comparable to those of nonexperimental settings.

Critical attitudes do not imply behavior change. In fact, HMO members tend to be generally more aware of and more vocal about their medical care. This leads me to be cautious in interpreting these satisfaction findings. HMO members may be more dissatisfied, but their behavior suggests that they have found the best option available to them. I tend to discount the use of satisfaction measures for absolute comparisons, although they are extremely useful in a relative sense. For instance, the scheduling of appointments has advantages and disadvantages. It makes the administration of a large medical practice much easier and also reduces waiting time for patients. Members like the short waits but are dissatisfied with the amount of time it takes to get an appointment, not seeing their usual physician for urgent visits, and feeling that there is not enough doctor-patient communication and warmth. People would like the plan to improve all these characteristics that bother them *and* maintain its low cost position.

TWELVE

Physician Satisfaction

As an article in a trade journal headlined, "The Two Barriers to HMO Success Are the Doctors and the Patients" (Anonymous in *Modern Healthcare*, 1974). Consumer satisfaction can be appropriately included as a performance measure, or as an index of success, but physician satisfaction with HMOs is a prerequisite to their development. In fact, a major difficulty in a national health insurance strategy relying on HMOs is that physicians have little incentive to establish such alternative delivery systems (McClure, 1976, p. 49).

By tradition and law, physicians are the pivotal element in medical care delivery. Their satisfaction with the work environment, broadly defined, is crucial to the success of the delivery system. This is generally not considered to be the case for other health care professionals. For instance, there are no discussions contrasting the satisfaction of such professionals as nurses, nurses aides, and social workers in HMOs as opposed to other settings. There are several reasons for this exclusive focus on the physician. First, only the physician can legally provide or direct medical care delivery. Thus HMOs must be able to attract a sufficient number of physicians. Second, the very idea of prepayment, which is at the core of the HMO concept, is diametrically opposed to the traditional medical reliance on FFS payment. In fact, even the now generally accepted role of third party insurers was bitterly opposed by much of the medical profession. Consider, for example, this statement in a 1934 professional journal, "No third party must be permitted to come between the patient and his physician in any medical matter" (American Medical Association, 1934; Numbers, 1978). The HMO concept goes further, and as we shall see, it may well lead to important changes in the traditional doctor-patient relationship. Third, unlike other health care professionals, for most physicians independent private practice is a viable, attractive alternative to a formal organizational framework. Fourth, because HMOs enroll consumers and, in essence, remove them from the traditional medical care market, they pose a potential economic threat to non-HMO physicians and hospitals in the area. This perceived threat led organized medicine to react with boycotts, refusal of hospital privileges, charges of violation of professional ethics, and other measures (Palley, 1965; Kessel, 1958; Yale Law Journal Editors, 1954). Several bitter lawsuits resulted in the cessation of such practices, and by the late 1950s an AMA report (written by the Larson Commission) could describe HMOs in relatively neutral terms (AMA Commission on Medical Care Plans, 1959). However, many battle scars remain.

These factors help to explain why the focus on provider satisfaction is essentially limited to physicians; they also reappear as key issues in determining physician satisfaction with HMOs. The first two points, the physician as the central deliverer of care and the resulting doctor-patient relationship, are crucial to the sections that follow. The second two points are important in terms of background and need to be recognized as subtly shaping people's views. For example, satisfaction is appropriately viewed as a continuum ranging from preference, to satisfaction (or acceptance), to dissatisfaction, to rejection (Rivkin and Bush, 1974, p. 305). Obviously, physicians who reject HMOs either never practiced in them or, if they have practiced in them, have left. Thus a survey of HMO physicians will be biased by leaving out those who reject the HMO model. Surveys of providers in traditional systems are similarly biased in the other direction. So information from those who decide to switch systems can be particularly valuable.

The concept of choice is important because of the readily available alternative of private practice. Thus for physicians to work within an HMO setting suggests that, at least at some point, they *chose* to do so. However, the situation is more subtle than the economist's traditional view of simple "revealed preference." Hirschman's concept of exit, voice, and loyalty (see Chapter 3) is particularly appropriate when discussing physician satisfaction with HMO practice (Hirschman, 1970). The transition from one form of practice to another is not easy. There are financial costs in moving and setting up new office arrangements, and the medical profession's disapproval of HMOs, particularly PGPs, raises the psychic costs of switching as well. Problems of status and professional ostracism were not uncommon in the early days of HMOs, and some of those issues linger. Hirschman's model suggests that, because entrance and exit are costly, HMO physicians are more likely to voice their dissatisfaction and attempt to change the system, rather than merely to leave. Furthermore, the model suggests that those who are most likely to complain are the physicians who are more sensitive to the qualitative aspects of their position.

The first section of this chapter reviews physician satisfaction with workload and income in various settings. Adequate payment is a necessary although certainly not sufficient condition for long-term satisfaction. Of course, adequacy is self-defined; for some, $20,000 in one job may be worth more than $100,000 in another job. A substantial part of what causes such different evaluations can be lumped under the heading of practice style, which is discussed in the second section of the chapter. This includes issues of professional ethics, physician control of medical care, and the doctor-patient relationship. The third section examines the entrance-exit, or recruitment-turnover issues. In most cases the discussion is limited to prepaid group practice, although in some instances general group practice issues are examined. Very few studies relate to satisfaction in individual practice associations, but when possible, they are included in the discussion.

WORKLOAD AND INCOME

Among the major advantages claimed for groups is that practice with a relatively large number of other physicians allows a work schedule with fewer night calls and longer vacations (American Association of Medical Clinics, AMA, 1970, p. 9; Center for Research in Ambulatory Health Care Administration, 1976). Paid vacations are sometimes over a month long, and some groups even offer sabbaticals of up to four months (Reynolds, 1972). The cash value of such benefits is probably less important than the flexibility of schedule and relief from patient care responsibilities. Prepaid groups offer similar advantages.

The physician's income depends upon the particular group's internal arrangements. Some provide for equal sharing of income, some have variations for certain specialties, some have an age profile for their salaries, and some essentially base income on productivity (Eisenberg, 1977; Beck and Kalogredis, 1977). The implications of the various forms will be discussed in Chapter 14. In almost all cases joining a group guarantees a comfortable starting salary, without the uncertainty and difficulty involved in developing a practice (Owens, 1973).

These references about reasonable workloads, income, and fringe benefits come largely from recruiting literature and general descriptions of group practice. Mechanic (1975) offers a valuable set of data from a national sample of pediatricians and general practitioners in solo, group, and prepaid group practice.* Table 12-1 presents data relevant to questions of workload and income. The general statements about shorter, less variable work weeks are partially borne out by the data. The key variable, however, seems to be *prepayment*, not *group practice*. General practitioners in both solo and group practice work an average of fifty-nine hours per week, while GPs in prepaid groups work a significantly shorter week—forty-nine hours. For pediatricians the results are similar. The differences in work week between group and nongroup pediatricians are not significant, while those between group and prepaid group pediatricians are statistically significant. Furthermore, although the coefficient of variation measures the variability of the work week *across* practitioners, rather than for a single practitioner *over time*, it is consistent with the hypothesis that PGP physi-

---

*The data for group practice include a small number of physicians in prepaid group practice.

Table 12–1   Workload and Income of Physicians in Varying Practice Settings

	General Practitioners			Pediatricians		
	Nongroup	Group	Prepaid Group	Nongroup	Group	Prepaid Group
Number of cases	(606)	(113)	(108)	(136)	(43)	(154)
Total practice related hours per week						
Less than 40	9%	6%	15%	7%	19%	21%
40–49	14	17	47	15	14	40
50–59	27	29	19	28	33	29
60–69	22	26	15	27	21	9
70 or more	28	22	4	23	14	2
Mean	59	59	49	59	54	47
Coefficient of Variation	39	32	22	28	35	23
Reported income group						
$50,000 or more	15%	16%	6%	21%	5%	5%
$40,000–49,999	21	20	14	15	9	17
$30,000–39,999	30	35	38	26	44	39
Less than $30,000	34	28	42	38	42	39
Average number of patients per hour in previous day[a]	3.4	3.3	4.0	3.2	3.0	3.8
Measures of satisfaction						
With amount of income						
Very satisfied	46%	47%	47%	37%	47%	45%
Not satisfied	12	11	10	20	12	16
With amount of time practice requires						
Very satisfied	35	33	47	27	42	52
Not satisfied	30	28	16	35	26	15
With amount of leisure time						
Very satisfied	25	30	41	26	35	44
Not satisfied	47	36	23	45	30	26
With amount of time for each patient						
Very satisfied	25	19	10	18	26	23
Not satisfied	38	39	49	43	23	31
Proportion agreeing that						
One should not become a doctor unless he is willing to work long and irregular hours	87	76	55	83	77	66
One should not become a doctor unless he is willing to sacrifice his own needs for those of the general welfare	55	37	31	49	51	27

SOURCE.   Mechanic, March 1975, Tables 1, 2, 4, 7, 8.
[a] These figures are derived from Tables 2 and 4 in the following manner. The numerators are from Mechanic's Table 2, which gives the mean number of patients seen during the previous day in the office and the distribution of practitioners, by whether they had 0, 1, or 2+ home visits. The proportion in the last category ranged from 1 to 9 percent with the exception of general practitioners in nongroup practice, 22 percent of whom had 2+ home visits. These solo GPs also had, by far, the lowest proportion with no home visits. Therefore, when computing the total number of office and home visits, the 2+ visit category was coded as four visits for all but solo GPs, who were given credit for six visits. (None of the overall findings are sensitive to these values.) The denominators in our ratio are drawn from Mechanic's Table 4 and refer to the amount of time in the previous day spent seeing patients in the office, talking to patients or doctors on the telephone, house calls and related travel, and administrative and paper work. Supplementary data in Mechanic's Table 3 indicate that, regardless of setting or specialty, the physicians spent from 80 to 83 percent of their practice time seeing patients. Thus the inclusion of administrative time in the hours data should not bias our conclusions.

cians have more stable work schedules. While PGP physicians tend not to work long hours, they also do not earn high incomes. Most prepaid groups have an income-sharing arrangement that results in a general leveling of income differences across specialties. This is most clear in the comparison between pediatricians in all groups and those in prepaid groups; the latter seem to benefit by such sharing. In fact, general practitioners and pediatricians in PGPs have similar incomes; these results are unlike those for non-PGP physicians (American Medical Association, 1974).

In summary, physicians' estimates of their work weeks suggest that PGP practitioners work substantially fewer hours, while income distributions indicate that they earn correspondingly less (Mechanic, 1975, p. 192). How do they feel about these levels of work and income? There is no difference across provider types in the proportion of general practitioners very satisfied or not satisfied with their incomes. Among pediatricians, there seem to be few differences between those in FFS groups and prepaid groups, while nongroup pediatricians seem less satisfied with their incomes. These results are initially surprising, given that nongroup pediatricians have the largest proportion in the top income category, and that PGP general practitioners earn substantially less than their counterparts in other settings.* The explanation apparently lies in the physician's evaluation of the time required by the particular practice. There is a relatively clear pattern of PGP physicians being the most satisfied with the amount of time their practice requires (and their leisure time). Nongroup practitioners are the least satisfied, and FFS group practitioners are in the middle. Thus nongroup pediatricians are dissatisfied with their high (objective) incomes because they see themselves working so hard for them, while PGP doctors are satisfied with relatively low incomes because they perceive themselves as having reasonable work weeks. This pattern is again visible in the low proportion of PGP physicians who think a doctor should be willing to work long, irregular hours and make great sacrifices for the general welfare. Furthermore, these results suggest that when physicians are asked about income satisfaction, they implicitly include an evaluation of their workload. In other words, some respond as if the question were: Are you satisfied with the income you receive for the work you do?†

Another important aspect of workload involves the intensity of work. An objective measure of this is the average number of patients seen per hour. For both general practitioners and pediatricians, physicians in PGPs see substantially (about 25 percent) more patients, indicating a greater

---

*The income figures are not precisely comparable, because the PGP survey was conducted in October 1972–April 1973, two years after the survey of the other physicians. However, the income changes in that period are not large enough to vitiate our comparison. Furthermore, in this case the bias is toward overstating the relative earnings of PGP physicians, thus strengthening the argument.

†This interpretation should not surprise economists, who have long considered the trade-off between income and leisure. However, the choice is particularly relevant and visible to professionals, such as physicians, who have an above-average normal work week and can directly control their hours.

work intensity. This is reflected in opinions about the amount of time available for each patient, a matter with which PGP physicians express dissatisfaction. The one anomaly seems to be nongroup pediatricians, who see a moderate number of patients per hour, yet feel overworked. This estimate does not include a heavy load of telephone consultations with patients (Mechanic, 1977).

A general ambivalence about the issues of workload and income is present in Mechanic's surveys, and it appears in a broad overview of the available studies on physician satisfaction. In some studies it is not seen to be a problem (Lum, 1975; Vayda, 1970; Dutton 1976; Ross, 1969), while in others it is the focus of substantial discontent (DuBois, 1967; Freidson, 1973, 1975; Freidson and Mann, 1971; Maloney, 1970; Prybil, 1971; and Ross, 1969). A closer look at the studies suggests some important patterns that explain at least part of the variation. However, with one major exception (Dutton, 1976), the studies deal only with a particular setting or type of setting. Thus comparisons across provider types are difficult.

Dutton's data are drawn from interviews with physicians who work in different practice settings and care for a sample of children living in the Washington, D.C. area. Two questions are particularly relevant for comparison with Mechanic's results: the level of satisfaction with (a) the total amount of time the practice requires and (b) the amount of time for each patient. The patterns of satisfaction for FFS providers in solo and in group practice are similar. For the total amount of time, about two-fifths are satisfied and less than one-fifth are very satisfied, while the remainder are dissatisfied. A similar pattern exists for the amount of time per patient; in this case more are very satisfied and fewer are not satisfied. Physicians in the prepaid group show a strikingly different pattern; none express dissatisfaction on either measure. With respect to the total amount of time, about the same proportion as the FFS providers are very satisfied, and essentially none are very satisfied with the amount of time per patient. The first result is contrary to Mechanic's (more would be expected to be very satisfied), and the second is also surprising (many more would be expected to be dissatisfied).

The other three studies indicating that workload or income are not problems have one thing in common; they all take the perspective of the plan or clinic administrator. Lum (1975) fielded a national survey of HMO directors in 1973. Over 85 percent expressed disagreement with the statement: "Physicians are reluctant to join an HMO because of high caseload volumes." Vayda (1970) provides a detailed discussion of causes of turnover in the Community Health Foundation of Cleveland during its initial five years. (Subsequently, this PGP was taken over by Kaiser.) Vayda notes that income apparently was not a problem in explaining the fact that thirteen of forty physicians left in that period, an annual turnover rate of 13 percent (1970, p. 164). His explanation is based on the fact that incomes in the group were comparable to those of physicians in the community and rose at about the same rate.

Ross (1969) surveyed clinic managers who were members of the western section of the Medical Group Management Association. (Most of the 134 clinics represented are FFS group practices.) They were asked questions about every physician who had left in the previous three years. Similar questionnaires were sent directly to each of those physicians. As viewed by the clinic managers, economic factors, such as low income, were only the fourth most important reason, after personal reasons, practice arrangement, and professional conflict. (See Table 12-2.) The second half of Ross's study provides a useful introduction to reports that not all is well with income and workloads as viewed by group practice physicians. When the physicians who left gave their reasons, economic factors ranked first. Ross theorizes that the clinics might feel threatened if economic factors were the main reasons for discontent, and therefore, they charge the termination off to professional conflict or practice arrangements. From the physician's point of view, relative income may be taken as a symbol of professional rankings within the group. Thus the income-workload concept may include a measure of relative worth, as well as intensity of effort. In fact,

Table 12–2   Reasons for Leaving a Group Practice as Seen by Clinic Managers and the Physicians Involved[a]

Rank	Primary Count ×5	Second ×3	Third ×1	Total
Termination Cause as Seen by the Clinic				
1. Personal, family, etc.	275	75	12	362
2. Practice arrangements	185	102	19	306
3. Physician relationship	185	102	5	292
4. Economic, low income, etc.	185	63	12	262
5. Other, miscellaneous	165	15	4	184
6. Future practice	75	24	5	104
7. Environmental	15	39	2	56
Termination Cause as Seen by the Physician				
1. Economic, low income, etc.	240	72	8	320
2. Personal, family, etc.	215	57	8	280
3. Physician relationship	185	57	8	250
4. Practice arrangements	115	66	11	192
5. Other, miscellaneous	145	6	1	152
6. Future practice	65	39	6	110
7. Environmental	25	21	5	51

SOURCE.   Ross, July 1969, p. 16. Reprinted with the permission of the Medical Group Management Association, 4101 E. Louisiana Avenue, Denver, Colo. 80222.
[a] Reasons cited as "primary" causes were given a weight of 5; those cited as "secondary" causes were given a weight of 3; and other reasons were assigned a value of 1. Unweighted responses give exactly the same rankings within each respondent group.

given the generally high level of physicians' earnings, typically in the top 1 to 2 percent of the nation's families, it is unlikely that the absolute level of income is a problem (U.S. Bureau of the Census, 1978; Dyckman, 1978). Instead, such economic evaluations are more likely to be made with respect to what physicians think they *should* be earning and the work they *should* be doing.

In a similar study Prybil (1971) obtained responses from a national sample of male physicians who left large, multispecialty group practices and remained in civilian medical practice. Their reasons for leaving are given in Table 12-3.* The most common reason was "income and/or income distribution," given by 42 percent of all the physicians. The next two most important reasons were "too much supervision" and "lack of personal control over working hours and/or workload," supporting the hypothesis that it is not so much the level of income as the working conditions that cause problems.

Various studies support these findings. For example, distribution of income was a major problem in a number of groups that failed (Dubois, 1967; Martin, 1953). The problem of too much work is not limited to physicians in groups. National surveys of physicians show substantial dissatisfaction with the lack of free time, and they indicate that there is a movement toward reducing practice size and taking more time off (American Medical News, 1976; Owens, 1977, 1978). Among a sample of physicians who left primary care, by far the major reason was overwork (Crawford and McCormack, 1971). In this instance workload seems to include both long hours (more than two-thirds worked sixty or more hours per week) and intensity (36 percent saw more than forty patients daily). This interpretation is supported by the new activities that they chose; nearly half went into psychiatry, anesthesiology, or radiology. Furthermore, 96 percent felt that group practice would be a useful strategy to enhance the viability and attractiveness of primary practice, and about one-half thought that prepayment or a guaranteed income would help. While the suggestions about group practice may be correct in leading toward a reduction in work week, there is some evidence that salaried practice does not necessarily lead to more satisfaction. Maloney (1970) examined an intensive survey of ninety-four clinical faculty in nine prominent medical schools. He found that nonsurgeons on a strict, full-time salary were the most dissatisfied with their incomes (relative to those whose incomes were partially dependent on clinical activities), despite the fact that they work fewer hours per week and earn the most per hour.

The most in-depth studies of physician satisfaction have been done in various New York City prepaid groups (McElrath, 1961; Freidson, 1973,

---

*Prybil also summarizes these responses using categories that are essentially the same as Ross's, and the patterns of responses are similar.

Table 12-3   Reasons Given by Physicians for Leaving Large, Multispecialty Groups

Response	Number of Responses	Percent of Responses	Percent of Physicians Giving Response
1. Income or mode of income distribution or poor retirement program	82	19.6%	41.6%
2. Too much supervision and control	62	14.8	31.5
3. Lack of personal control over working hours or workload	44	10.5	22.3
4. Impersonal patient care within clinic	37	8.9	18.8
5. "A better opportunity"	32	7.7	16.2
6. Conflict with other physicians	28	6.7	14.2
7. Did not like city or region or climate	28	6.7,	14.2
8. Disagreement over department or clinic administrative policies	22	5.3	11.2
9. Excessive numbers of allied health workers or equipment, resulting in high overhead	19	4.5	9.6
10. Constraints on patient referrals or consultations with nongroup physicians	17	4.1	8.6
11. Disagreement over clinic goals or objectives	16	3.8	8.1
12. Lack of opportunity to concentrate on specialty or subspecialty	16	3.8	8.1
13. Personal or health related factors	10	2.4	5.1
14. Hostility toward multispecialty group practice by nongroup physicians	5	1.2	2.5
Total Responses	418	100.0	197
Total number of physicians giving responses	—	—	—

SOURCE.   Prybil, September 1971, pp. 6, 24. Reprinted with permission from the Medical Group Management Association, 410 E. Louisiana Avenue, Denver, Colorado 80222.

1975).* Both report substantial physician dissatisfaction with work overload (Freidson, 1973, p. 475; McElrath, 1961, p. 602). McElrath found that those physicians who worked full-time or nearly full-time in the group were more likely than part-time physicians to say they did not have enough time to handle patients. (In part, this may be a reflection of specialty differences, a point to be discussed below). McElrath summarizes the physician's perspective in the following way: "For doctors with a high level of participation [in prepaid group practice] subscribers are viewed as demanding, complaining too often, and occasionally needlessly utilizing the services of physicians who feel pressed for time" (1961, p. 602). Freidson

*Both McElrath's and Freidson's data are drawn from interviews with and observations of physicians. McElrath's data are from several HIP groups in the late 1950s, and Freidson's data are all from one group in which all physicians were salaried. Although most of Freidson's results were published in the 1970s, the study data are from 1961–1963. And while he never identifies the group, it is likely that it is one of the HIP group practices.

(1973) expanded the concept of the "demanding patient" into a more comprehensive discussion of physician satisfaction; this is addressed below.

This review suggests one major point: physician satisfaction with prepaid group practice is dependent on much more than salaries and hours of work; instead, the style of practice is paramount. As is the case with most conclusions, once stated it appears to be obvious. After all, physicians' earnings are such that they are not likely to be sensitive to small income variations. Increased leisure, while a major plus, still does not satisfy many physicians. Nor is the patient load sufficient to explain their dissatisfaction. Instead, we must examine the more subtle factors involved in medical practice and professionalism.

STYLE OF PRACTICE

Many studies show that job satisfaction is related to factors other than economic reward, in particular, the amount of control over and the content of one's work. (See Stamps, 1978; Mechanic, 1976b). Physicians are among the workers most subject to such noneconomic considerations. Not only are their incomes generally high, implying that the marginal utility of an extra dollar is low, but medical training emphasizes the professional role of the physician (Menke, 1969; Vahovich, 1977; Seldin, 1977). Among the most important aspects of this professional role are the service ideology, autonomy, and rationality or quality.

The service ideology suggests that a physician's primary concern is for the patient, not economic gain or the fulfillment of personal needs. A key aspect of the service ideology is the relationship of mutual trust between physician and patient. The relationship is not one-sided; while the physician implicitly gives up economic gain and self-interest, the patient relinquishes power and initiative. (See Waitzkin and Stoeckle, 1976; Freidson, 1960). Whether or not the physician-patient relationship is appropriate, changes in it are not easily accepted by most physicians.

Physician autonomy and individualism are based upon the perceived need to respond creatively to the particular problems of each patient. The resulting challenges and stimulation provide the physician with opportunities for self-actualization and validation (Guze, 1979). Furthermore, the physician-patient relationship requires the exclusion of outsiders. This is demonstrated most clearly in the profession's adamant stance against "lay control," or the involvement of the uninitiated in medical matters.

The emphasis on rationality stems from the scientific orientation of modern medicine. Despite major biomedical advances, much in medicine still is based on tradition, intuition, and faith. (Engel, 1977; Seldin, 1977). In fact, the value the profession attaches to medical care quality seems inversely related to our ability to measure quality.

Despite the difficulties in evaluating quality, it is an important aspect of physician satisfaction. The remainder of this section examines physician satisfaction with three aspects of practice: the physician-patient interaction, autonomy, and the ability to practice good medicine.

Physician-Patient Interaction

Freidson (1973, 1975) presents the concept of the "demanding patient" as a problem for physicians in prepaid group practices. Although his data are from the intensive observation of one New York City group, and Freidson provides substantial evidence that the group was atypical (1975, pp. 19-23), his analysis offers valuable insights into group practice in general. (McElrath, 1961; Hetherington, Hopkins, and Roemer, 1975, p. 179; Lum, 1975, p. 1199; and Zako, 1976, p. 83, all discuss the problem of the demanding patient.) Freidson outlines three types of demanding patients: (1) those with complaints for which the physician can find no cause or cure; (2) those who attempt to use political influence or threaten to leave to support their demands; and (3) those who emphasize the contractual agreement with the HMO to support demands for service. The first type of patient is typically a supplicant and commonly appears in medical discussions as the "crock" or the "worried-well." Such patients are often seen as frustrating, because they do not get better. However, they do not represent a major threat to physician satisfaction. The second type of patient is relatively rare and also appears in various guises in traditional FFS practice. It is the third type, the bureaucratic or contractual demander, who was found to be particularly galling to the physicians. These patients did not conform to the usual patient role, and instead, argued forcefully that certain services were due them; if they were not forthcoming, formal complaints would be submitted. Freidson offers the caricature of the demanding patient as a "schoolteacher, sufficiently educated to be capable of articulate and critical questioning and letter writing, of high enough social status to be sensitive to slight and to expect satisfaction, and experienced with bureaucratic procedures. In the physicians' eyes, they were also neurotically motivated to be demanding" (1973, p. 484).

The key difficulty with this type of patient is that the contractual nature of the relationship with an HMO implies that the patient *does* have the right to medical care; but the physician is the gatekeeper in the system. Such patients cannot be easily shuffled off to other physicians. They remain within the system. Neither difficulty appears very often in FFS practice, if only because dissatisfied patients move to other physicians. But it may be that patients are becoming increasingly dissatisfied and demanding, especially as they perceive themselves as paying (or having insurance that pays) the full cost of care.*

---

*The traditional sliding scale of fees and perception of the overworked physician led people to cherish what they received. As public opinion toward physicians has become more negative, it is reasonable to expect patients to view medical care more as a commodity and physicians more as businesspeople, and thus be more demanding.

Freidson suggests two strategies for managing demanding patients. The simplest and most common is to give in to their requests, as long as this is not too expensive. Laboratory tests and X-rays typically cost nothing in terms of physician time, and they are not too expensive for the system; hospitalization, on the other hand, is not likely to be dispensed on request. The second strategy would require physicians to invest time in educating these problem patients in order to develop a relationship of trust. This method requires a greater initial effort, and some physicians are unwilling to play the role of educator or persuader (Heagarty and Robertson, 1971). Furthermore, the strategy, even if truly superior, requires changes in organization and incentives that may not be forthcoming.

While Freidson focuses on the bureaucratically demanding patient in the prepaid group, Mechanic (1975, 1976) emphasizes the importance of the more common neurotic patient with "trivial" problems, as a source of physician dissatisfaction. His national surveys suggest that pediatricians and general practitioners in prepaid groups are much more likely than either group or nongroup FFS physicians to perceive a large fraction of their patients' visits as trivial, unnecessary, or inappropriate. In fact, the PGP physicians' responses are more similar to those of British general practitioners than they are to other physicians in this country, suggesting that the financing scheme is the underlying explanation. Although it is possible that the better ambulatory coverage of HMOs induces patients to present complaints that are truly more trivial, Mechanic persuasively argues that there is little evidence to support that view. On the other hand, there is substantial evidence that a large proportion of patients normally seen by practitioners in both PGPs and traditional settings are not seriously ill (Garfield et al., 1976; U.S. National Center for Health Statistics, Series 13, No. 21, 1975). Furthermore, differences in specialization across provider types do not adequately explain the perceptions of triviality. Instead, Mechanic suggests that two key predictors of triviality are: (1) dissatisfaction with the amount of time per patient; and (2) physicians' low tolerance for dealing with psychosocial problems, such as alcoholism and obesity (1975, p. 202).

Unlike Freidson's bureaucratically demanding patient, the problem of trivial complaints seems to be associated with fixed payments to the physician, not full insurance coverage of the patient. A physician paid a salary or capitation, rather than FFS has little incentive to expand hours to meet increased patient demand. This leads to considerable time pressure and a reduced ability to deal with root problems. According to Mechanic:

The primary care physician sees many patients whose problems are diffuse or vague and who cannot be processed quickly by providing a discrete technical service. With many of these patients, the physician requires time to explore their complaints and to allow them to express their feelings and concerns. The willingness of the physician to do so depends on both his social orientations to practice and the time pressures he faces. Under conditions where the physician feels under considerable time pressure, and where he feels uncomfortable and ineffective in dealing with more diffuse complaints, he is more likely to treat the patient symptomatically. Doctors are often aware of these failures in dealing with patients, and feel frustrated by pressures that do not allow them to take the time to explore a problem with greater depth. The attribution of triviality is probably in part a reflection of this feeling and of the primary care physician's lack of comfort in dealing with many psychosocial issues for which he feels he cannot do a great deal. I believe that much of the feeling that patient visits are trivial is a consequence of the physician treating the patient's complaint as if it is trivial. (1975, p. 203)

However, not all of the small number of available studies support the Freidson and Mechanic models. Dutton's (1976) data from Washington, D.C. physicians indicate that PGP doctors are substantially *less* dissatisfied than either FFS group or solo doctors with the amount of time for each patient, taking care of patients with social or emotional problems, and the manner in which patients related to them. Darsky, Sinai, and Axelrod (1958) present physicians' perceptions of problems with patients. These perceptions are then compared to the proportion of each physician's patients who are covered by the Windsor Medical Services prepayment plan. There are strong relationships between plan involvement on one hand, and both less patient delay in seeking care and more doctor shopping on the other. While the first perception is supported by patient utilization data, the second is not, suggesting that physicians' responses may be unduly weighted by a few incidents. (This concentration on the exception to the rule is also noted by Freidson, 1973, p. 482.) Weaker perceived relationships were found between the plan and unnecessary home and night calls, demanding unnecessary services and treatment, and an overconcern with illness. The first two are similar to Freidson's demanding patient; however, patients in this study had the free choice of any physician in the community, all of whom worked on a solo FFS basis. Thus the nature of the contractual relationship was different, in that Windsor Medical Services merely guaranteed payment. The last point, overconcern with illness, while not strong, is reminiscent of Mechanic's trivial complaint, yet the fees should have provided the standard incentive to see more patients.*

The above studies strongly suggest that in at least some HMOs, physician-patient interactions are the cause of provider dissatisfaction. Although there are a few counterexamples, the weight of evidence and associated descriptive explanations indicate that the design of the new HMOs should be sensitive to such issues.

---

*There is a suggestion by Darsky, Sinai, and Axelrod (1958, p. 180) that Windsor Medical Service patients accounted for a somewhat smaller proportion of physician income than would be expected by their share of patient load. If true, this could explain a reluctance on the part of physicians to spend more time on them. However, the question was asked in an indirect fashion, and the differences were small.

Autonomy and Organizational Responsiveness

The solo physician in FFS practice is the epitome of autonomy. Such a physician deals with patients on a one-to-one basis, and while hospitals may be large bureaucratic organizations, they are usually set up to be responsive to physicians' needs. One would imagine that prepaid group practices, with their organizational structures, compromises among physicians, and inter-position of a health plan, would threaten physician autonomy. For exam-ple, "too much supervision and control" was the second most frequently mentioned reason for termination in Prybil's sample (1971). (See Table 12-3 above.) Zako (1976) also complained about the unresponsiveness of the health plan organization. Lum's survey of HMO directors found two-thirds agreeing that physicians prefer private practice to PGPs because of minimal restrictions in the former (Lum, 1975, p. 1199). Carnoy and Koo (1974) report that some Kaiser physicians think that the medical group is controlled by an autocratic executive committee. In a survey of large group practice administrators, however, Freidson and Mann (1971) found that bureaucratic organizations, with a high degree of formal supervision and prepayment, were only slightly negatively related to physician satisfac-tion. The surprisingly small relationship is partly explained in Freidson and Rhea's 1964 study of physicians in a subsample of these groups. They found that a majority highly valued certain aspects of autonomy, for example, regulating one's own time and managing patients without inter-ference. At the same time 87 percent felt that the group should insist that doctors keep strict office hours. Those to whom abstract autonomy was most important were most prone to agree. Substantial majorities also contended that a lay administrator is justified in reprimanding a physician for technical inadequacies and that a medical director should be allowed to reprimand a physician for being impolite to a patient.

Engel's study (1969) of perceived autonomy in solo, prepaid group, and government medical practice supports the Freidson findings that au-tonomy is not a major problem. Autonomy with respect to clinical practice is perceived to be highest in PGPs. She explains that government organiza-tions are so highly bureaucratic that they interfere with a physician's practice, and that the nonbureaucratic nature of solo practice implies an absence of the physical and professional supports that are often required by modern medicine. Thus the solo practitioner loses autonomy (relative to the PGP physician), not because of roles but because of isolation. Engel's analysis supports the hypothesis that an optimal (middle) level of bureau-cracy maximizes a physician's autonomy. This may explain the relative lack of complaints about autonomy by group practitioners.

The "ideal" world of the independent solo practitioner outlined at the beginning of this section no longer exists. While traditional practice continues without groups or foundation arrangements, it is rare that a physician is not required to deal with private insurance companies and government agencies for at least some reimbursements. For instance, 88 percent of office-based practitioners accept assignment under Medicare (American Medical Association, 1973, p. 619). Such third-party payers exercise increasing control over fee schedules; they also determine the appropriateness of certain types of care. Physician reaction is both predictable and vocal. A survey of California practitioners who either refuse or have cut down on their treatment of Medicaid enrollees indicates that 46 percent consider "bureaucratic interference with patient care" a "critical problem" (California Medical Association, 1975, p. 3). This interference is likely to increase over time.

HMOs and group practices may help to improve physician acceptance of this loss of autonomy. A 1973 survey of the entire American Medical Association membership indicates that group practice physicians are significantly more accepting than other office-based physicians of third-party (private and federal) authority in certain aspects of medical care delivery, such as utilization review of ambulatory and inpatient services, establishment and monitoring of quality standards, and fee setting (American Medical Association, 1973). Of course, such differences may be accounted for by physician self-selection in terms of who chooses to join a group practice, but it should be remembered that these groups are small, and the survey was limited to AMA members. An alternative explanation is that a group can insulate individual practitioners from direct confrontation with third parties. Similar findings are reported by Mechanic (1974). Berkanovic et al. (1974) also provide evidence that physicians practicing in an IPA-type plan are more favorably disposed to both the HMO concept and peer review than practitioners in a neighboring county without an IPA.

Further support for the advantages of local control of HMOs is seen in the study of Windsor, Ontario, physicians. Over 80 percent preferred local direction of voluntary plans over provincial or national direction. The major reasons given for this preference were that a community-centered organization is more responsive to local conditions that affect a physician's practice and that physicians have easier access to a local plan's personnel (Darsky, Sinai, and Axelrod, 1958, pp. 205-206).

Thus the weight of evidence suggests that the autonomy issue is largely a nonproblem. While physicians still value autonomy, they reluctantly accept numerous restrictions, and they often find organizations helpful. Group practices seem to offer valuable clinical supports that are seen to be necessary for good practice. Organizations also seem useful as physician-controlled intermediaries between the practitioner and distant third-party financing bodies (Sheridan, 1978).

Ability to Practice Good Medicine

There are two major aspects to physicians' satisfaction with their ability to practice good medicine in a certain setting. The first is the general impact of the setting in terms of such factors as incentives for quality, availability of facilities, and removal of impediments. The second refers to the extent to which physicians feel that an organization helps or hinders the full realization of their abilities, particularly in terms of specialization.

There is general agreement that most HMOs and group settings help promote good quality care. Cook points out that among the major reasons expressed by physicians for joining a Kaiser group is the ability to practice high quality medical care without having to be concerned about a patient's ability to pay (1971, p. 104). This view is strongly supported by the perceptions of physicians treating patients covered by different types of health insurance. Physicians in Kaiser and Ross-Loos were much less likely than other physicians to feel that insurance limits adequate diagnosis and treatment and were much more likely to think that it helped promote preventive medicine (Hetherington, Hopkins, and Roemer, 1975, pp. 111, 158). The impact of the improved insurance coverage offered by HMOs is repeated in a study of Windsor Medical Services in which 87 percent of the physicians felt that it helped to provide necessary diagnostic and treatment procedures, without cost considerations (Darsky, Sinai, and Axelrod, 1958, p. 190). Seventy percent of the physicians in the large group practices surveyed by Freidson and Rhea felt that the group was responsible for an increase or improvement in the scientific quality of their work. Furthermore, 46 percent felt that the group increased their "sensitivity to the psychological needs of the patient" (1964, p. 834).

It may be asked, however, whether 70 percent is high or low. Mechanic's comparative study offers some insight into this question. In terms of incentives for high quality in one's practice, 66 to 70 percent of group and nongroup general practitioners and pediatricians were very satisfied. Smaller proportions of PGP general practitioners and pediatricians (57 and 64 percent) were very satisfied. (In the decade between Freidson and Rhea's and Mechanic's surveys, health insurance coverage markedly improved, probably reducing the relative advantage of the comprehensive coverage offered by HMOs. Somewhat lower levels of satisfaction were also expressed by the PGP physicians with respect to their office facilities and hospital privileges (although the latter difference is primarily for general practitioners) (Mechanic, 1975, p. 199).* Even among the Windsor physicians, all was not well. While 51 percent thought that Windsor Medical Services helped their practice to maintain a high quality of care and 33 percent thought it made no difference, 16 percent thought it hindered (Darsky, Sinai, and Axelrod, 1958, p. 293). Furthermore, specialists were more likely than general practitioners to think that WMS hindered rather than helped the quality of care.

The Windsor case is interesting because it involves an IPA-type plan with all physicians in independent practice on an essentially FFS basis. Because the plan does not directly intervene in practice patterns, it is difficult to see

---

*The dissatisfaction of the GPs may be a reflection of either problems with community physicians or the structure of the group itself, which may seek to limit inpatient care to specialists.

how it has an effect on quality, except through the fee schedule, which does appear somewhat disadvantageous to specialists.* The extent of intervention in practice is much greater in group practice. A prepaid group must set itself up to provide essentially all the care for its enrollees. FFS groups, while having no such contractual requirements, try to refer only within the group. Both forms of groups may find themselves caught in a conflict between the type of medicine physicians are taught to practice and the type of problems presented to them by patients. Most training programs are hospital based and subspecialty oriented, though there is some evidence of a change in this pattern toward a primary care orientation (Fox, 1974). The bulk of patient problems, however, require only ambulatory care from a nonspecialist (Aiken et al., 1979). Thus the groups find themselves with too many specialists and not enough generalists, or more precisely, given the predominance of specialists entering practice, there is more general-practice ambulatory care to be done than the specialists would like to do.†

This role incongruence has been a major source of instability in some group practices and has caused some physicians to leave groups (DuBois, 1967, p. 265; Prybil, 1971; Egger, 1977). The problem seems to be more prevalent in medical than in surgical specialties, probably because the day-to-day work of surgeons is more akin to their training. Pediatricians and internists, in particular, seem dissatisfied with the largely ambulatory practice required in groups (Vayda, 1970, p. 165; Tilson, 1973a, 1973b; Perkoff, 1977b).

There seem to be a number of different approaches to this issue. In some Northern California Kaiser hospitals the division of labor is carried even further, so that in 90 to 95 percent of the cases, the hospital attending physician is not the patient's usual physician (Somers, 1971, p. 115). Southern California Kaiser has followed the strategy of establishing small neighborhood medical offices, which are staffed primarily by general practitioners who serve as day-to-day family doctors, with internists and pediatricians as consultants (Kaiser Foundation Medical Care Program, 1964, p. 12). The Oregon region presents yet a third pattern in which physicians' assistants do many general-practice-type tasks, making it easier for the internists to specialize (Record and Greenlick, 1975). GHCPS relies primarily on family practitioners for medical care.

*The linkage may occur in the following manner: specialists earn less per visit under the WMS fee schedule than would otherwise be the case; therefore, they may tend to give somewhat less time or effort, reducing quality. The reverse may also be true: GPs may give more than their usual time to WMS patients. Both specialists and GPs, however, report lower earnings from WMS patients, but the shortfall is greater for the former (Darsky, Sinai, and Axelrod, 1958, pp. 181-182).

†The problem is not so acute in the independent FFS or IPA setting. In such cases specialists receive referrals from the "pure generalists" and from other specialists for problems outside their area. Because groups typically do not get referrals from nongroup physicians, they do not have this source of patients, and unless they are very large, they have problems simulating it internally.

Practicing "good medicine" in the manner to which one is accustomed is an important aspect of physician satisfaction. A key distinction between successful and unsuccessful group practices is their commitment to professional objectives (DuBois, 1967, p. 268). Although the better insurance coverage of HMO members is seen as a definite advantage in practicing good medicine, there is some evidence that HMO physicians are less satisfied with their incentives for quality. Freidson and Rhea's survey found that 58 percent of the group practice physicians surveyed agreed with and 38 percent disagreed with the statement: "One of the dangers of an incentive system of payment in a group is that the doctors are likely to sacrifice quality to quantity so as to make more money" (1964, p. 833). Such statements both ignore the incentives of FFS practice and assume that more care is better. However, satisfaction is based on perceptions, not on how things ought to be, or even on how a clear-thinking analyst describes them.

One measure of such perceptions is the change in the status of PGP physicians. In the 1940s and early 1950s organized medicine actively and vocally attacked PGPs and physicians who worked in them (Palley, 1965; Kessel, 1958; Yale Law Journal Editors, 1954). In 1958 low status in the community and identification as a "group doctor" were important issues to physicians (McElrath, 1961). By 1972 only a small percentage of the PGP physicians in a national survey were not satisfied with their community status and esteem (Mechanic, 1975, p. 199). These changes are probably due more to attitudes in the larger medical community than to changes among physicians in prepaid groups. Similarly, some of the internist and pediatrician dissatisfaction with patient mix is the result of inappropriate emphases in medical education, not HMO policies. In fact, to the extent that an HMO includes a microcosm of the population, many problems experienced by physicians inside a plan eventually will be felt by those in traditional practice.

RECRUITMENT AND TURNOVER

The expressed satisfaction of physicians refers directly to those who are current members of the organization. The intensity of feelings, however, is reflected in the organization's ability to recruit new physicians and keep turnover to a reasonable level. Recruitment and turnover are important issues for prepaid groups; thus some data are available. The issue never seems to have been addressed by IPAs, although physician participation is by no means guaranteed. In the three IPAs for which data are available, participation rates among eligible physicians exceed 95 percent (Berkanovic et al., 1974, p. 7; Darsky, Sinai, and Axelrod, 1958, p. 31; Sasuly and Hopkins, 1967). However, eligibility is often limited to medical society members, so it is impossible to tell how many physicians in the area refuse to participate in either the medical society or the IPA. A key aspect of IPAs is the claim to offer essentially free choice of any physician in the area. If a substantial minority of physicians refuse to participate initially, an IPA is unlikely to get started. A substantial number of IPAs have been initiated and subsequently failed because of insufficient physician enrollment (Lubalin et al., 1974).

Prepaid groups were known to have difficulty recruiting physicians in the late 1950s and early 1960s, probably because of opposition by the medical establishment (Saward and Greenlick, 1972, p. 161). The picture has changed somewhat. The groups basically see little difficulty in hiring physicians, except in certain subspecialty areas in which there are national shortages and physicians can command exceptionally high incomes (Saward and Greenlick, 1972, p. 161; Lum, 1975, p. 1199; Smillie, 1976). This is a particular problem because many groups try to maintain relatively equal salaries across specialties (Newman, 1972, p. 211; Cook, 1971, p. 105). A more general problem is the rapid rise in overall physician incomes in the post-Medicare era; this has made it difficult for the groups to keep pace (Eisenberg, 1970, p. 270; Smillie, 1972, p. 319). Surveys of hospital house staffs indicating that over half feel that prepaid group practice is the best way to practice suggest that, unless a tremendous expansion occurs in PGPs, there is a sufficient pool of potential recruits (Bahn, 1970, p. 66).

If groups can recruit adequate numbers of new physicians, can they also keep them? Of course, some turnover not only is expected, it is desirable, so that quality can be maintained. The question is: how much is a reasonable rate? Comparison data indicate a 10 percent turnover among the Veterans Administration full-time physician staff and a 12 percent rate among career officers in the U.S. Air Force Medical Service Corp (Prybil, 1971, p. 8). Turnover rates for group practice physicians range from 3.6 to 6.5 percent in various studies from 1953 to 1968 (Prybil, 1971, pp. 8, 9; Ross, 1969, p. 15). Ross indicates that the turnover rate falls with group size. Two other points are worth noting: nearly half of those who leave do so within their first two years in the group, and 18 percent of the terminations are involuntary (Ross, 1969, pp. 17, 18). The first suggests that while much of the turnover occurs during the traditional probationary period, many of those who leave are full partners. The second point probably understates the extent to which a group can pressure a physician to leave "by mutual arrangement."

Data from individual prepaid group practices are consistent with these general findings. The group Freidson studied exhibited a 25 percent turnover rate, but he notes the many problems of that particular group (Prybil, 1971, p. 8). In the first four years of its existence, the Community Health Foundation had a 13 percent average turnover rate, despite careful recruitment (Vayda, 1970, p. 163; Yedidia, 1968, p. 66). Larger groups, such as the Northern and Southern California and Oregon Kaiser groups and Group Health Cooperative of Puget Sound, have turnover rates of less than 5 percent among partners and rates of about 10 percent for employed, usually probationary, physicians (Cook, 1971, p. 105; Newman, 1972, p. 108; Kaiser Foundation Medical Care Program, 1964, pp. 8, 13, 15). For the Permanente Medical Group (Northern California Kaiser) the termination rate among employed physicians ranged from 7.7 percent to 16.2 percent between 1968 and 1975, with an average of 12.0 percent. For partners the rates ranged from 1.3 to 4.8 percent, with a mean of 2.6 percent, two-fifths of which was due to death or disability (Smillie, 1976, pp. 24-25). Some Kaiser data offer an insight into the organization's perspective on physicians who leave. In twenty-one of forty-eight cases the physician-in-chief would reject the return of physicians who resigned, if they wanted to come back. Another eleven physicians would be accepted back reluctantly because of department staff needs. Of the forty-eight who left, in thirteen cases resignation was requested or instigated by the group, thirteen physicians wanted more income or wanted to try FFS, and twenty were satisfied with Kaiser but left for personal reasons, such as a residency, academic appointment, or to move to another region (Smillie, 1976, p. 23). Thus it is clear that zero terminations is not the goal of these organizations. Furthermore there seems to be no evidence that established PGPs have had substantial difficulty either recruiting physicians or keeping most of them once they have joined the group.

SUMMARY

Any HMO strategy is doomed to failure if it cannot produce reasonable levels of satisfaction among physicians. Physicians control the medical process, and while other personnel and educational programs can reduce the number required, they will continue to be central figures. At a gross level the evidence is reassuring. IPAs generally have been able to retain the involvement of their physician members. Most FFS and prepaid groups have little trouble recruiting new physicians and experience notably low turnover rates. When more subtle measures are considered, however, several problem areas appear. These relate to workload and various aspects of the style of medical practice.

Few HMO physicians are unhappy with the amount of money received for the work they do; in fact, the stable and shorter working hours in PGPs are a great attraction. The problems occur through a combination of minimal incentives to expand hours, the resultant overwhelming patient load, the lack of medically interesting cases, and a loss of control. When faced with increases in patient demand, the salaried physician has no incentive, except genuine concern, to work longer hours. However, HMO patients are less likely to know when their physician is working overtime and thus are less appreciative. They cannot be consistently shuffled off to someone else because of the plan's responsibilities to treat enrollees. Overworked physicians do not have enough time to devote to their patients, and this often means that psychosocial problems are treated symptomatically. This is frustrating for the physician who is trained to cure rare diseases, rather than deal with such problems as alcoholism, stress, and poor diet. Such major problems, because they cannot be easily cured, are labeled trivial, rather than recognized as areas in which traditional medical care breaks down.

The patient is not passive in this little drama. As discussed in Chapter 11, some see the organization as unresponsive to their needs and begin to demand attention and treatment. These demands can be pursued through formal complaint mechanisms, a valuable source of recourse not available to an individual patient in an FFS setting; there they merely leave and are labeled doctor-shoppers. Furthermore, there may well be a trend over time to increase consumer questioning of the medical profession. While affecting everyone, it may be more apparent among HMO enrollees, who both chose to leave traditional settings and have formal channels for voicing their complaints.

The typical responses of a group may also be counterproductive. Faced by heavy demands for ambulatory care, they hire newly trained physicians, and in order to increase productivity, they concentrate responsibility for inpatient care among a small number of physicians. The typical young physician, however, is trained not for ambulatory care but for sophisticated inpatient treatment. Efforts to increase output reduce the possibility of getting to the root of the problem, and they seriously threaten the physician's need for control. Some HMOs are experimenting with different practice patterns that emphasize caring for psychosocial problems and include a greater role for general or family practitioners as primary providers (Harrington, Burnett, and Korenoff, 1974; Thompson, 1979). Whether such settings can also be designed to meet more of the physician's needs remains an area for future research.

THIRTEEN

Can HMOs Serve the Poor?

In the mid-1960s the federal government rediscovered the existence of poverty in the United States and the large fraction of the poor who had little or no protection against medical care costs. The ensuing Great Society legislation resulted in a number of medical care programs for the poor, in particular Medicaid and various Neighborhood Health Centers. These programs for the poor, as well as Medicare for the elderly, were associated with, and to some extent caused, a large increase in medical care prices and expenditures. Thus many people have turned to HMOs, with their track record of cost containment, as a means of providing care to the poor at minimum cost.

HMOs, however, were initially developed as a means of providing medical care to workers and their families. Many of the earliest HMOs were developed to serve employees of specific companies or were organized with the close assistance of one or two labor unions (see American Medical Association, Commission on Medical Care Plans, 1958; Weinerman, 1956; Blumberg, 1977). The continued growth of established HMOs generally has been through the enrollment of employee groups. Whether they can effectively serve the poor is thus a question of some concern.

This chapter examines the issues and reviews the evidence concerning HMO delivery of care to the poor. An introductory section outlines the problems of medical care for the poor and alternative strategies to solve them. A review of HMOs designed to enroll the poor suggests that there are two types: demonstration projects and real-world situations. Some of the latter have been associated with various abuses; these are discussed in the third section. The fourth section reviews the evidence on whether the poor are able to use HMOs, when given the opportunity. The final section raises the question of whether HMOs and the poor are a viable combination.

MEDICAL CARE AND THE POOR: A FRAMEWORK FOR DISCUSSION

There are two major issues concerning medical care for the poor: (1) the rising expenditures in public programs for the poor; and (2) even with such increases, the question of whether the poor are receiving what they should. Karen Davis argues persuasively that the growth in Medicaid expenditures can be attributed to three factors: (1) the increase in the number of Medicaid recipients covered under the Aid for Families with Dependent Children Program; (2) the general rise in medical care prices; and (3) the high cost of nursing home care for an impoverished aged and disabled population (Davis, 1976, p. 124). As will be discussed below, while there may be some waste and outright fraud in Medicaid, there is no evidence that it is substantially worse than that in the rest of the medical care system. It is also likely that some of the Medicaid abuses can be traced directly to the structure of that program.

Before the Great Society programs in the 1960s, there was ample evidence that the poor used certain types of medical care substantially less than the nonpoor. Generally, there was a uniform positive gradient relating utilization to income. (See Covell, 1967; Kosa, Antonovsky, and Zola, 1969). More recent data exhibit a different pattern, showing an approximately equal number of physician visits per person across income levels, or a U-shaped pattern, with fewer visits by middle-income people than either the rich or poor (Bice, Eichhorn, and Fox, 1972; U.S. National Center for Health Statistics, Danchik, March 1975). Moreover, in 1975 persons in families earning less than $3000 per year had 6.4 visits per year versus 4.9 for those in families earning $15,000 and over (U.S. National Center for Health Statistics, "Physician Visits," April 1979, p. 21).

However, these aggregate statistics are misleading, because they conceal three important aspects of utilization data. (See Dutton, 1977, for a more complete discussion of these issues.) First, different age groups show substantially different utilization patterns. For children there is still a clear positive relationship between income and use. Second, there are different types of visits: elective, preventive, and follow-up. In general, there is a clear positive income relationship for preventive and patient-initiated visit, in contrast to a negative relationship for follow-up services. Thus much of the apparent high utilization by the poor is the result of a larger proportion of people who do not receive any services, while those who do enter the system receive well above the average. Third, utilization should be measured in relation to need. If one corrects for disability levels, it becomes clear that the poor use fewer services than the affluent (Aday, 1975, 1976; Fox and Bice, 1976; Davis and Reynolds, 1976). Thus the apparent equality in overall utilization data is a mirage.

One must ask if equal utilization is the real goal. Some argue that the poor, by definition, have less to spend on everything, and therefore, will consume less medical care, other things being equal. This implies that we should even out the income distribution, rather than focus on medical care. The Congress, however, seems more willing to provide in-kind assistance, such as housing, food stamps, and medical care. Within this context, it is clear that, at the very least, equal *access* is more important than equal *usage*. So the medical care system should be responsive to the greater prevalence of health problems among the poor.

Barriers to Utilization by the Poor

Strategies to ensure equity depend upon the factors that are called upon to explain the different utilization patterns between the poor and nonpoor. There are three major explanations: (1) sociocultural barriers, (2) financial barriers, and (3) systems barriers.* In economic terms, the first two factors deal with demand, and the last aspect, which is often neglected, concerns supply. The sociocultural barrier explanation stems from the culture of poverty concept formulated by Oscar Lewis (1966). In brief, it contends that social and psychological traits passed from generation to generation among the poor serve to perpetuate the poverty cycle. Such traits include alienation, crisis orientation to life, lack of future orientation, and failure to define symptoms as illness. While there is some evidence that such attitudinal variables have an effect on utilization, they hardly seem to be the dominant influence (McKinlay and Dutton, 1974; Kravits and Schneider, 1975; Riessman, 1974).

The financial coverage explanation is based on the argument that, because the poor cannot afford medical care out-of-pocket, their lack of health insurance coverage is all the more burdensome. In its simplest terms, this implies that complete health insurance coverage for the poor, such as that ideally provided by Medicaid, should overcome the barrier. While it is clear that complete coverage does not eliminate access barriers, it does go a substantial part of the way. This can be seen most clearly in the very low utilization of the poor and near poor who are *not* covered by Medicaid, in contrast to those with coverage (Davis and Reynolds, 1976; Skinner et al., 1978).

A simple market solution to the utilization issue seems to derive from the financial coverage model; if the poor initially demand too few services, give them coverage to buy what they need. If physicians are relatively scarce in urban poverty areas, increased demand will draw in new providers. But this may occur only at prices above the Medicaid fee schedule; so the supply problem is not solved. (In some states Medicaid pays only half what Medicare allows, which, in turn, is below usual fee levels (Burney et al., 1978).) If Medicaid administrators were willing to let fees rise substantially, there would be many more physicians serving the poor (Holahan et al., 1978; Sloan, Mitchell, and Cromwell, 1978; Garner, Liao, and Sharpe, 1979). The "physician shortage" in poverty areas is manifested in longer travel and waiting times for the poor (Robert Wood Johnson Foundation, 1978). Furthermore, there are consistent differences in the types of providers available to the poor. They are more likely to see physicians in clinics, hospital outpatient departments, and emergency rooms (U.S. National Center for Health Statistics, "Physician Visits," April 1979, p. 31). These settings tend to make it more difficult for the poor to seek care.

*I am indebted to Diana Dutton's work for much of this discussion. However, we do not agree on every point.

Thus the poor also face structural or systems barriers because of the providers available to them.

Alternative Strategies to Overcoming the Barriers

Two major strategies were undertaken to overcome these barriers. The relatively complete coverage offered by Medicaid was aimed at eliminating financial barriers and indirectly at improving the supply situation by attracting medical resources to poverty areas. Neighborhood Health Centers were directed at all three barriers. They were designed to make services available without charge and, more importantly, to bring new resources into poverty areas. To overcome sociocultural barriers, special emphasis was given to community participation and outreach programs, as well as innovative forms of team medical care delivery. (See Zwick, 1972.) However, together these strategies have failed to provide equity of access. Both programs are underfunded relative to the tasks at hand, and there has been no substantial flow of medical resources into poverty areas. The overall picture is one of great unevenness. Many poor people are not covered by Medicaid or are living in states with minimal Medicaid benefits. Those who are covered often find it difficult to obtain providers willing to care for them. If they do get into the system, they often find it fragmented, impersonal, and biased toward offering many services of questionable quality.

It is with this background that people ask whether HMOs offer a solution. After all, they have a record of delivering quality care to large populations at reasonable cost. They offer complete ambulatory coverage so that financial access barriers are minimized. Block payments to the provider would eliminate the massive problems of claims payments under Medicaid and allow state governments to set fixed budgets.* Furthermore, prepaid group practices are similar in concept to the Neighborhood Health Center, in that a group of physicians and other providers offer comprehensive and continuous services as a group. In more sparsely populated rural areas, the IPA types of HMO could provide care for the rural underserved populations. Such was the promise. What is the record?

ENROLLING THE POOR IN HMOS: EXAMPLES OF TWO DIFFERENT SITUATIONS

The available evidence concerning the experience of the poor in HMOs comes from a wide range of accounts that represent two distinct situations. The first is that of the demonstration project or semiexperiment in which a

---

*Although the use of HMOs to serve the poor is often justified in terms of cost, a survey of eighteen states indicated that few had realized substantial savings. In part this is because premiums were based on local FFS costs (Vignola, 1977).

small number of poor people are given incentives to enroll in an HMO, and their experience is carefully monitored and evaluated. The second may be termed the "real world," in which an HMO option is made available without special incentives or an evaluation design. In order for such situations to be reviewed here, data must have been collected and published, but in these real-world cases it is always after the fact. As will be seen, the differences extend far beyond the question of who does the evaluation.

The key distinction between a demonstration project and a market test lies in the incentives for participation. The major difficulty in providing HMO coverage for the poor is the lack of continuous financial coverage. The poor obviously cannot afford to enroll on their own; their only chance is for the state to use Medicaid funds to pay their premiums. Unfortunately, many of the poor continually move in and out of eligibility for such assistance (D'Onofrio and Mullen, 1977; Wollstadt, Shapiro, and Bice, 1978). Even when not eligible, most are still effectively, although not technically poor; so the option of continuing coverage out-of-pocket is not available. Thus the usual Medicaid population presents the HMO with a group of people whose enrollment status is uncertain from month to month, requiring extensive bookkeeping and patient orientation. Moreover, some states are notorious for determining eligibility retroactively, further adding to the HMO's risk.

From the Medicaid recipient's perspective, the HMO option has an important drawback: it severely limits freedom of choice of provider. Medicaid typically offers complete coverage with no copayments for services rendered by any provider. If a recipient has identified a set of providers willing to provide care (which is often difficult), then joining an HMO usually entails surrendering the Medicaid card that will pay for treatment by those providers. A particularly difficult situation arises when a provider that does accept FFS Medicaid patients, such as a Neighborhood Health Center, attempts to convert to a prepayment scheme. Refusing to enroll allows the Medicaid recipient to use both the center *and* any other providers (Borsody, 1972; Hester and Sussman, 1974).

Two situations can overcome these problems and lead to enrollment of the poor in HMOs. In the first, special inducements are provided to improve the option for both consumers and providers. This has generally been the case in the demonstration projects listed in Table 13-1. The Office of Economic Opportunity projects in Kaiser Portland, Kaiser Fontana, GHCPS, and HIP Suffolk are clear examples. In each case the HMO was given Neighborhood Health Center grant funds to enroll low-income people in certain neighborhoods. Harvard Community Health Plan had similar programs. Because Medicaid coverage was not required, month-to-month eligibility problems were eliminated. Extra funds were also available for services not normally provided, such as outreach, social services, and child care. The plan was attractive to consumers, because it

Table 13-1 Demonstration Projects Enrolling the Poor in HMOs

HMO	Number of Poor	Enrollment Factors and Incentives	References
Kaiser-Portland 1967–	6800 as of 1972 ~4% of total enrollment ~3300 as of 1975 ~2% of total	OEO-NHC coverage for low-income families meeting specific eligibility criteria in selected neighborhoods; OEO bore medical care costs plus special outreach services	1,2,3,4,5,6
Kaiser-Fontana 1970–	2800 as of 1972 ~2% of total	OEO-funded project, includes transport and outreach services; about 40% are also covered under Medicaid contract	5,6
Kaiser-Hawaii 1971–	1300 as of 1972 ~1% of total	Medicaid contract with the state includes extra funds (about 30% of total) for outreach program	6,7
Kaiser-Harbor City/ PCC 1969–	472 as of 1969 ~.5% of total	Families associated with the Parent-Child Center; membership costs borne by Kaiser; about 48% eligible for Medicaid	6,8
Group Health Cooperative of Puget Sound			
OEO 1971	2150 as of 1972 ~1.5% of total	OEO-NHC coverage for low-income families; includes transport and outreach	5
Model Cities 1971–74	~1300 ~1% of total	Project funded through Model Cities, open to individuals in target area, under age 65, not on public assistance, but with incomes no more than $2,000 above federal poverty line; offered a choice of GHC or complete coverage through BC	9
HIP-Suffolk 1970–	2300 as of 1972 (753,000 in HIP total, Suffolk membership unknown)	OEO-NHC coverage for low-income families; includes transport and outreach	5
Group Health Association, Washington, D.C. 1971–73	1000 ~1.3% of total	Medicaid eligibles in one service area were invited to enroll; free dental services offered (not in Medicaid) as well as waiver of eligibility redetermination for up to 3 years	10
Harvard Community Health Plan 1970	1750 as of 1974 ~4% of total	Medicaid eligibles in surrounding neighborhood; outreach program, transport, childcare funded 314e Public Health Service grant; additional program for low-income, nonwelfare recipients, with PHS funds to supplement family-employer contributions	11,12

REFERENCES.

1. Colombo, Saward, and Greenlick, 1969, pp. 641–650.
2. Phelan, Erickson, and Fleming, 1970.
3. Greenlick et al., 1972, pp. 187–200.
4. Hurtado, Greenlick, and Colombo, 1973, pp. 189–198.
5. Sparer and Anderson, 1973, pp. 67–72.
6. Kaiser Permanente Medical Care Program, 1973.
7. Worth, 1974, pp. 91–96.
8. Shragg et al., 1973, pp. 52–60.
9. Richardson, et al., January 1977.
10. Fuller and Patera, January 1976.
11. Birnbaum, 1971, pp. 42–46.
12. Gaus, Cooper, and Hirschman, 1976, pp. 3–14.

offered more services and an eligibility guarantee that was unavailable elsewhere. For example, the Group Health Association contract with Washington, D.C., Medicaid included free dental care (not covered by Medicaid) and a three-year waiver of eligibility redetermination (Fuller and Patera, 1976). A notable exception to this package sweetening for HMO enrollees was the Group Health Cooperative-Model Cities Project. It offered comprehensive coverage to low-income persons in certain neighborhoods, and once enrolled in the project, they could choose between GH and individual providers through a King County Medical-Blue Cross plan (Richardson et al., 1977).

The second situation is one in which the existing environment makes the advantages of enrolling Medicaid recipients outweigh the disadvantages. From the provider's perspective, this usually means that enough Medicaid eligibles can be enrolled to compensate for the costs of monthly enrollments and protracted negotiations with the state. In some instances supplemental funds were available to cover those above the Medicaid line (Skinner et al., 1978). (For a discussion of some of the problems in developing Medicaid contracts, see Levin, 1971.) From the consumer's perspective, the medical care alternatives are often bleak. The urban poor are often concentrated in areas characterized by an unavailability of physicians, so a new HMO that offers needed services can be very attractive (de Vise, 1973; Dewey, 1973; Sullivan, 1977; Guzick and Jahiel, 1976). This is particularly true if an HMO establishes a new clinic and "imports" physicians, thus adding substantially to the available resources. A different situation exists with an IPA type of HMO. Physicians who form IPAs are usually enticed by prospects of regaining control and forestalling competition. Patients are attracted because there is no change in practice patterns. And physicians who were unwilling to accept Medicaid patients directly may accept them through the IPA, which then handles all the negotiations with the state, thus adding to the effective supply.

Table 13-2 lists some nondemonstration projects. Several of these are restricted to Medicaid enrollees. Others, such as the Family Health Program, established separate clinics in poverty areas, and they draw a substantial fraction of their enrollees from the Medicaid population (Gumbiner, 1975). HIP of New York is a special case. It began serving the indigent aged under contract with the city in 1962 (Shapiro et al., 1967). The association was readily converted to cover Medicaid eligibles in 1966. This led to a massive increase of enrollees in certain areas, with most of the Medicaid eligibles in ten of the twenty-nine HIP groups (Shapiro and Brindle, 1969, p. 635).

In most cases Medicaid enrollees in HMOs are racially and ethnically similar to nonenrollees in the same area (Gaus, Cooper, and Hirschman, 1976, p. 7). The high proportion of blacks and Spanish-speaking people in these groups is consistent with the hypothesis that they are in ghetto areas with minimal medical resources. A different situation is revealed if one

Table 13−2   Nondemonstration Project Examples of HMOs Enrolling the Poor

HMO	Number of Poor	Population	References
HIP	69,000 as of January 1974 ~8% of total	Began serving welfare recipients in 1962, Medicaid eligibles in 1966; of these, 59% are Black, 30% Spanish-speaking; most are concentrated in 10 of 29 groups	1,2,3
Central Los Angeles Health Project, Calif.	8700 as of January 1974 100% of total	Medicaid enrollees, 91% Black, 6% Mexican-American	3
Consolidated Medical System California	52,000 as of January 1974 49% of total	Of Medicaid enrollees, 41% are Black, 23% Spanish-speaking; other enrollees through union and other contracts	3
Family Health Program, Calif.	15,000 as of January 1974 32% of total	Of Medicaid enrollees, 58% Black, 13% Spanish-speaking	3
Harbor Health Services, Calif.	6200 as of January 1974 100% of total	Medicaid enrollees; 41% Black, 23% Spanish-speaking	3
Temple Health Plan, Pa.	11,000 as of January 1974 100% of total	Medicaid enrollees; 94% Black, 6% Puerto Rican	3
Redwood Foundation, Calif.	29,000 as of January 1974 100% of total	Medicaid enrollees; 2% Black, 8% Spanish-speaking; the Foundation also performs peer review and claims management but is not at risk for other patients	3
Sacramento Foundation	36,300 as of January 1974 100% of total	Medicaid enrollees; 28% Black, 14% Spanish-speaking; the Foundation also performs peer review and claims management, but is not at risk for these other patients	3
Kaiser-Oakland		Comparison of utilization of pediatric services by socioeconomic class of regular enrollees	4
Kaiser-Portland		Comparison of utilization patterns by socioeconomic class of regular enrollees	5,6
Group Health Cooperative of Puget Sound 1969	~4500 enrollees April 1974 ~2.3% of total	Medicaid enrollees; unclear whether there is an outreach program	7
East Baltimore Medical Plan	1900 Medicaid, 1880 PHS low-income eligibles, 300 FFS	All inner city residents	8

REFERENCES.

1. Shapiro and Brindle, 1969, pp. 635−641.
2. Hester and Sussman, 1974, pp. 415−444.
3. Gaus, Cooper, and Hirschman, 1976, pp. 3−14.
4. Nolan, Schwartz, and Simonian, 1967, pp. 34−47.
5. Weiss and Greenlick, 1970, pp. 456−462.
6. Freeborn et al., 1977, pp. 115−128.
7. Hall, 1974.
8. Skinner et al., 1978, pp. 1195−1201.

examines non-Medicaid enrollees of different socioeconomic levels in an HMO. Such people generally are employed and have a choice of health insurance plans. Their expectations and evaluations of HMO performance are likely to be different from those for whom the HMO is essentially the only choice. Using this framework, it is important to examine HMO performance with respect to the surrounding system. While there may be differences between HMO and FFS providers in poverty areas, they are probably more like each other than similar organizations in markedly different settings. A number of issues drawn from this framework will be discussed in turn: alleged abuses by HMOs serving the poor, utilization of services, accessibility, outreach, and patient satisfaction.

ABUSES BY HMOS SERVING THE POOR

In 1970 California began a policy of encouraging the development of HMOs to serve its Medicaid population. These HMOs, called prepaid health plans (PHPs), were supposed to save state money by reducing unnecessary utilization and administrative costs of claims reimbursement. The conservative governor, Ronald Reagan, also attempted to control utilization of FFS providers by limiting office visits and requiring prior authorization for hospital admissions. (See Goldberg, 1975; California Department of Health, 1975; Chavkin and Treseder, 1977). This strategy was also designed to make HMO enrollment more attractive to the Medicaid population, because no such external restrictions on utilization would be imposed. In fact, the Medicaid agency termed the plan a "carrot and stick approach" (California Department of Health, 1975). (Of course the PHPs have their own incentives to control costs.) In succeeding years criticism of PHPs has grown, and most observers agree that the initial program was poorly designed (Goldberg, 1975; D'Onofrio and Mullen, 1975; Moore and Breslow, 1972; California State Legislative Analyst, 1973; U.S. Senate Committee on Government Operations, 1975, 1978; Anonymous, "HEW's Dual Option Regulations," 1973; and Health/PAC, 1974). The major problems appear to be marketing abuses, excessive administrative costs and profits, and poor quality of care. While there has been little focus on problems in other states, there is evidence that problems with "Medicaid HMOs" are not limited to California (Spitz, 1979; Chicago Daily News, 1976). There is little doubt that many of these charges are true. It is essential to identify the causes of the problems, in order to determine whether the basic HMO concept is at fault.

Marketing Abuses

The principal charges concerning marketing stemmed from PHP use of door-to-door salespeople to enroll Medicaid eligibles. These people often posed as physicians or Medicaid officials and rarely explained fully the options available to consumers. Promises often far exceeded reality. These marketing abuses were at least partially attributable to the intense competition for enrollees among plans, which in turn, was fostered by the ground rules laid down by the state (U.S. General Accounting Office, 1974). The PHP signed a contract allowing it to receive a fixed monthly capitation fee of no more than 90 percent of the average FFS cost of similar enrollees. No funds were available for startup or fixed costs, so it was imperative that the PHP enroll members as quickly as possible. In an effort to encourage competition and promote choice for Medicaid eligibles, the state took a laissez-faire attitude and authorized many plans to operate in the same service areas. While creating a situation in which there was a rush to enroll people, the state refused to release the names of Medicaid eligibles, so the PHPs had to use door-to-door salespeople paid on commission. There was also little control over PHP attempts to enroll only the healthy and to keep dissatisfied members from disenrolling. The situation was almost perfectly designed to lead to the abuses that followed.

Administrative Costs and Profits

A second major criticism concerned excessive administrative costs and profits. For example, an audit of fifteen PHPs found that 52 percent of Medicaid payments either were spent by the PHPs or their subcontractors for administrative costs or resulted in net profits (California Office of the Auditor General, 1974). Similarly, a study of five PHPs showed extensive subcontracting relationships between nonprofit PHP contractees and for-profit subsidiaries owned by the same principals. In some, nearly all funds went to the for-profit subcontractors (U.S. General Accounting Office, 1976). Again, the design of the program and its setting largely determined the result. Long before the PHP experiment, the poor had essentially been abandoned by true not-for-profit hospitals and the traditional dedicated physician (Roemer, 1966). There are opportunities, however, for profit-seeking individuals and firms to enter the Medicaid market, as is amply evidenced by the "Medicaid mills." (See U.S. Senate, Special Committee on Aging, 1976, 1977; Bacon, 1979.) It may be possible for responsible for-profit providers to offer quality services to the poor (Gupte, 1976). The California Department of Health, however, preferred form to substance and refused to contract with for-profit firms, thus encouraging the establishment of dummy organizations. At least the attempts at deception would have been eliminated had the state been open about its priorities. Furthermore, the notion of profit and administrative costs is fuzzy. About 75 percent of nationwide health care expenditures go to physicians, dentists, other employees, drugs, and medical supplies; the rest are labeled administrative costs (Luft, 1976, p. 358). But how does one compare an independent practitioner who nets $100,000 (none of which is counted as profit) with one who receives a salary of $30,000 and a profit share of $70,000?

Quality

The quality issue is even more complex. As outlined in Chapter 10, quality is impossible to measure in ways that everyone agrees upon. But there was almost no concern for even minimal quality audits in the early years of the PHP program, and only after June 1973 were medical professionals assigned by the state to audit PHPs (California State Legislative Analyst, 1973). The following testimony by a physician member of the audit team raises an important issue:

May I cite one case? In this particular case while the patient was a Medi-Cal patient, the patient had been hospitalized eight 'times within one year with a rule-out diagnosis of myocardial infarction.

Once she became a PHP enrollee, a letter was written to the hospital:

"This dear, sweet lady has been hospitalized eight times in the past year with a diagnosis to rule out myocardial infarction. In fact she has had no major episode of this disease in the past three years. Fifty milligrams of Demorol will suffice in quieting her pain or until she can see me in my office." This is signed by the doctor.

Apparently when they were on fee-for-service, these people did get good care, as good care as one can possibly get under the system. Once they became enrollees of the prepaid health plan system, their care declined measurably. The quality of care, per se, both for Medi-Cal and for the PHP enrollee is poor at best, but is worse under the PHP plan. The quality of care is really unacceptable. (U.S. Senate, Committee on Government Operations, 1975, p. 262)

In truth, it is not clear whether the quality was unacceptable in the FFS system, with eight hospitalizations, or in the PHP, with none. The FFS versus PHP contrast under Medicaid is likely to create the widest extremes in utilization and, therefore, invalidate any quality assessment based on comparisons of process measures.

A detailed investigation in 1974 of five PHPs in operation prior to December 1972 showed substantial variability in quality, with some significantly better than FFS Medi-Cal and some significantly worse. Plans with a high proportion of non-Medi-Cal enrollees scored consistently better (Louis and McCord, 1974).

Thus, while the record of abuses in the California PHP experiment is clear, the lessons to be learned are not so obvious. The state has reacted with attempts to regulate and monitor the PHPs in order to eliminate the most flagrant abuses (California Department of Health, 1975). It also has made it easier for dissatisfied members to disenroll. The press and local welfare rights organizations have also created pressure for improvements (Health Law Newsletter, 1976). None of these approaches, however, penetrates to the root problem—the limited availability of resources for the poor. There is a two-tier system in which the poor get poor-quality care (broadly defined) in PHPs *and* in Medicaid mills, but in both cases such care is probably better than the available alternatives (Nathan, 1976). The cause of the PHP abuses lies not in the HMO incentives, but in the failure of the surrounding system.

IS IT MORE DIFFICULT FOR THE POOR TO USE HMOS?

The issue of the difficulties the poor face, once enrolled in HMOs, is complicated because of self-selection and the absence of well-defined evaluative measures. For instance, the simplest approach is to examine utilization rates, but with what group should the study population be compared? One can argue that the poor have more health problems than the nonpoor, so the poor in an HMO should be compared to the poor in the traditional system. Alternatively, one might reason that the FFS system is not meeting the needs of the poor. Thus the experience of the poor in an HMO should be compared to that of the middle class in the same organization. Studies of both types are available.

Utilization

Chapters 5 and 6 reported most of the findings concerning utilization of comparable groups of the poor in HMOs and FFS settings. The major studies are those of Gaus, Cooper, and Hirschman (1976) on ten HMOs; Fuller and Patera (1976) on Group Health Association; and Richardson et al. (1977) on the Seattle Model Cities Project. For ambulatory care, the results are mixed; in half, there are more visits by the poor in HMOs, and in half, the results are reversed. There is reason to believe, however, that these averages are misleading. The Seattle Model Cities Project offers by far the most detailed analysis. It shows nearly equal annual rates (452 per 100 for GH, 450 for KCM-BC enrollees), but substantially different distributions. Only 25.8 percent of the GH enrollees had no visits, in contrast to 35.8 percent of those with FFS physicians. This suggests that access is easier for GH enrollees. Similar findings are reported by HIP. (See Shapiro et al., 1967.) Two additional studies using multiple regression analysis support these general conclusions. Holahan found that the San Joaquin Foundation had no effect on the proportion of visits by Medicaid eligibles, the number of visits per year, or the cost per visit. This analysis used counties as the unit of observation and controlled for the availability of providers in the area (1977). Salkever et al. (1976) found that enrollees in the East Baltimore Health Plan were more likely to see a physician if they had an episode of illness than people with other usual sources of care.

For hospitalization, the results are markedly consistent: lower admission rates for HMO enrollees in all twelve cases. The prevailing opinion is that this generally is not due to an inability of patients to gain admission. In fact, somewhat lower utilization is probably good because of the presumed excessive hospitalization in conventional settings. While exceedingly low utilization rates may not be good practice, more detailed studies are necessary in order for us to determine if this is the case.

The second type of comparison involves the poor and nonpoor in the same organization. In general, the poor are underserved. The question is: does enrollment of the poor in the same plan with the middle class, and with the same financial coverage, eliminate the difference? Sparer and Anderson cite this as the major reason for the Office of Economic Opportunity buy-in arrangements with existing group practices: "If the same utilization results could be achieved for low-income families as for regular-plan members, the arrangement could provide a satisfactory alternative model to deliver and finance health services for the low-income persons" (Sparer and Anderson, 1973, p. 67). In support of their argument they present data showing ambulatory utilization of OEO enrollees to be about the same or slightly above that of regular members. But these data are almost impossible to interpret because of different age-sex distributions.

Of the four OEO demonstration projects, only Kaiser Portland performed extensive studies comparing regular and OEO members. (See Greenlick et al., 1972.) Overall utilization patterns are markedly similar: 77 percent of both the Health Plan and OEO populations received some services in the year, and there were 4.8 to 4.9 services per person in each group. The figures, however, mask some important differences by demographic subgroups. Persons aged 0 to 18 used about the same number of doctor office visits in both groups, but older OEO members used substantially more services. This, plus the fact that a somewhat smaller proportion of the OEO visits were for preventive care, supports the argument that the poor are more likely to be sick and thus *should* use more services in an HMO. Priority was given to enrolling low-income people with health problems, so these results cannot be generalized (Colombo, 1969). Other differences appear in the *types* of utilization. The poor are much more likely to walk in or use the hospital emergency room than they are to make a regularly scheduled appointment. The former results in fragmented care but may better fit the life circumstances of the poor. (The differences are only partially attributable to location, because they remain even when the OEO group is compared to Health Plan members living in the core city.) Further adding to the fragmentation was the fact that when appointments were made, the OEO group failed to appear 25.5 percent of the time, in contrast to 8.5 percent for regular members. Even the institution of special coordinators for the indigent population resulted in no lowering of this rate over a two-year period (Hurtado, Greenlick, and Colombo, 1973, p. 197).

Another example of utilization patterns by the poor and nonpoor is provided by the Kaiser Harbor City-Parent Child Center (PCC) project

(Shragg et al., 1973). The PCC provides a range of social services to 100 poor families. Kaiser contributes dues to provide coverage for these families who live in a city housing project across the street from a major Kaiser facility. The experience of the PCC families is contrasted with that of a sample of 100 regular Kaiser families in the Harbor City area. Unfortunately, the samples are substantially different. The PCC group has more children and fewer adult males, and 48 percent are covered by Medicaid, which provides full coverage through other providers. Although PCC members were more likely not to use any Kaiser services, regardless of Medicaid status, overall they had about the same number of doctor office visits per person. The similarities remain after age-sex adjustment.

Coltin, Neisuler, and Lorie (1978) have compared the use of services in Harvard Community Health Plan by Medicaid recipients, a low-income Medicaid-ineligible population (the "near poor"), and nonpoor regular enrollees. Age-sex standardized visit rates were 4.2 per year for the poor, 3.8 for the near poor, and 3.5 for the nonpoor. Almost identical proportions of each group had at least one contact in the preceding year. Hospital days per 1000 members were 337 for the poor, 506 for the near poor, and 286 for the nonpoor. Preventive visit rates were the same or higher for the poor. Process measures of quality indicate equal or better care for the low-income groups. The cost of serving the poor was 8.8 percent less than for the nonpoor, and their capitation payments were 33 percent less than Welfare Department estimates of FFS care. The near poor, however, were significantly more costly, in part because of adverse selection. Adding the costs of outreach services brings the cost for Medicaid recipients above that of the nonpoor, but still below that of FFS estimates.

These studies examined the behavior of special subgroups of the poor who were introduced to an ongoing HMO as part of a demonstration project. Such an arrangement requires adjustments by both the HMO staff and the new enrollees. An alternative research design examines whether different utilization patterns occur by socioeconomic group within the regularly enrolled population. While this approach is limited to employed people with an HMO option (and thus omits the very poor), it provides better measures of long-run equilibrium. If differences appear, they are likely to be larger if coverage is extended to the poor.

Again, much of the work has been done by the Kaiser Portland Research Center. Freeborn et al. (1977) summarize their results concerning outpatient utilization with respect to socioeconomic status. Health status measures appear to be the dominant factors, and once they are held constant, education, income, and socioeconomic class have little effect on utilization. The one exception is preventive service, which is not related to health status but, for women, is positively related to education and income. Socioeconomic status does have an indirect effect. The poor are more likely to have health problems and thus to need more medical care. Therefore, actual utilization is the net result of two opposing factors; people with a low income and a limited education need more care, but they may find access more difficult. *If* this were a major problem in the Kaiser Portland setting, it would appear in the form of positive income-education coefficients, once health status was held constant. This was not the case.

The Kaiser Portland data suggest some differential patterns of care. For example, members with higher levels of education, income, occupation, and social class were more likely to use the telephone for reporting symptoms of a new morbidity and less likely to walk into the clinic (Pope, Yoshioka, and Greenlick, 1971). In contrast to these results, once age and sex are held constant, education, income, and social class are not significantly related to unscheduled use of ambulatory care (Hurtado et al., 1974, p. 507). The major differences in utilization by social class among regular members are the much greater telephone use by the middle class and their higher use of walk-in services. It is only among emergency room services that the working class demonstrates higher rates (Weiss and Greenlick, 1970, p. 460). A separate study by Nolan, Schwartz, and Simonian (1967) in the Kaiser Oakland pediatrics clinic suggests that those in lower social classes are more likely to use drop-in clinics. This is related to transportation problems and to a greater proportionate use of preventive services by the middle class.

Hetherington, Hopkins, and Roemer argue that in PGPs people with more education and higher incomes can more easily "work the system" (1975, pp. 116-117). Combined with an earlier version of their study purporting to show substantially higher out-of-pocket costs for lower-income people in PGPs, these findings deserve careful attention (Roemer et al., 1972). The higher out-of-pocket expenditures were attributed by Roemer et al. to maternity cases and difficulty in "working the system" (1972, p. 45). These results have played an important role in other studies. (See Carnoy, Coffee, and Koo, 1973.) Hetherington, Hopkins, and Roemer present data (reproduced in Table 13-3) concerning ambulatory use per person by families with incomes above and below $11,000. This is about the mean income in their sample and is hardly at the poverty line. It is true that higher-income enrollees in Kaiser and Ross-Loos have more visits per year than lower-income enrollees, but this is also the case in the other plans. Hetherington, Hopkins, and Roemer focus their discussion on the differences between plans before and after controlling for income. In doing so, they seem to miss the important points in their data. For instance, they note that the effects of income should be greatest when comparing the plan having the least comprehensive coverage (the hospital-sponsored plan, or Blue Cross) with the plan having the most comprehensive coverage (the large group, or Kaiser). In the first part of the table, this is $4.70 - 3.94 = 0.76$. When controlling for income the differences hardly change, 0.71 for low-income and 0.74 for high-income families. Hetherington, Hopkins, and Roemer then repeat this analysis with the proportion of people receiving no services. The difference is $38.8 - 18.2 = 20.6$ percent for

Table 13–3   Doctor Visits per Person per Year by Plan and Family Income (Annual)

Doctor visits per person per year	Plan						
	All Plans	Large Comm[a]	Small Comm[a]	Blue Cross	Blue Shield	Kaiser	Ross-Loos
None (%)	28.4	47.4	39.1	33.2	19.3	18.8	9.8
Fewer than four	32.5	28.4	22.6	32.1	34.5	36.6	41.9
Four or more	39.1	24.3	38.2	34.7	46.1	44.6	48.3
Mean	4.06	2.77	4.26	3.94	4.09	4.70	4.61
SD[b]	5.29	4.36	5.76	5.10	6.69	5.01	4.59
N[c]	809	137	146	147	109	142	128
Less than $11,000							
None (%)	31.9	52.0	35.8	38.8	18.6	18.2	15.8
Fewer than four	36.0	25.4	28.6	31.9	41.6	46.1	48.7
Four or more	32.1	22.6	35.5	29.4	39.8	35.6	35.4
Mean	3.54	2.66	3.25	3.58	4.18	4.29	3.65
SD	5.43	4.57	4.19	5.46	7.93	5.69	3.89
N	468	104	61	100	69	69	65
$11,000 or more							
None (%)	20.8	31.5	31.6	23.5	15.0	20.9	4.1
Fewer than four	29.6	38.7	21.0	36.9	22.9	29.8	34.0
Four or more	49.5	29.8	47.4	39.7	62.1	49.2	61.9
Mean	4.97	3.16	5.94	4.26	4.24	5.00	5.74
SD	5.08	3.70	6.85	3.98	3.73	4.38	5.21
N	306	32	70	42	37	67	58

SOURCE.   Hetherington, Hopkins, and Roemer, 1975, pp. 92, 99.
[a] Commercial
[b] Standard deviation
[c] Number of cases

low-income families and $23.5 - 20.9 = 2.6$ percent for high-income families, in contrast to a combined gap of $33.2 - 18.8 = 14.4$ percent. When repeated for combinations of plans, with similar results, "[t]hese findings reveal that the gap widens for low-income families and is reduced for high-income families. . . . The impact of comprehensive plans on the low-income famiies is relatively small" (Hetherington, Hopkins, and Roemer, 1975, p. 100).

Instead, the reverse seems to be true. The usual case in utilization studies is that low-income people are much more likely not to use any services. Those enrolled in Kaiser are no less likely to receive services than higher-income people (18.2 versus 20.9 percent used no services). While access may be more difficult for the lower-income group, scheduling multiple visits seems to be more of a problem than learning how to use the system. Although Hetherington, Hopkins, and Roemer present similar results with respect to education, these data are also difficult to evaluate, because there are no controls for such standard variables as age and sex. And in the 1975 version there is no evidence or discussion of higher out-of-pocket expenses by lower-income people, suggesting that the initial results were in error.

Taken together, these studies suggest important differences in utilization patterns among regularly enrolled HMO members. While overall use of ambulatory services does not differ very much, especially when factors such as age, sex, and health status are held constant, the types of services vary. The middle class is much more likely to use the telephone to report symptoms. Walk-in visits and appointments, both of which are held during normal working hours, also appear easier for the middle class. While the unemployed may have a low time cost, the working poor probably have less flexible schedules than the middle class. (For discussions on the value of time, see Acton, 1975, 1976.) Thus the poor are more likely to use the emergency room, and they are more likely to miss appointments without cancelling them.

Perceived Accessibility, Patient Satisfaction, and Outreach Services

Utilization measures are only one aspect of medical care accessibility—whether and how often the enrollee actually gets to the provider. As has been seen, there appear to be more differences between the poor and nonpoor in utilization patterns and in visit time and content than in the total number of visits. Thus a second and perhaps more important dimension is the enrollee's perception of access.

It is important to note that the poor often have very limited access to the traditional FFS system. In mid-1972 less than 20 percent of Orange County, California, Medicaid eligibles obtained care through mainstream providers (Auger and Goldberg, 1974, p. 355). Thus the alternatives, such as public clinics and the few physicians willing to treat the poor, may set a standard of difficult access. This may partially explain the similarities in ease of access reported by the poor in HMOs relative to those in the traditional system. There is, however, a pattern of differences. If a person has an illness episode, it is easier for an HMO enrollee to contact a physician (Gaus, Cooper, and Hirschman, 1976, p. 13; Salkever et al., 1976). This seems related to the group practice mode of organization; the results are mixed for IPA enrollees. Other studies (for example, Tessler and Mechanic, 1975) suggest that HMOs tend to structure their office time so that, while patients have a shorter wait in the office, it is necessary for them to wait longer for an appointment. This is borne out in the Seattle Model Cities data (Richardson et al., 1977) and in four of nine settings in the Gaus, Cooper, and Hirschman (1976) survey. There are, however, a number of settings in which both waits are shorter for HMO enrollees (Fuller and Patera, 1976). Furthermore, the times to wait for an appointment show much greater variability (5 to 20 days in HMOs and 3 to 18 in

FFS) than office waiting times (19 to 42 minutes in HMOs versus 21 to 46 in FFS). The situations with extreme differences in the same area appear to depend on relative availability of FFS practitioners for the poor. They are relatively abundant in Seattle and parts of New York, resulting in easy appointments, while they are relatively unavailable in the poverty areas of Los Angeles and Philadelphia. (See Roemer, 1966.)

Many people held the theory that the ability to use the HMO system would be a major problem for the poor. There were at least two reasons for this: (1) the PGP type of HMO tends to be centralized and bureaucratic, and thus may present various structural barriers to utilization; and (2) there are HMO incentives to minimize services rather than to encourage them; thus there is always a potential for underserving people, especially the poor, who might not know what to expect. Therefore, most demonstration projects included special outreach workers to help the poor appropriately use the HMO. The Seattle Model Cities Project included an experimental evaluation in which only a randomly selected sample of enrollees in each plan received outreach services (Diehr, Jackson, and Boscha, 1975). Those in the outreach sample were slightly more likely to use certain services, but the differences were small and concentrated among those seeing FFS providers. Surprisingly, outreach had no effect on GH enrollees. Furthermore, while the outreach group reported more medical care for the preventive visits, these differences are not corroborated by medical records data. This suggests that the major impact of outreach may be on perceptions rather than behavior.

While access measures indicate few consistent differences, measures of satisfaction seem even more dependent on alternative sources of care. Richardson et al. (1977) report that GH enrollees were less satisfied than those in the FFS system on all dimensions. When one considers the alternatives, however, this result is hardly surprising. The Model Cities FFS enrollees had free choice of almost any physician in a county with a high physician-population ratio. All services were completely covered, so GH offered no financial advantages. Gaus, Cooper, and Hirschman (1976) report few differences in satisfaction across a broad list of measures, but unfortunately, they do not provide any data. Fuller and Patera (1976) report that significantly more Medicaid enrollees in GHA were very satisfied with their overall care (39 percent) than was the case for Medicaid recipients in the FFS system. On the other hand, more of the GHA enrollees were dissatisfied. This pattern of more extreme feelings by HMO enrollees is repeated for specific measures. For instance 31 percent of GHA enrollees liked its personalized service, in contrast to 1 percent of the control group, but 12 percent of GHA enrollees complained about impersonal service, versus 4 percent.

Only two major studies compare levels of satisfaction across income and education levels among regularly enrolled HMO members. Pope, Greenlick, and Freeborn (1972) found that people with higher incomes were more satisfied with the range of services, costs, and facilities and were less satisfied with system characteristics, such as making appointments and location of physicians. These results are not striking, and many apparent relationships are due to age and sex differences rather than socioeconomic factors. Similar problems arise in interpreting the Hetherington, Hopkins, and Roemer results (1975).

Enrollee views of accessibility and satisfaction present the same wide range that is found with utilization data. In some settings access and satisfaction appear to be worse in HMOs, while in others they are better. Availability of physicians and other health personnel is generally better in an organized setting. Some other patterns that might be expected are only partially borne out. While it is often more difficult to get an appointment, the office waiting times are less for HMO enrollees. There are, however, several counterexamples. Similarly, when financial coverage in the two systems is equivalent, there is less satisfaction for HMO enrollees. But this is true in one case, and the reverse is true in another. Thus the key variable seems to be, not HMO incentives, but the structure and performance of the local FFS system.

HMOS AND THE POOR: HOW VIABLE A COMBINATION?

This review of the evidence concerning HMOs and the poor should temper great hopes, calm overwhelming fears, and lead to careful thinking about the future. It is clear that HMOs per se cannot solve the problems of medical care for the poor. These problems are primarily the result of the poor being poor. They simply cannot command the same resources as the rich. This is especially true in medicine, which has been characterized by a sellers' market for the last few decades. Medical providers can do well treating the middle class, who are generally seen as more desirable patients because they share similar values and priorities and are reasonably compliant (Berkanovic and Reeder, 1974). The few physicians who choose to practice in poverty areas find themselves quickly overwhelmed with work, and they can easily be sucked into an assembly-line type of practice. While Medicaid coverage helps, its fees are too low to induce the supply that is necessary to provide mainstream medicine to the poor. The result is the worst of all possible worlds: high costs because services of poor quality are often provided to those who can get care, and many people who are still outside the system.

In theory, the HMO, particularly the PGP model, could provide comprehensive, one-stop care to the poor at lower cost. The gap between theory and reality has already been described. Currently, the only way that the poor can afford HMOs is through Medicaid or a limited and shrinking number of demonstration projects. Medicaid enrollment often entails monthly uncertainty about eligibility and turnover rates two to three times that of employed HMO members. From the recipient's perspective, the HMO's attractiveness is inversely related to the availability of other providers. If other good sources are available, the freedom to choose among them is desirable; if there are few alternatives, the pressure to join an HMO is greater, but its incentives to perform well are reduced.

New regulations at both the federal and state levels have been designed to curb some abuses that occurred in the early California prepaid health plan program (Chavkin and Treseder, 1977). Among these are the requirements that HMOs receiving Medicaid funds meet federal HMO qualification requirements. This includes provisions that at least half the enrollees be private (that is, not Medicare or Medicaid) and that there be substantial consumer representation on the board of directors. The first is by far the most important. (For a discussion of consumer representation see Chapter 14.) Its intent is that middle-class enrollees, who have good alternative sources of care, will be able to force the HMO to maintain appropriate levels of quality and accessibility. The effect of the restriction, however, may be to substantially hinder the development of HMOs. The crucial problem is not only that the poor generally lack medical care coverage but that they often live in economic ghettoes. Thus a single location for a PGP is unlikely to serve the poor *and* the middle class conveniently. Furthermore, although poverty areas usually include many employed people, they often are in low-wage jobs with few fringe benefits and no concentration in a small number of companies. Marketing to employee groups becomes exceedingly difficult. Spitz (1979) argues that in most areas, HMOs serving the poor will become "Medicaid HMOs." In such cases special policies must be instituted to counter problems created by the Medicaid program.

A possible alternative model is an HMO composed of facilities in suburban and inner-city locations, thus meeting the 50 percent limit on publicly funded enrollees. One problem is that separate but equal often implies separate but unequal (Roman, 1975, p. 130). While the dual system may not be ideal, it may be substantially better than the alternatives. There has been some experience with such multisite organizations through the Office of Economic Opportunity Health Networks. These were designed to enroll both the poor and the middle class in the same organizations, albeit in different locations. The program can hardly be called successful, but Penchansky and Berki (1976) persuasively argue that it would be foolish to conclude that the experiment has failed, because it was never really tried. In addition to the problems in implementing the program at the federal level, there was a multiplicity of goals, overfunding, geographic service area boundaries, state resistance, and attempts to develop programs without competitive advantages. Some of these problems potentially could be overcome with better planning. Others would require some form of national health insurance coverage that would allow, if not encourage, HMOs and include not just the very poor, but people at all income levels, without regard to group employer-based contracts.

Another alternative approach is to interpose an intermediary agency between the Medicaid agency, the providers, and the enrollees. The purpose of such a health plan office is to assume responsibility for marketing, enrollment, coordination of services, consumer advocacy, and quality control (Bosch et al., 1979). While the primary difficulty with such a plan is that it does not address the fluctuating eligibility of Medicaid recipients, a similar and more encompassing plan is in operation in Portland, Oregon (Lewis, 1979; Multnomah County, Oregon, Project Health, 1977a,b). Project Health was originally designed to guarantee services for the near and working poor, who are not eligible for Medicaid and who rely heavily on county hospital services. It uses local tax funds previously earmarked for the county hospital to subsidize insurance premiums for low-income families. A family's share is based on income, family size, and the cost of the plan. This sum ranges from $1 to $53 per month. Project Health then serves as an insurance broker to enroll its clients in any of six prepaid health plans, including three HMOs. Each plan is required to offer a standard benefit package and thus compete for enrollees by lowering premiums. Enrollment counselors are provided by Project Health, thus reducing the potential for marketing abuses. Project Health is now responsible for Medicaid recipients in the county and will be able to guarantee coverage in prepaid plans as these families move in and out of Medicaid eligibility. In essence, Project Health serves as a low-income version of Enthoven's Consumer Choice Health Plan (Enthoven, 1978b).

Problems of supply maldistribution still exist. The turnover rate of Neighborhood Health Center physicians has been discouragingly high (Tilson, 1973a). There is also evidence that many of these physicians were recruited from other poverty areas (Reynolds, 1976, p. 77). When there is a real shortage of physicians in an area, group practice may be the only way to assure physicians that they will not be overwhelmed by patient demands (McLaughlin, 1978; Orso, 1979; Leff et al., 1977). The group allows a sharing of responsibilities. Prepayment helps to limit the population for which the physicians feel responsible. Many physicians, however, find the socioeconomic problems of ghetto patients overwhelming even when there is an effective gatekeeper. One possible scheme would involve a split practice for physicians in an HMO serving middle-class and poverty populations in two locations. The physicians might spend half-time at each, providing both a balance for their practice and a broader understanding of health problems (Peebles, 1977).

Problems in rural areas are often very different. Population density is insufficient to sustain a large prepaid group, and unattractive cultural surroundings cannot be solved by a simple commute to the suburbs. There is, however, some evidence that physicians are beginning to locate in nonmetropolitan areas again, and that group practice and other organizational arrangements are encouraging this shift (Evashwick, 1976; Mattera, 1978). Such groups tend to be small, and rural HMOs are likely to be IPAs. There are some rural PGPs, such as the Bellaire, Ohio, Medical Group. These generally are dependent on a single large employee group, like the

United Mine Workers, and they obtain much of their income from FFS practice (Neil, Goldstein, and Birmingham, 1974). IPAs are unlikely to add substantially to the physician supply in a rural area, but they can increase the willingness of available physicians to accept Medicaid eligibles (Sheridan, 1978). In practice, however, Holahan found no evidence that the San Joaquin IPA had any effect on utilization patterns or the proportion of Medicaid eligibles seeing physicians (1977a). Indeed, Havighurst (1974) argues that a major aim of IPAs is to prevent competitors from entering their market area. Thus it appears that the major problems in rural areas are attributable to long-term trends in physician location patterns that are unlikely to be easily reversed by HMO incentives.

The medical care delivery problems of the elderly poor are very different from those of ghetto and rural populations. Medicare was designed to offer health insurance coverage to the elderly, but it included coinsurance and deductibles to help control demand. There is some evidence that they do reduce demand (Peel and Scharff, 1973). Even with Medicare, however, out-of-pocket costs for the elderly are well above those of other ages (U.S. National Center for Health Statistics, "Personal Out-of-Pocket Health Expenses," November 1978, p. 18). The covered costs of the Medicare program have also been growing rapidly, largely because of hospitalization. These issues of out-of-pocket costs and hospitalization are problems that HMOs are better designed to tackle. The elderly are much more likely to live in areas with medical resources, so supply is not such an overwhelming issue. A major constraint seems to have been the resistance of the Social Security Administration to contract with HMOs on anything but FFS or very unfavorable risk-sharing arrangements. On their part, HMOs seem to have been afraid of massive selective enrollment of high-risk beneficiaries. While difficult, these problems are more likely to have administrative solutions than the others discussed in this chapter (see Luft, Feder, Holahan, and Lennox, 1980). The Health Care Financing Administration is currently undertaking some capitation experiments for Medicare beneficiaries (1978). Legislative changes will be required to allow more general capitation payments in the Medicare program.

A strategy for encouraging HMOs to serve the poor is unlikely to have a major effect unless other policies are also initiated. If the poor already have reasonable sources of care, HMOs are likely to provide another good alternative. If the poor are currently mistreated by the system—either underserved or overserved by Medicaid mills—competing HMOs are likely to do the same. HMOs may have an impact on the location of physicians in urban poverty areas, but much stronger incentives are necessary for rural areas. The one area in which HMOs may have a major effect is in serving the elderly, but that experiment has not been pursued. Thus major improvements for the poor depend upon broad initiatives, not on the activities of a small number of HMOs. As will be discussed in the next chapter, the environment in which HMOs exist is crucial to their performance.

FOURTEEN

Organizational and Environmental Factors in HMO Performance

The preceding chapters have relied upon the heroic assumption that only three types of medical provider-insurance systems exist: prepaid group practices, individual practice associations, and "conventional providers." Differences within each type have been deemphasized. This gross simplification was necessary for two reasons. First, policy-makers usually approach HMOs as if all such organizations were the same. Second, as will be outlined in this chapter, HMOs differ along so many dimensions that our state of knowledge and the data are insufficient to provide an understanding of why they differ in performance. In contrast to previous chapters, the focus here is on describing these more subtle dimensions that affect HMO performance.

HMOs are composed of physicians, administrators, staff, directors, and consumers, and these organizations exist within a larger environment that may be supportive, neutral, or antagonistic. In order to understand the performance of a given HMO, one must consider two crucial areas: (1) *internal factors* of the organization, such as sponsorship and goals, financial support, organizational structure, and individual personalities; and (2) *external factors,* such as the health insurance market, legal restrictions, and competitive responses of conventional providers.

Successful performance may be measured in terms of enrollment growth, financial viability, or consumer or provider satisfaction. Regardless of the measure, however, it is likely to depend on a complex combination of internal and external elements. While HMOs can probably succeed with certain factors working against them, other factors must be able to compensate. A truly dedicated group of consumers and providers may be able to survive in a hostile environment, but a poorly organized group can fail in even the most supportive environment. These factors are also likely to interact with each other. For example, an HMO that is sponsored by groups interested in producing fundamental change in the delivery of care is more likely to face opposition by local providers than one that has more circumscribed and conventional goals.

These issues are examined under four broad headings within the remainder of this chapter. The first section examines the influence of the sponsorship and goals of the organization. This issue includes the importance of profit versus nonprofit orientation and the impact of consumer involvement. The second section covers the general area of organizational structure, management, and internal incentives. In addition to the issues of administrative structure, centralization, and managerial skills, this section addresses questions of how physicians are paid, whether they are full- or part-time, whether an HMO should control a hospital, and how access to specialists is controlled. The third section is concerned with external or environmental factors that affect HMO performance. These include legal and regulatory constraints, general sociodemographic factors, and the influence of the medical care market. The fourth section expands the discussion from the influence of external factors on the organization to the impact of the HMO on its environment through teaching and research and the effects of HMO competition on other providers. A final section offers a brief summary.

SPONSORSHIP AND GOALS OF THE ORGANIZATION

The sponsorship and goals of HMOs are often thought to be major variables in determining performance. Many states refuse to sign Medicaid contracts with HMOs that are organized on a for-profit basis. The HMO Act requires HMO boards to have substantial consumer representation (U.S. Department of Health, Education, and Welfare, 1974, p. 37,315). Also one can expect differences among HMOs sponsored by consumer cooperatives, labor unions, employers, FFS group practices, county medical societies, and insurance carriers. Because the type of sponsorship often conditions the goals and structure of the organization, this section first explores the range of sponsorship and its implications. The remaining two subsections examine the importance of profit and nonprofit structures and the implications of consumer involvement.

Sponsorship

HMOs have been developed by a wide range of groups for various purposes. In some cases sponsorship and goals have had a clear impact on the organization's development and success. Many of the precursors to modern HMOs were developed by industry during the late nineteenth century to serve isolated groups of railroad, mining, and lumber company employees (Weissman, 1962; Blumberg, 1977; American Medical Association, 1959; Schwartz, 1967). These often included medical and surgical care of employees and their families through providers under contract to the health care program. Such programs have been criticized, often justly, for poor-quality care geared more toward cost minimization than enrollee needs (MacColl, 1966, p. 11). Some of these employer-sponsored programs, however, have a long history of providing quality care, although in a paternalistic environment. The Hawaiian sugar plantations, for example, traditionally offered cradle-to-grave medical coverage with an emphasis on easy access and a personalized physician-patient relationship (Bailey, 1971, p. 42). Recently, industry has again begun to sponsor HMOs in an effort to control the costs of employee health benefits (Katz, 1978; Stacey, 1978; Halenar, 1979).

In a parallel fashion, union-sponsored plans have provided benefits for their members either through indemnity reimbursement plans or directly through union-controlled clinics. The United Mine Workers of America (UMWA) program is one of the oldest and largest of such industry-wide organizations. Reflecting its rural bases, the UMWA plan has used a retainer system for 6000 individual physicians across the country (Kerr, 1968). Other unions, such as Garment Workers in Chicago, Teamsters in St. Louis, and United Farm Workers in California, operate health centers to service their members and families (Simon and Rabushka, 1956; MacColl, 1966; Chamberlin and Radebaugh, 1976).

Some HMOs began with employer or union sponsorship and have since changed. Kaiser-Permanente was begun by Kaiser Industries as a method of providing medical care for its workers on isolated construction projects. During World War II it expanded to serve workers in Kaiser shipyards in Richmond, California and Portland, Oregon and in Kaiser steel mills in Fontana, California. When the shipyards closed in 1945 the health plan, which was headed by Dr. Sidney Garfield, chose not to close but to attract enrollees from employee groups and local unions. Although still informally linked to Kaiser Industries, the Kaiser Foundation Health Plan is now an independent, nonprofit organization with the goal of providing medical services to the community (Williams, 1971). The Community Health Foundation of Cleveland, now Kaiser Cleveland, was begun on the initiative of the Meat Cutters and Retail Clerks Unions (Banta and Bosch, 1974). The Community Health Association of Detroit was developed with the support of the United Auto Workers and is now under local Blue Cross sponsorship.

In addition to single employer-union sponsors, some HMOs have been sponsored by a more broadly based community effort. GHCPS is the largest and best known of these and still retains its cooperative structure. (It is interesting to note that even in this case 55 percent of the subscribers enroll through large groups and do not have full cooperative membership; Mercer, 1973, p. 46.) Other well-known community-sponsored plans are Community Hospital Association of Elk City, Oklahoma, and GHA of Washington, D.C. (MacColl, 1966).

HMO sponsorship has also come from the provider side. The Ross-Loos Medical Group was founded by two Los Angeles physicians in order to deliver prepaid care to employees of the Department of Water and Power (Kisch and Viseltear, 1967). The partnership has grown to include over 100 physicians and now controls its own insurance company and hospital. The San Joaquin Foundation for Medical Care and the Physicians Association of Clackamas County were both founded by local medical societies (Sasuly and Hopkins, 1967; Haley, 1971). Group Health Plan of St. Paul, Minnesota was founded in 1956 by a local insurance company (MacColl, 1966). In the 1970s health insurance-sponsored programs became more common, particularly those backed by Blue Cross and Blue Shield (Gossett, 1972; Blue Cross and Blue Shield, 1978). The 1977 *Census of HMOs* listed forty-two carrier-sponsored plans; these were second only to fifty-three consumer-sponsored HMOs (U.S. Health Maintenance Organization Service, 1978).

Several medical schools have sponsored HMOs with the goals of teaching and research, as well as provision of medical care for the community. Among those established in the late 1960s and early 1970s were the Harvard Community Health Plan, Community Health Care Center Plan (Yale), Columbia Medical Plan (Johns Hopkins), and Medical Care Group of Washington University (Pollack, 1969; Falk, 1969; Heyssel and Seidel, 1976; Perkoff, Kahn, and Haas, 1976). Other new HMOs have been sponsored by hospitals (Light and Match, 1976; American Hospital Association, 1975; Simler, 1977; Shortell, 1978).

It would be surprising if the different types of sponsorship were not reflected in the goals and performance of the various organizations. In order to examine the evidence surrounding this conjecture, it is necessary to consider first the issues of sponsorship and goals in a historical perspective (Blumberg, 1977). The late nineteenth century saw the development of the railroad and mining company-sponsored plans in isolated areas, as well as those of mutual aid societies and fraternal orders. The spread of workers' compensation laws between 1910 and 1920 shifted responsibility for medical care following accidents to the employer. Particularly in the Pacific Northwest, this led employers of miners and loggers to contract with physicians and hospitals for such care. Over time, these contracts were broadened to cover nonindustrial accident care and also workers' families. In the 1930s the depression led to increased concern about people's inability to obtain and pay for medical care. During that period a lack of purchasing power left physicians and hospitals idle. The Committee on the Costs of Medical Care then suggested the development of voluntary health insurance and prepaid group practices (Andrus and Mitchell, 1977). Even prior to those recommendations, 1929 saw the founding of the Farmers Union of Elk City, Oklahoma and the Ross-Loos Clinic. World War II caused major population shifts and shortages of physicians for the civilian population because of military demands for medical personnel. This led to the development of the Kaiser plans for Kaiser shipyard and steel workers. During the postwar period fringe benefits were exempted from the general wage and salary freeze. This special exemption and the defeat of President Truman's national health insurance proposal led to a particularly rapid growth of voluntary insurance and prepaid group practices in the late 1940s and early 1950s (Vial, 1975). Even after the elimination of controls, the exclusion of fringe benefits from income and payroll taxes has provided a substantial incentive to expand health insurance coverage (Feldstein and Allison, 1972; Comanor, 1979). A recent study indicates that employee benefit costs increased 173 percent between 1967 and 1977, almost twice the expansion rate for annual earnings—98 percent. Moreover, health insurance fringe benefits increased 284 percent in the same period (National Chamber Foundation, 1978, p. 4). The rapidly escalating costs of medical care in the last decade have shifted the emphasis from improving access and coverage to cost control. Thus it is not surprising that recent interest in HMOs is based largely on their potential for controlling utilization. This is reflected in the specific aims of new HMOs sponsored by various firms (Walsh and Egdahl, 1977; Egdahl and Walsh, 1977; Salmon, 1975). The thrust of such organizations can be expected to differ from those founded in earlier periods, when the goal was toward the expansion of services, rather than their contraction.

There is some evidence that sponsorship affects the structure and performance of HMOs. Lum (1974) surveyed a sample of 173 PGPs and obtained usable responses from 66 (38 percent). While the low response rate limits our ability to draw firm conclusions, the results are still illustrative. Provider-sponsored plans, which include those of hospitals, physician groups, private corporations, medical schools, and IPAs, tended to have large-scale operations. They were more likely to control their own hospitals than other sponsors. These plans tended to cater to employed groups, and they offered most services, with the exception of treatment for alcohol and drug abuse and dental care. Carrier-sponsored plans tended to have a single clinic facility with hospitalization arrangements at existing institutions. Their governing boards tended to have little control over budgets and contract approvals. Enrollees in carrier-sponsored plans were generally from employed groups and an employed-unemployed mix. (The latter group is composed of public welfare, Medicaid, and Medicare recipients.) Preventive services, alcohol and drug abuse treatment, and dental care were typically not covered. Carrier-sponsored plans tended to be highly decentralized and traditional in orientation. Consumer and union-sponsored plans were characterized by strong and active governing boards that maintained budgetary control and contract approval authority. Their enrollee mix was weighted toward employed groups but also included the unemployed. These PGPs tended to own their primary care facilities, and they offered the most comprehensive range of services. A final group, identified as "the independents," seemed to be composed largely of Neighborhood Health Centers and other public facilities. Their enrollment was heavily weighted toward the unemployed. Their governing boards had policy-making powers but not budget control. These organizations generally had their own primary care centers and arrangements with other facilities for hospitalization. Services included dental care but not alcohol and drug abuse treatment or long-term care.

A few other reports also indicate differences in performance based on sponsorship. Data from the 1977 *Census of HMOs* suggests that among PGPs in operation for eight or more years, which are the older, more stable plans, the hospital utilization rate for carrier-sponsored plans was 784 days per 1000, in contrast to an overall average of 482 (Morris, 1978). (These data are not adjusted for enrollee age-sex composition and thus should be treated with caution.) Strumpf and Garramone (1976) found that insufficient sponsor commitment was a major reason for termination of HMO development. This seemed to be a particular problem for plans sponsored by hospitals and medical schools. Physician-sponsored groups were often found to have goals inconsistent with those of the HMO Act and of long-term success (Zelten, 1977). In reviewing the problems encountered in the early years of the Columbia Medical Plan, Heyssel and Seidel (1976) suggest that some difficulties can be attributed to the complex arrangements stemming from dual sponsorship by a medical school and a commercial insurance carrier.

Profit-Nonprofit Orientation

The question of profit-nonprofit orientation is clouded by the absence of a clear relationship between the legal status of an organization and its true orientation. In fact, the profit-nonprofit distinction is largely a legal fiction (Starkweather, 1970). For many HMOs the decision to have for-profit or not-for-profit status is primarily dependent on (1) state laws concerning for-profit medical groups, (2) federal restrictions on grants to for-profit organizations, and (3) the trade-off between the tax advantages of the not-for-profit model and access to capital markets of the for-profit model. As discussed in the Chapter 13 section on HMOs serving the poor, a major example of the arbitrariness of legal distinctions is seen in the prepaid health plans designed for California's Medicaid population. When the state resisted contracting with for-profit firms, many of the same organizations established nonprofit corporations to contract with the state, while draining off substantial profits through subsidiaries (U.S. General Accounting Office, 1976; California Department of Health, 1975; U.S. Senate, Committee on Governmental Affairs, 1978).

Four major groups can sponsor, finance, and profit from HMOs: enrollees, physicians, other providers, and outside investors. It is the last group that is often considered to be in it "just for the profit," and in one sense, this is true by definition. On the other hand, the long-run interests of such investors might be best realized by HMOs that effectively serve their communities and offer a reasonable return on investment. The best model for comparison is that of proprietary hospitals, but the evidence concerning their efficiency and mode of operation relative to community hospitals is inconclusive (Eamer, 1971; Johnson, 1971; Steinwald and Neuhauser, 1970; Ferber, 1971; Kushman and Nuckton, 1977; Ruchlin, Pointer, and Cannedy, 1973; Rafferty and Schweitzer, 1974). (In fact, some proprietary hospital chains are beginning to enter the HMO field; Federation of American Hospitals Review, 1978.) Few people would be concerned if an HMO earned "profits" that were then returned to enrollees in cash, lower premiums, or increased benefits. Yet what if these "profits" were achieved through unfair labor practices? Similarly, it is difficult to distinguish profits from salaries or bonuses for physicians.* In particular, many not-for-profit HMOs, such as Kaiser, contract with medical groups that must be understood as for-profit partnerships (Etzioni and Doty, 1976).

It is probably impossible to separate the structure and goals of an organization from the preferences of the people who work for it. For instance, a consumer-run HMO is unlikely to attract or hire physicians whose primary motivation is income maximization. Similarly, it is not surprising that the for-profit (de facto) prepaid health plans in Southern California had a disproportionate number of young and part-time physicians (Moore and Breslow, 1972). Such physicians are likely to be less interested in long-run stability than in short-term gains. Thus much more emphasis should be placed on the horizon of the organization than on its apparent corporate structure. A for-profit HMO formed by local physicians seeking long-term growth and stability in the community would be preferable to a not-for-profit HMO that maintains a for-profit subsidiary that offers investment opportunities based on an expectation of very high short-term growth rates and earnings. The latter is much less likely to make long-term investments in quality equipment and personnel, provide preventive care for its enrollees, and seek to maintain enrollee satisfaction.

Consumer Involvement

A potentially important factor in discussing the goals of an HMO is the nature and extent of consumer involvement and control. Unfortunately, the situation is much like that of the profit-nonprofit distinctions; what appears on the surface to be consumer involvement may just be tokenism (Arnstein, 1969). The federal requirements are that "(A) at least one-third of the membership of the policymaking body of the health maintenance organization will be members of the organization, and (B) there will be equitable representation on such body of members from medically un-

---

*The issue of whether physicians earn an excessively high rate of return on their educational investment has been widely debated, but there is no definitive answer to this question. See Lindsay (1973, 1976); Mennemeyer (1978); Sloan (1976); Fein and Webber (1971); Dyckman (1978).

derserved populations served by the organization" (U.S. Congress, 1973, Section 1301, c(5)). This can obviously be implemented in many ways. The true nature of consumer involvement can probably only be known by undertaking a careful case study of each plan.

Before further discussing consumer involvement in medical care, it may be useful to identify the consumer. The director of member relations for Southern California Kaiser identifies two important types of consumers: (1) members, including existing or potential subscribers and dependents; and (2) third-party purchasers, those representatives who purchase or negotiate contract coverage on behalf of a group of employees or union members (Slayman, 1973). He explicitly excludes "'professional consumers'—concerned health care observers and students who believe because they are concerned they are 'consumers' and as such should have a voice in the operation of *all* health care organizations" (1973, p. 52). While most others would not make the distinction with such vehemence, voluntary enrollment makes it easy for an HMO to concern itself only with people who choose to belong to the organization. The ease with which dissatisfied members can leave an HMO, however, may have a substantial impact on the quality of the organization (Hirschman, 1970). The focus on members and their contracting groups also implies that an HMO need not be concerned about people who are not in eligible groups or cannot afford the basic package. Thus an HMO may take a stance of pleasing its overall membership to the exclusion of some specific members and of groups and individuals who are unable to join. Such an organization may quite reasonably justify its position with the claim that it cannot be responsible for the ills of society but that its greatest service is to maximize the benefits for its members and their negotiating groups.

Consumer members of an HMO may find themselves in conflicting roles—as responsible members and as individual patients. For example, as a patient, an enrollee may support the position of the organization financing second opinions from outside consultants. As a member, however, the same consumer may be concerned about the costs of such an option and the HMOs' potential risk of professional liability (Ladimer, 1977, p. 15). As a patient, one may be unconcerned with the financial implications of extra services. Direct consumer involvement, however, makes the trade-offs and their implications explicit and puts a greater part of the decision-making responsibility on the consumer. Enrollees vary in their interest in such involvement. While some pursue it, others prefer to make as few decisions as possible.

While there is extensive literature on what consumer involvement should be, there are almost no data on current experience. There is even less evidence on the effects of consumer participation on HMO performance. In part, this may be because it is difficult to maintain a high level of participation. For instance, less than 1 percent of the Group Health Cooperative membership actively participates in its operation (Mercer,

1973, p. 46). Harrelson and Donovan (1975) identify some of the difficulties faced by the Columbia Medical Plan in involving consumers and in actually achieving an effective consumer role in the plan. One difficulty seemed to be a lack of broadly based interest on the part of the enrollees, so that only a small, self-selected group of members served as consumer council members. Steinberg (1977) examined the development and role of consumer councils in HIP. Largely because they were not integral parts of and valued by the organization, they had little power and were essentially ineffective. This is also the case in United Mine Workers of America clinics (Goldstein, 1978).

The potential for consumer influence is greatest in the consumer cooperative health plans. Members own the plan and are generally constrained from involvement only in medical decision-making. At the other extreme are physician-sponsored plans that vest control of both medical and nonmedical decisions in the physicians. Schwartz (1965, 1968) examined six plans of each type in order to test the hypothesis that greater consumer control leads to differences in services, benefits, staffing, enrollment policies, health education, and methods to assess consumer satisfaction. Surprisingly, the two types of plans were similar in many respects. All plans offered broad coverage of basic medical services and most preventive services. Consumer plans offered more extra benefits, such as eyeglasses and prescription drugs, in their packages. These extra benefits often reflected an expressed willingness on the part of cooperative members to bear extra premium costs. Group enrollment policies were the same in both types of plans, but the consumer cooperatives all allowed individual enrollment, in contrast to only two of the six physician plans. This reflects a greater commitment to the community at large, even at the risk of some adverse enrollee-selection. Neither type of plan devoted much attention to health education, information programs, evaluation of clinic care, or assessment of consumer satisfaction. The consumer plans, however, had much more clearly defined grievance and complaint mechanisms. The consumer plans were weaker in two areas: they were more likely to be staffed by part-time physicians, and they had greater difficulty offering coverage in medical specialties. These results are based on data fifteen years old, but they offer the only objective comparison of the influence of consumer control.

Consumer ownership of HMOs is controversial because of the different experiences of two highly visible cooperatives—GHA, Washington, D.C. and GHCPS. GHA has been plagued by a dispute with its physicians that erupted in a strike in 1978 (Meyer, 1978; Cohn, 1976; Peck, 1978). The major issue was not physician salaries, but the extent to which GHA could control physician activities. The GHA board of trustees, committed to consumer control, was unwilling to allow more physician autonomy. The physicians charged that the structure fostered a nine-to-five, civil-service mentality among its physicians. Some of these problems may underlie the relatively slow growth in GHA membership. Quite the opposite set of experiences can be found a continent away in Seattle, where GHCPS has grown rapidly and relations are congenial between the physicians (who are employees, as is the case at GHA) and the board. Thus it is unlikely that consumer control per se is responsible for either the severe difficulties at GHA or the success of GHCPS.

In summary, the goals of an organization are likely to have an important effect on its performance, especially on those aspects that deal with subtle issues such as quality, ambience, and satisfaction. It does not seem to be the case that the obvious identifiers, such as type of sponsor, profit-nonprofit status, or consumer involvement, are effective in measuring the goals of the organization. Instead, more detailed studies are necessary in order to assess the impact of these factors on performance. Such studies should be designed to avoid a tautological relationship in which, for instance, consumer orientation is determined by examining the extent of proconsumer activities.

ORGANIZATIONAL STRUCTURE, MANAGEMENT, AND INTERNAL INCENTIVES

For any given set of goals, an organization can adopt a wide range of structures, management styles, and internal incentives. While a substantial body of literature has developed concerning organizational style and behavior, there is little addressed to HMOs in particular. There are two major exceptions to this generalization. Mechanic (1976) and Freidson (1975) consider the implications of group practice and prepayment on the behavior and roles of physicians. Chapter 12 discusses some of these results with respect to physician satisfaction. In this section, however, the focus is on the effect of organizational structure on the performance and long-term success of the HMO itself. Under this broad heading, several variables are of interest, and each is discussed in a separate subsection. The first deals with the general administrative structure, the level of centralization, and the importance of managerial skills. The second concerns methods of paying physicians and the extent of their participation in the HMO. The third section explores the issues surrounding HMO control of hospitals and access to specialists.

Administrative Structure, Centralization, and Managerial Skills

All forms of medical practice require some degree of administration. Even a solo FFS practitioner must be concerned with billing and control of office expenses. A 1975 survey indicates that administrative costs amounted to 15 percent of gross revenue, and that these costs ranged from $2.66 per visit for solo practitioners to $1.91 in physician groups of five or less (Abt

Associates, 1977, pp. 26-27). As the size of a group increases, physicians spend less time performing administrative tasks, because full-time personnel are assigned these duties. HMO administrations perform the combined functions of regular office practices and the financial and enrollment activities of insurers.*

The issue at hand, however, is not how much administration is necessary, but how the administration is carried out. It appears that a high degree of centralization is necessary only for those functions that are most closely akin to HMO insurance and enrollment functions. This seems related both to the inherent nature of those tasks and the fact that the models for these activities in the non-HMO sector are centralized. The delivery of medical care is a different matter; both centralized and decentralized models can succeed in terms of enrollment growth and financial viability.

Some large prepaid group practices are highly centralized and structured. Even Kaiser, however, allows substantial regional autonomy, and individual clinics within each region exercise some control over their own procedures. (There is some evidence that hospital chains that allow greater local autonomy are more efficient than their centrally controlled counterparts. (Coyne, 1978).) At the other extreme are the highly decentralized IPAs. Chapters 4, 5, and 11 suggested that while IPAs were less effective than PGPs in obtaining lower hospitalization rates and medical care expenditures, they were more successful in achieving consumer satisfaction. Whether any of these results is due to the greater decentralization in IPAs is unknown, but the findings are consistent with the expected results of less control. Between the two extremes are the network HMOs, such as HIP of New York with its nearly thirty group practices relating to a central insurance payment plan. Some of HIP's problems have been attributed to its lack of control over the part-time physicians in independent groups, and a major financial crisis was precipitated by its attempt to buy out the groups and convert its physicians to full-time practice. (Group Health and Welfare News, 1972; Schwartz, 1972; Hicks, 1972a,b; Bird, 1975; Steinberg, 1977.)

Wasserman (1976) reported that two factors could discriminate between plans that failed (eleven of twelve) and those that succeeded (six of six). The factors are: (1) the legal structure of the organization and its board of directors; and (2) administrative and managerial staffing. While these results seem impressive, they must be treated with caution. The weights used by Wasserman in setting his scales were arbitrary, and more importantly, the data were collected ex post facto. It is not surprising that a

---

*Some HMOs can eliminate the need for billing, but this seems to be a smaller saving than might be expected. The Abt survey indicates that of the average $2.45 per patient visit, $.43 was for making appointments and preparing insurance forms, and $.42 was for accounting, billing, and cashiering. Thus, at most, one-third of the administrative costs could be saved. On the other hand, because of its fixed revenues, an HMO probably has to maintain more careful control over the utilization of services, and thus requires more information of a different variety.

description of a plan's management, drawn up just one month before the organization failed, would indicate substantial chaos. The important question is whether it is possible to predict a plan's success rate based on information gathered at its inception.

The lack of clear evidence makes a comprehensive analysis impossible. However, there is support for the conjecture that an organization's formal structure is less important than the nature of the individuals who run it. In part, this statement is based on the observation that structure alone is a poor predictor of HMO performance. Insufficient managerial expertise is a variable that consistently appears in case studies of HMO failure (Strumpf and Garramone, 1976; MacColl, 1966; Lubalin et al., 1974; Lane, 1979). Intuitively, this makes sense. (An attempt at scoring various aspects of managerial competence could not demonstrate a correlation with overall performance [Jurgovan and Blair, 1979], but this may be a reflection of problems in scoring "competence.") Getting an HMO started is similar in many ways to setting up a small business, and the failure rate for new businesses is extraordinarily high (Dun and Bradstreet, 1978). While a physician can generally set up a new practice and begin to turn a profit within a year, an HMO must be concerned with marketing, enrollment, cost control, long-range planning, and meeting various regulatory requirements (Owens, 1973; Birnbaum, 1976; Kress and Singer, 1975). All of these items require expertise that is often not possessed by HMO founders (Biblo, 1972; U.S. General Accounting Office, 1975).

Payment of Physicians

Perhaps the most critical variable to be considered is the method of paying the key HMO decision-makers—the physicians responsible for ordering and providing medical services. The definition of an HMO implies that the organization has an incentive to contain costs and reduce utilization. One cannot assume, however, that the organization's goals will necessarily be carried out by the people within it. In particular, some internal incentives can be in conflict with the goals of the organization. (While this does not seem rational on the surface, it is not uncommon. See Whipple, 1977.)

Pauly (1970) provides an extensive discussion of the incentives operating at the margin under salary, capitation, and FFS payment of physicians. Pure salary arrangements, without bonuses tied to performance, afford no extra incentives for greater effort in order to promote patient satisfaction. Under a capitation system, the HMO pays the physician a fixed amount for a specified group of enrollees, in order to provide an incentive to attract patients. For a given patient load, physicians tend to reduce the amount of care they provide, either through less utilization (follow-up visits, procedures, inoculations, and so on) or more referrals to other providers. Clearly, the latter behavior does not result in a net savings to the HMO and may increase costs. One way to prevent overuse of referrals is to make the primary physician responsible for the referral costs, as in the SAFECO plan (Gregory, 1978; Moore, 1979). This does not solve the former problem, however, and may lead to "skimping" by the primary care physician. FFS payments to physicians, such as those in many IPAs, are likely to increase the number and costs of physician procedures. Even with a fixed fee schedule, the provider can increase the effective income per procedure by reclassifying marginal procedures into more complex (expensive) categories.

Bonuses, or the mechanism by which salaries are revised, tend to alter the incentives to approximate those of capitation or FFS. For instance, bonuses based on crude measures,of productivity or services rendered will produce salaries similar to those in FFS, while bonuses based on caseload tend to approximate a capitation scheme. In short, there is no single optimal way of paying physicians. (For a proposal on a three-part plan, including payments in recognition of special skills and activities and incentive payments, see Lee and Butler, 1974.)

Thus, regardless of the method of payment, there is likely to be some tension between providers and the organization. It is useful to examine the structure of HMO payment schemes that are designed to achieve the appropriate balance of incentives. There are very few pure salary arrangements. In most cases physicians are salaried for a brief probationary period and then receive substantial bonuses that are based on some measure of merit (Cook, 1971, p. 105; Group Health Association of America, 1972). The use of bonuses may be an attempt to prevent staff physicians from becoming bureaucrats, to avoid the development of the kind of impersonal, unsympathetic approach that often characterizes public clinics and government facilities. The FFS Marshfield Clinic, on the other hand, has developed a straight salary, equal sharing system.

Capitation payments to individual physicians are rare in the United States, with the exception of some plans that provide capitation payments to primary care physicians (Gregory, 1978; Moore, 1979; Health Maintenance Organization of Pennsylvania, 1978). Prepaid group practices often arrange health plan contracts with a physician group on a capitation basis. In such cases there are also negotiations to determine staffing ratios and other performance measures (Handschin, 1971, p. 51). HIP of New York developed an extensive list of incentive payments to its physician groups, in order to counteract the tendency to underserve enrollees; this often exists under a standard capitation plan. These payments were designed to influence ambulatory and hospital utilization, augment office hours, reduce patient turnover, and meet time-per-service standards. The incentive allowances could increase the basic capitation payments by 40 percent (Health Insurance Plan of Greater New York, 1970, p. 19. See Gintzig and Shouldice, 1971, for descriptions of similar plans in other HMOs). Morever, by making capitation payments to the physician group, which is typically small enough to police itself, the costs of excess ambulatory referrals are borne by the group (Whipple, 1977; Sloan, 1974). Wisconsin Physician Service (1977) has a similar arrangement, with capitation payments to groupings of independent physicians. Within each county there are from one to twenty-two pools, and risks are borne collectively by the physicians in each pool.

Within an IPA the FFS method of paying physicians, combined with a fixed budget, presents a potential problem at the end of the fiscal year. If there is a budget overrun, all parties suffer a proportionate cutback. This procedure has obvious disadvantages, the most important of which is illustrated by the following equation. If there were n physicians in the IPA, an extra service that went beyond the budget would still return $(n - 1)/n$ times the charge to the physician providing the service. The physician receives the full charge, but then is responsible, along with the other physicians, for 1 nth of the overage. IPAs have instituted peer review systems in order to reduce unnecessary utilization and excessive charges as they occur, rather than wait for the budget constraint (Egdahl, 1973; Steinwald, 1971). In the San Joaquin Foundation, cost review, which examines the reasonableness of the fee, has led to a 2 percent savings, while utilization review has resulted in an 11 to 15 percent savings (Morozumi, 1971, p. 26). Although IPAs generally are less successful than PGPs in achieving lower utilization, those IPAs that have done reasonably well seem to have had unusually effective peer review (Egdahl, Taft, and Linde, 1977, p. 339; Meier and Tillotson, 1978; Jensen, Warren, and Seigal, 1975).

In addition to their base payment method, physicians can share to various extents in the HMO's potential gains and losses. This can be accomplished by making each physician's bonus (or the total amount of the physicians' budget in an IPA) dependent on the overall net revenue of the HMO. Sometimes such profit sharing is limited to ambulatory and inpatient physician services and does not apply to hospital costs (Schlenker et al., 1974, pp. 35-46). When this is the case physicians may substitute hospital services for ambulatory services, resulting in a conflict between personal incentives and the administrative goal of minimizing hospital costs (see Ting, 1975). If this merely results in a bargaining game to allocate costs, then it is of little overall interest. Of course, because inpatient services are more expensive, the substitution will reduce overall plan efficiency. It may be argued, however, that even if bonuses are not directly affected by hospital costs, in the long run they will reflect overall cost savings through the process of annual negotiations. Given the loosely competitive nature of the relevant markets for health professionals and health services, it is likely that internal bargaining power, information, and negotiating skill will be of primary importance.

The focus of this discussion, however, is on factors that lead to successful or unsuccessful performance, not those that will eventually dominate. Thus explicit sharing schemes and schemes in which risk and surplus are handled symmetrically are likely to accelerate efforts to improve performance. Some HMOs allow physicians to share the profits of the hospital side but do not penalize them for the losses (Schlenker et al., 1974, Tables 13, 16; Egdahl, Taft, and Linde, 1977, p. 339). As long as the hospital operates with a deficit, physicians in such plans are likely to be indifferent to the size of the deficit. A similar problem exists with quasi-HMOs, such as HIP of New York, in which the organization has no financial responsibility for hospitalization costs, which are covered directly by Blue Cross (Greenberg and Rodburg, 1971, p. 914).

Meier and Tillotson (1978) conducted intensive interviews with physicians and administrators in nine HMOs to examine the role of physician reimbursement patterns on hospital use. In general, they found that the level of financial risk borne by physicians was small (always less than 10 percent of income) and not directly related to lower hospital utilization. In some instances bonus payments were viewed as effective positive incentives. The potential risk can have an indirect impact by leading to the implementation of peer interaction and cost-effective orientation, under the direction of active medical leadership. These responses, however, seem conditional upon the perceived threat of competition that initially induced the physicians to accept the risk and restrictions. Discussions at a conference of PGP medical directors also support the notion that, from the physician's perspective, the role of financial incentives is indirect (Newman, 1973, pp. 73-77).

Some issues related to physician payment schemes are peculiar to IPAs, because IPA enrollment in most areas is so small that physician members derive most of their revenue from non-IPA enrollees (Egdahl, Taft, and Linde, 1977, p. 339). As the proportion of their revenue from the IPA grows, physicians may become less enchanted with the concept. When most of a physician's income is obtained from uncontrolled FFS practice, the lower fees and peer-monitored practice associated with IPA enrollees may be appealing, because the additional revenue from the IPA patients exceeds the additional costs. As the fraction of IPA patients grows, their fees may no longer cover their marginal costs. IPA patients will become less attractive, and more costs will be shifted to the FFS patients, making that physician less competitive. This appears to be the case for hospital care when hospitals receive Medicare reimbursements at less than their average cost, and an ever-increasing "deficit" (or overhead cost) is shifted to a smaller number of private patients. The end of this story appears to take place when all patients are in the IPA (or government Medicare), and providers are faced with negotiated budgets.

Even very large PGPs, such as Kaiser, need to contract with outside physicians on a part-time or FFS basis. For example, Kaiser Northern

California contracts with Stanford University for open heart surgery. Many HMOs allow their primary care physicians to maintain active private practices. These HMOs generally fall into two groups: (1) stable HMOs that are large enough to maintain a full-time staff but, by reasons of design or historical negotiations, allow their physicians to maintain FFS practices; and (2) newly developing HMOs that are not yet able to support a full-time staff.

There are some particular problems associated with the use of part-time physicians. First, physicians who maintain private practices have greater bargaining power vis-a-vis the HMO: they can more readily leave and therefore may be able to increase their relative share of the profits or savings achieved by the HMO. Second, part-time physicians are likely to prefer a lesser degree of risk sharing with the HMO, because their FFS practice can offer more substantial income-generating possibilities, and the HMO work may be seen as a stable source of base income. Thus part-time physicians are likely to prefer a straight salary or capitation, and this gives them an incentive to minimize their efforts for the HMO. Third, part-time physicians will be tempted to shift costs from their private practice to the HMO and be less responsive to their HMO patients. This cost shifting is easier to do and less noticeable if the same office is used for both practices. It is worth noting that HIP was plagued by the fact that most of its medical groups were only part-time (Hicks, 1972b; Levy and Fein, 1972).

In summary, the design of the physician payment scheme must contend with the inherent conflicts that exist in transactions among independent parties. The conflict is not unique to medicine. In any commercial transaction one expects the consumer to demand as much as possible and the supplier to offer as little as possible, with each weighing the long-run consequences of their acts. Medicine is different in that the physician serves both as the patient's agent and as a major supplier of services. FFS, salary, and capitation schemes all have advantages and disadvantages. The choice among them depends in part upon one's values and assumptions about how the medical care system works.

It is possible, however, to point to some schemes that have definite disadvantages and should probably be dropped from consideration as viable alternatives. Without some risk sharing, FFS payments to physicians within an HMO (either IPA or PGP) seem to generate substantial conflicts in incentives and the need for cumbersome utilization controls (Whipple, 1977; Egdahl, Taft, and Linde, 1977). (As will be seen below, fear of PGP competition may enable such schemes to work in the short run.) Risk sharing should apply equally to all types of services so as not to induce distortions in resource allocation. Furthermore the risk should be borne by relatively small pools of physicians. It also seems to be the case that part-time practice leads to conflicts of interest among physicians in terms of time and effort allocations. This major issue stems from the very high incomes available to specialists in private practice and has caused serious controversy among a number of medical groups (Group Health and Welfare News, 1972; Sullivan, 1977; Steinberg, 1977).

Organizational Control of Specialists and Hospital Services

The HMO maintains responsibility for providing or assuring provision of the complete range of medical care, including specialist treatment and hospital services. The question is: how should the HMO control access to services? Specialist treatment and hospital care, although required relatively infrequently, account for a large fraction of total expenditures. Decisions to employ both types of services require the technical training of a physician, and patients do not make these judgments independently. The major issue with respect to specialists is the extent to which an HMO limits member access to specialists through maintenance of control through the primary care physician. As for hospital services, the issue for HMOs is whether they should directly control hospitals or purchase services from local hospitals.

Control of Hospital Services.   Whether an HMO should control its own hospital has been a major issue for several decades. Of the large HMOs, Kaiser and GHCPS are hospital-based, while HIP and GHA are not. A review of the literature suggests that controlling one's own hospital is generally considered a major advantage (Gumbiner, 1975, pp. 32-36; Rothenberg, Pickard, and Rothenberg, 1949, pp. 231-234; MacColl, 1966, p. 116). The primary reasons advanced are: savings in physician time; concentration of consultants in one location; avoidance of duplication of equipment and personnel between hospital and clinic; better control of bed usage; and the assurance of adequate patient volume so that the hospital is not compelled to compete for physicians with expensive and underused equipment. The primary reason for not maintaining a hospital is related to scale; to fill a moderately sized hospital requires an enrollment of 50,000 to 80,000 people. Unless an HMO can achieve a very high market penetration within a densely populated area, travel time to the hospital facility can be a major deterrent to enrollment.

Both HIP and GHA have blamed their excessive costs on the lack of hospital control and have made attempts to gain more direct control over hospital service provision (Greenberg and Rodburg, 1971, p. 911; Steinberg, 1977, p. 67; Schwartz, 1972; Barker, 1976; Cohn, 1976). The Columbia Medical Plan explicitly recognized the problems faced by HIP and GHA when in 1968 it chose to build, own, and operate its own hospital (Heyssel and Seidel, 1976, p. 1226). HIP also purchased a hospital (La Guardia) and is increasing its ties with other hospitals (Steinberg, 1977). In the face of currently increasing surpluses of hospital beds, it is less likely that an HMO will obtain approval by planning agencies to build its own hospital. HMOs have thus consistently fought for exemption from such health planning regulations. Partly because existing providers may attempt to use certificate-of-need as an anticompetitive device, new regulations have been issued to exempt HMOs from certificate-of-need requirements (Havighurst, 1970, 1973; U.S. Department of Health, Education and Welfare, 1979). It may be useful, however, to reconsider the potential advantages and disadvantages of hospital control.

The advantages claimed for hospital control actually fall into two categories: those related to proximity and those related to hospital technology and efficiency. An HMO can locate its clinic adjacent to a hospital and achieve most, if not all, of the following advantages: saving physician time; access to consultants; and avoiding duplication of equipment for inpatient and outpatient services, such as laboratory and X-ray. In fact, many conventional hospitals have constructed medical office buildings that achieve these purposes. Controlling hospital technology and efficiency is a different matter. The physician has control over patient admissions and discharges but exerts less authority over such matters as the speed with which laboratory tests are returned and operating rooms are scheduled. As was seen in Chapter 7, HMOs controlling their own hospitals do not seem to have achieved substantial savings per patient day. Thus the potential for efficiencies may be small. The major alternative to controlling a hospital is for an HMO to contract with a local hospital for services and be able to negotiate lower rates (Meier and Tillotson, 1978). The HMO is then in a position to threaten to pull out if costs get out of line, which may be a more effective incentive for cost savings than direct control. (A wholly owned hospital has little fear of losing its "customer.")

The primary disadvantage in using local hospitals is that they often feel compelled to compete for FFS physicians by adding underused equipment and services. This inevitably results in higher costs. There is some evidence that, controlling for bed size and distance to the nearest hospital, Kaiser hospitals regionalize their services and have fewer specialized facilities (Luft and Crane, 1979). The differences, however, are not large and may not be significant in terms of total costs. If an HMO develops a substantial amount of bargaining power in a local hospital, it is likely to have much more influence than the FFS physicians, with their diverse interests and requests for a wide variety of equipment. Moreover, Health Systems Agencies require increasingly convincing justification from hospitals seeking to add equipment, thus strengthening the HMO's position.

In sum, the question of HMO control over hospitals probably depends on the HMO's bargaining power. If it merely buys hospital days passively on an average cost basis, it will pay for all of the inefficiencies of community hospitals. If the HMO approaches hospitals with excess capacity and offers to guarantee a certain number of bed-days, but only on the condition that they negotiate costs and decisions on new equipment, then there may be little further advantage to be gained by the HMO in the outright purchase of a hospital. Alternatively, an HMO may choose to use a hospital with a high occupancy rate in which pressure for space leads to more efficient utilization (Meier and Tillotson, 1978). Group Health in Minneapolis negotiated lower hospital rates by switching facilities in 1971 (Christianson and McClure, 1978). Furthermore, sharing facilities is likely to be less costly from the perspective of the community (Ramsay and Wright, 1978).

Control of Specialists. The issue of who controls access to specialists has not been addressed very often, yet it may have substantial implications for HMO performance.* While patients cannot admit themselves to the hospital, in most cases they can see a specialist without going through their primary physician. More importantly, even if a patient is initially referred to a specialist, most systems—whether FFS or HMO—make little attempt to return the patient to the primary physician (Wescott, 1976). Perkoff (1978) notes that in many settings the proportion of visits to specialists is substantially higher than the referral rate, suggesting that patients continue to see specialists with some freedom. Specialists tend to rely more heavily on tests and procedures, many of which have not been demonstrated to be diagnostically superior to careful history taking and physical examinations, but all of which are costly (Marton, 1979; Marton, Rudd, and Sox, 1979; Schroeder and Showstack, 1978).

Within an HMO excessive use of specialists can be costly. In small HMOs specialists are often hired on an FFS basis because the patient load is too small to justify full-time specialists. Unless the HMO physicians exercise special care to assure that the referrals are appropriate and that the patients are promptly returned to the referring physician, the costs can be substantial. In response, the HMO may shift to a capitation arrangement with specialists, but that too has its drawbacks (Reimers, 1973). If the HMO is large enough to hire full-time specialists, they will tend to provide more specialty care than is absolutely necessary, because that is what they have been trained to do. Such care is more exciting to them than primary care, or it is necessary in order to justify their position. Thus it may be necessary to recruit an initial core of HMO physicians who strongly believe in primary care and practice cost-conscious medicine, and then establish the necessary procedures so that they maintain control over the use of specialists (Perkoff, 1978; Zelten, 1977; Gregory, 1978).† It is difficult for IPAs to exclude physicians who do not fit this model. This is especially true when the IPA is sponsored by a local medical society that is composed of too many specialists and too few primary practitioners.

*Some specialists, such an internists and ob/gyns, function as primary care physicians (Aitken et al., 1979). As will become clear, the distinction here is between the primary physician and the more costly consultant services. In fact, the same person may be primary physician to some patients and consultant to others.

†In part, this was the intent of the Hunterdon system, even though it was operated on an FFS basis (Wescott, 1970). Recently, however, the specialists rebelled and regained the right to practice outside the hospital and see patients directly, without referrals from family practitioners (Rosenberg, 1978; Sullivan, 1977).

EXTERNAL FACTORS INFLUENCING HMO PERFORMANCE

While various internal factors, such as financial support and managerial competence, may explain the success or failure of specific organizations, external or environmental factors are likely to have a greater influence on the long-term success and performance of HMOs as a generic way of providing health care. In a hostile environment even the best-designed HMO will have difficulty succeeding, but in a conducive environment, even if some poorly designed organizations fail, other HMOs will succeed. Three groups of environmental factors will be considered: the local legal and regulatory constraints faced by the HMO; the sociodemographic and economic characteristics of the population; and the local medical-care market situation.

Legal and Regulatory Constraints

Strumpf and Garramone (1976) discuss the importance of an adequate population base, a positive legal climate, and a nucleus of supportive physicians. Legal restrictions, however, cannot always be classified in the same category as other environmental factors. It is necessary to explore these issues and to ask: (1) are they exogenous or endogenous? and (2) is it the letter of the law or the spirit that matters? Over a period of years legal constraints, which have generally been state rather than federally imposed, can be locally modified. Thus they are really endogenous to the area and reflect a strong antipathy to, or at least a lack of strong support for, HMOs. This certainly does not deny the importance of the legal setting in the history of HMO development. Two major court battles were won in the 1940s, GHA versus the American Medical Association and Group Health Cooperative versus King County Medical Society. Furthermore, the 1959 Larson Commission report of the AMA found no legitimate basis for opposing group health plans, and advised local medical societies to exercise caution in their responses to HMOs and to resist harrassment of such plans (American Medical Association, 1959). While restraints on "corporate medical practice" continue to exist in some states, the legal bases per se for HMO prohibition have largely disappeared.

The letter of the law is probably less important than how it is applied. For instance, MacColl (1966) notes that even after the Larson Commission report and the successful suits by Group Health Cooperative, the King County Medical Society ignored HMO requests for evaluation. Kissam (1978) and Havighurst (1978) outline an extensive series of anti-HMO actions that are possible within the law. Extralegal activities still take place; a boycott of prepaid group physicians by Spokane Blue Shield was recently lifted by Federal Trade Commission order (U.S. Federal Trade Commission, 1976). A civil antitrust suit has been filed against a hospital and a Florida county medical society for conspiring to inhibit the development of an HMO by denial of hospital staff privileges (Cowan, 1978). Evidence in the opposite direction is also available. McNeil and Schlenker found little difference between states with and without HMOs in the frequency of laws restricting such plans (1975, p. 199).

Historically, legal restrictions on types of medical practice have fostered diversity in organizational structure among plans (Gintzig and Shouldice, 1971: MacColl, 1966). For example, New York state insurance laws require HIP to set aside substantial financial reserves. In addition, until it obtained a change in the state law, HIP was forbidden to own and operate hospitals (Greenberg and Rodburg, 1971, p. 970). Similarly, until 1976 under Massachusetts law, Harvard Community Health Plan was required to maintain insurance company linkages (Bruzelius, 1976). State legislation has also been changed because of pressure by sponsors of potential HMOs (Vayda, 1968; Falk, 1969; Downey, 1974). There is no evidence that legal problems have posed major barriers to the establishment of HMOs in the last few years (McNeil and Schlenker, 1975; Strumpf and Garramone, 1976).* However, legal technicalities can hinder or prevent HMO development (Epstein and Kopit, 1977; Seabrook, 1979).

Usually, the focus has been on state laws prohibiting HMOs. In some instances, however, laws designed to regulate or even promote HMOs have become major hindrances. For instance, many states require extensive financial, utilization, and quality audits that monitor HMO performance (Lipton, 1978). But state requirements often differ from federal regulations, so new HMOs can be swamped by reporting requirements. While such requirements may be merely nuisances to an established HMO, they can pose crippling overhead costs for a fledgling organization. The original 1973 HMO Act, which was designed to promote the HMO concept, included so many restrictions and required such an extensive range of benefits that few HMOs sought to qualify. The difficulty was that similar conditions were not placed on conventional health insurers. Similarly, for some time the federal benefits package was considered a maximum, and when New Jersey required HMOs to offer additional services, plans were faced with the choice of federal or state qualification, but not both.

General Sociodemographic Factors

A wide range of environmental factors can hinder or promote HMO development. While some of these are measures of the market available to the HMO, others are more subtle, such as measures of openness to change or preferences for particular styles of medical practice. Table 14-1 offers an overview of some of these factors and how they differ among three sets of Standard Metropolitan Statistical Areas (SMSAs). The first set is

*The latter observation may be biased by the fact that if laws are so restrictive that an HMO never begins to develop, there is no one to complain. Nonetheless, it appears that legal problems have been overdrawn and that they can be changed or circumvented if there is sufficient support to do so.

composed of the twenty-four SMSAs that had an HMO in 1970 (HMO70). The second set (HMO76) is composed of those SMSAs that had HMOs in 1976 but not in 1970. (To be precise, the HMOs existing in the HMO76 SMSAs started after 1970.) The third group of SMSAs had no HMOs in 1976 (NOHMO). Simple comparisons of these data in Table 14-1 often show monotonic patterns across the three sets of SMSAs and suggest tentative conclusions. For example, HMO development seems related to higher socioeconomic levels as measured by median incomes, percent poor, median education, and percent black. However, while SMSAs in the HMO70 and HMO76 groups have proportionately fewer poor people, they have higher proportions on Aid to Families with Dependent Children (AFDC) and pay substantially more to such people. The proportion of Democratic voters in 1972 (not a good year for that party) is also correlated with HMO development, suggesting that liberalism may be a factor. Certain occupational and health insurance factors, such as the extent of unionization, white collar employment, and proportion with major medical health insurance, also seem related. Surprisingly, given the usual assumptions about HMO preferences for group enrollment, the presence of large manufacturing firms seems inversely related to HMO development. The differences in market size and density suggest that large, densely populated SMSAs allow HMOs to develop sufficient enrollments with relatively low penetration rates and travel times. Keller (1979) examined these variables in a multiple regression model of four aspects of HMO development and growth: (1) whether an HMO existed in the SMSA in 1970; (2) the market share achieved in those SMSAs; (3) the HMO enrollment growth between 1970 and 1976; and (4) whether the SMSA developed a new HMO between 1970 and 1976. In general, these multivariate findings are similar to those in Table 14-1. HMO presence in 1970 is associated with high income, Democratic voters, low proportion of large firms, market size, and low population mobility. SMSAs with new HMOs were primarily identified by large size and Democratic voting patterns.

The Influence of the Medical Care Market on HMO Performance

HMOs generally compete for enrollees in the health insurance market, and the generic definition of an HMO requires that enrollees have the choice of alternative health insurance schemes. The major market for HMOs and conventional health insurance is employee or union groups (Enthoven, 1979). HMOs have traditionally set their premiums at about the level of the conventional plan and then offered increased benefits to make the package more attractive. There is some evidence that HMOs with premiums of more than $10 a month above the competition have difficulty growing (ICF, 1976). Over time, however, the health insurance market has been changing. Employers have increased both the comprehensiveness of the conventional insurance packages and the proportion of the premium they

Table 14−1 Sociodemographic Measures and HMO Development

	SMSAs With		
	HMOs in 1970	HMO Development between 1970&76	No HMOs by 1976
Income measures			
Median income, 1969	10,989	9,898	9,175
% families below low income level, 1969	0.074	0.088	0.111
% population receiving AFDC, 1970	0.042	0.031	0.030
Average assistance per AFDC family, 1972	225	181	151
Social characteristics			
Median education, persons 25+, 1970	12.26	12.01	11.82
% black, 1970	0.079	0.081	0.100
% vote Democratic, 1972 (statewide)	0.416	0.368	0.347
% in each of 16 age-sex categories	*	*	*
Occupation/health insurance characteristics			
% nonagricultural employees in unions, 1970	0.315	0.272	0.245
% labor force in manufacturing, 1970	0.221	0.242	0.251
% manufacturing establishments with 100+ employees, 1967	0.093	0.122	0.133
% labor force white collar, 1970	0.538	0.496	0.473
% labor force in federal government, 1970	0.056	0.033	0.034
% population with major medical health insurance, 1975	0.735	0.714	0.680
Spatial characteristics			
Total population, 1970, in (000s)	2,368	734	327
% population change, 1960−70	0.266	0.241	0.173
Density, population per square mile, 1970	104	41	33
% of labor force working outside county of residence, 1970	0.177	0.116	0.130
% of population in HMOs, 1976	0.107	0.033	0.0
Number of SMSAs	24	39	194

SOURCE. Data drawn from the *County and City Data Book,* Area Resource File, and *1976 HMO Census.*

* Distributions by age and sex in the three groups are essentially identical.

pay (Walsh and Egdahl, 1977; Quigley, 1975). For instance, the proportion of wage and salary workers with hospital insurance rose from 49 percent in 1950 to about 69 percent in the mid-1960s and has fluctuated around that level ever since. In contrast, coverage for regular medical (that is, nonhospital) services has risen steadily from 16 percent to 67 percent in 1974, and major medical coverage went from zero in 1950 to 34 percent (Skolnik, 1976). This has been seen by some HMOs as squeezing their competitive advantage (Goldberg, 1969). In some cases, such as that of the United Auto Workers, employers pay the full premium, but it is $202 for BC-BS or $142 for an HMO (Peterson, 1979). In fact, the employer pays the full premium in most negotiated employee health plans in California (Vial, 1975). On the other hand, in recent years, employers have become acutely aware of the cost of health insurance for their employees and are beginning to increase copayments or actively encourage HMOs (Walsh and Egdahl, 1977; Goldbeck, 1978; Meyer, 1977).

As conventional plans increase their coverage and are unable to reduce utilization, they find their premiums rising substantially *above* those of HMOs, even without considering differences in out-of-pocket costs. For example, premium costs for family coverage in the University of California system are shown in Table 14-2. Blue Cross and Kaiser premiums maintained the same relationship to each other from 1968 to 1975. Since then, Kaiser's relative advantage has markedly increased, so that the Blue Cross package is now 56 percent more expensive. More importantly, after considering the fixed payment by the university, the employee's monthly out-of-pocket premium cost for Blue Cross is nearly four times that for Kaiser. With dramatic changes of this type in the last few years, the system is unlikely to be in equilibrium. This issue will be addressed more fully in the next section.

One important factor in the health insurance market is the mere availability of the dual choice option. A survey of 147 major employee health insurance plans in 1974 revealed that only 18 offered a choice of benefits (Quigley, 1975). A mid-1974 survey of the 1000 largest industrial firms in the nation showed that only 18 percent of the top 500 and 10 percent of the next 500 largest firms offered HMO options at any of their locations. Geographic limitations, however, were infrequently cited as HMO disadvantages. The most important negative factors involved increased administrative workload and increased cost of coverage (Fortune, 1975). (Fear of increased cost is likely to be expressed by employers who offer relatively limited packages and are concerned that a broader and more expensive HMO package will increase employee demands for better coverage.)

The HMO Act now requires that a dual choice option be made available by firms having twenty-five or more employees in areas with federally qualified HMOs. This can have a major impact on HMO growth by allowing organizations to market in firms that previously never allowed

Table 14—2 ,Monthly Health Insurance Premiums for Employee and Two or More Dependents
University of California

	Total Insurance Cost		Employees' Out-of-Pocket Premium Cost Net of Employer Contribution		Ratio of Blue Cross to Kaiser	
	Blue Cross North (1)	Kaiser North (2)	Blue Cross North (3)	Kaiser North (4)	Total (1)/(2)	Employee (3)/(4)
1968	$ 34.60	$29.43	$26.60	$21.43	1.17	1.24
1969	34.60	30.28	26.60	22.28	1.14	1.19
1970	43.18	39.18	35.18	31.18	1.10	1.13
1971	50.96	45.78	40.96	35.78	1.11	1.14
1972	53.81	50.57	41.81	38.57	1.06	1.08
1973	59.81	54.75	43.81	38.75	1.09	1.13
1974[a]	65.30	57.23	24.30	16.23	1.14	1.50
1975	77.28	66.53	30.28	19.53	1.16	1.55
1976	99.76	74.91	39.76	14.90	1.33	2.67
1977	113.82	79.98	53.82	19.98	1.42	2.69
1978	127.58	81.70	61.58	15.70	1.56	3.92

SOURCE.   Dyan Piontkowski, *Selection of Health Insurance By an Employee Group in Northern California*. San Francisco: University of California San Francisco, Health Policy Program, 1979.
[a] Note: In 1974 the University of California substantially increased its contribution for employees with dependents. The contribution, however, remained the same regardless of the health insurance coverage chosen.

dual choice (Dorsey, 1975). While dual choice provisions are no panacea, they do seem to have been of substantial assistance to some HMOs (Anonymous, "HEW's Dual Option Regulations," 1976, p. 23; Sleeth, 1976; U.S. Health Maintenance Organization Service, 1977). At the same time, firms that grudgingly offer a choice are successful at discouraging HMO enrollment.* The long-run effects of the dual choice provision and the changes that take place in relative benefits will depend, in part, on the responses by the conventional system to HMO development. Some of these competitive reactions will be discussed in the next section.

*For example, one information brochure concluded with "[Company X] is not recommending any program and cannot, of course, promise that you'll be more satisfied with services in the HMO. The choice is yours to make." It is not surprising that only 3.4 percent of the firm's employees joined an HMO. In contrast, over half the employees in some other major firms in the same city joined HMOs (Christianson, 1978).

In addition to the local health insurance market, other aspects of the local medical care system may affect HMO development and performance.* For example, if hospitals have low occupancy rates, they may be willing to negotiate more favorable contracts with new HMOs. An area with more physicians may have a greater proportion of physicians who find attractive the assured income and steady patient flow that an HMO can offer. HMOs may also find it easier to get started in areas with unusually high, rather than low, hospitalization rates. Some of these conjectures can be examined in Table 14-3, which utilizes the same three-way split of SMSAs as does Table 14-1.

The sociodemographic characteristics listed in Table 14-1 tended to fall into consistent patterns, with the values of HMO76 falling in between the other two groups. Many medical-care characteristics of the HMO76 and NOHMO groups are similar, whereas the values for HMO70 are substantially different. This new pattern is particularly apparent for factors related to hospitals. SMSAs with well-established HMOs have fewer beds per 1000, more hospitals with low occupancy, fewer voluntary hospitals, and substantially more nursing home beds per capita. They also have more physicians per capita and a greater proportion of doctors in multispecialty groups. The SMSAs with older HMOs also had fewer hospital days per 1000, shorter stays, and higher expenses per patient day.

Interpretation of these different patterns is difficult, but it should be remembered that the data generally relate to 1970. Thus, while HMOs may have influenced the observed patterns of medical care in the HMO70 group, they cannot have done so in the HMO76 group. The relatively clear patterns across the three groups for the sociodemographic characteristics listed in Table 14-1 suggest that they may, in fact, be causally related to HMO development. For the medical care system variables, the causation is more likely to be in both directions, with some factors contributing to HMO development and others reflecting the presence of HMOs. Keller's (1979) multivariate analyses indicated that a high ratio of physicians per capita is associated with HMO presence and development. This leads to the next section, which examines the impact of HMOs on the rest of the medical care system.

---

*The larger socioeconomic environment can also have a substantial impact. Ross (1977) provides two examples concerning HMO development in the South. While bowing to dual choice requirements, Duke Power Company of Greenville, South Carolina, refused to allow a payroll deduction for the HMO. Employers in the South have traditionally opposed the "check-off" or voluntary deductions because of their use for union dues. It may not be accidental that J. P. Stevens, a major textile firm with a long history of union opposition, has large plants in Greenville. In contrast, R. J. Reynolds has sponsored an HMO in Winston-Salem, North Carolina. This substantial fringe benefit may also be designed to lessen the likelihood of unionization (Stacey, 1978).

Table 14—3   Medical Care Market Measures and HMO Development

	SMSAs With		
	HMOs in 1970	HMO Development between 1970—76	No HMOs by 1976
Resource availability			
General hospital beds per 1000 population, 1970	4.439	5.147	5.078
% general hospitals with 0—69% occupancy, 1970	0.331	0.242	0.267
% hospital beds in proprietary hospitals, 1969	0.067	0.041	0.046
% hospital beds in voluntary hospitals, 1969	0.614	0.680	0.664
Nursing home beds per 1000 population, 1973	6.271	4.813	4.610
MDs per 1000 population, 1970	1.733	1.438	1.251
% MDs in multispecialty groups, state, 1970	0.203	0.131	0.130
% MDs belonging to AMA, 1976	0.567	0.545	0.565
Medical care utilization			
Inpatient days in general hospitals per 1000, 1970	1,241	1,476	1,450
Outpatient visits to general hospitals per capita, 1970	1.068	0.930	0.871
Average length of stay, 1971	7.588	7.919	7.769
Expenses per adjusted inpatient day, 1971	105.0	85.0	74.0
Medicare geographic index of reimbursement, 1969	1.171	1.046	0.910
Synthetic estimate: average length of stay, 1969—71	7.999	8.614	8.629
Synthetic estimate: % with 1+ hospital stay, 1969—71	0.102	0.103	0.105
% of population in HMOs, 1976	0.107	0.033	0.0
Number of SMSAs	24	39	194

SOURCE.   See Table 14—1.

THE EXTERNALITIES OF HMOs

The economic concept of an externality is important, but it is generally ignored in discussions of HMOs. An externality occurs when A does something that directly affects B without there being any market transaction, and the absence of such a transaction for compensation results in an underprovision of good externalities (see Bator, 1958). Two often-cited but relatively unimportant examples in public health illustrate the concept. Someone with a cold who feels well enough to continue working usually does not take account of the external costs imposed upon others who may catch the cold. In theory (and such payments are usually theoretical), one's coworkers could pay to have the cold victim stay home. In a second and related example, obtaining a rubella vaccination protects not only oneself but also others, and in a pure market world, there will be too little immunization. To correct that market failure, a social decision is made to require such immunizations.

Three general types of externalities are of interest with respect to HMOs. Two of these elements can be discussed jointly—education and research. Both types of activities are undertaken in HMOs in much the same manner as they are in other organizations. Certain HMO characteristics may warrant using them as special resources. However, without special incentives, HMOs will tend to offer fewer research and training opportunities than would be optimal. The third type of externality involves the HMO's competitive influence on the rest of the medical care system. Because the medical care system currently deviates so greatly from a competitive market, any steps in that direction may well be considered an externality. That is, the mere introduction of HMOs may have an impact on not only their enrollees, but everyone else as well. Whether this impact is beneficial or detrimental will be discussed below.

Education and Research

The comprehensive nature of an HMO suggests that it can be a useful setting for conducting medical education and research. Many observers contend that the United States medical care system is impossibly fragmented, with little coordination among providers and too much concern with episodic care. If a long-term, community-based approach is the goal, then the HMO can more closely approximate the ideal model (Lathem, 1976). Some HMOs offer residency programs, as well as student clerkships (Shearn, 1971, p. 126; Kaiser Foundation Hospitals, 1975; Heyssel and Seidel, 1976; Bosch et al., 1973; Dorsey, 1973). There is little evidence, however, that the existing training programs utilize, to any substantial degree, the HMO's potential for primary prevention and population-based care. Instead, they seem to be traditional programs that look very much like those available in conventional settings (Haggerty, 1973; Kaiser Foundation Hospitals, 1969). Moreover, such training is expensive, and the costs are unlikely to be borne by health plan enrollees (Paulson, Schroeder, and Donaldson, 1979).

The HMO's potential for undertaking research has been exploited to a greater degree. The availability of a defined population allows epidemiological and health services research studies that require known population bases (Collen, 1971; Studney et al., 1977; Greenlick et al., 1977; Friedman, Dales, and Ury, 1979). In some cases the very large and stable memberships of organizations such as Kaiser and HIP have made possible long-term follow-up studies of conditions with relatively low prevalence. (See Friedman et al., 1974; Shapiro, 1977.) HMOs have also served as test sites for evaluating innovations in medical care delivery, such as the use of multiphasic screening, nurse practitioners, and automated medical records (Collen, 1970; Barnett, 1976; Record and Cohen, 1972; Heyssel and Seidel, 1976). In some instances HMOs are beginning to promote healthy behavior through such methods as offering refunds for weight reduction (Collins, 1977). While the research output of many HMO-based groups is impressive, it does not seem substantially different from that of researchers in other settings. In particular, with the exception of epidemiological studies, few of the research projects could not and have not been done in non-HMO settings (e.g., Maccoby et al., 1977). What seem to be lacking are well-designed experiments and evaluations that examine how HMOs work and how various changes to the medical care system affect outcomes. What has been done is valuable, but the great potential for these endeavors goes largely untapped.

The Competitive Influence of HMOs

While the medical care market lacks many aspects of competition, there are some clear instances in which competitive behavior occurs. Hospitals often compete for physicians to provide them with patients. This competition takes place by offering physicians such carrots as new equipment, easier access to beds, and low-cost office space (Lee, 1971, 1972; Cohen, 1978). Insurance companies compete with each other in the packages they offer to various employee groups. Such competition, which is usually based on experience rating, has all but eliminated the use of community rating by the BC-BS plans (Richardson, 1977; Shain, 1966). In fact, one may argue that some inefficiencies and inequities in medical care delivery stem from the fact that competition takes place in such a limited number of areas. Either more *or* less competition might be better than what currently exists.

HMOs introduce a new competitive influence. They compete directly with conventional insurance companies and indirectly with local hospitals and physicians. The crucial question is the nature of this competition and its effect on the system.* Enthoven (1978a) outlines three models of competitive responses by the FFS sector. In Model I, Blue Cross, other third party payers, and perhaps hospitals and physicians respond by constraining utilization by their members in order to reduce per capita costs. In Model II the response by the FFS providers is perverse. Faced with excess beds and physician time, because HMOs have lowered resource use for part of the population, the FFS system responds by raising fees and performing more discretionary procedures. Thus, under Model II, per capita medical care costs could increase with the introduction of HMOs. Furthermore, Enthoven reasons that HMOs may have little incentive to try to take advantage of this response, and they may allow their costs to float up along with those of the FFS providers. Enthoven's third model breaks this comfortable relationship by introducing several competing HMOs within the same market. Because the HMOs compete by lowering premiums or increasing benefits, they have continued incentives for cost reduction and for expanding their market share.

Enthoven's Models I and III are desirable, and his Model II is relatively innocuous. It describes a situation in which HMOs accomplish little but do no harm. Furthermore, Model II is unstable; the mere entry of another HMO can lead it toward the beneficial Model III. I suggest the consideration of at least one more situation, Model IV, in which the benefits of competition are less clear. Chapter 3 discussed the potential for self-selection by people with an HMO option. Given the differences in consumer satisfaction discussed in Chapter 11, it is likely that HMO enrollees, particularly PGP members, have preferences for the lower HMO costs and may, in fact, be relatively low utilizers. For IPAs the situation may be reversed. Because an IPA enrollee can continue a relationship with his or her physician and probably receive better coverage, the IPA may attract high utilizers. Chapters 3 and 5 present some evidence supporting this conclusion. HMOs also can encourage selection through such marketing strategies as liberal maternity coverage, which encourages the young couples to enroll (Hudes et al., 1979). Even mandatory open enrollment can be overcome through subtle changes in the benefit package and, for PGPs, location of clinics in desirable neighborhoods. In Model IV HMO enrollment grows and utilization and cost differences widen, but at least part of these differences are attributable to selection effects.

While HMOs enroll relatively low-cost people, conventional carriers are left with an increasingly more expensive population pool, and it becomes more difficult for them to compete. The FFS sector may also become

---

*Other market-based externalities can occur inadvertently through the design of certain programs. The Federal Employees' Health Benefits Program bases its employer contribution on the average of six large health plans, including the two California Kaiser plans. Thus Kaiser premiums have an impact on the government's cost for all enrollees (U.S. General Accounting Office, 1978).

fragmented as certain carriers establish IPAs on the SAFECO model or Ellwood's health care alliance model (Gregory, 1978; Moore, 1979; Reynolds, 1979; Ellwood, 1976). Such organizations are designed to exclude FFS providers who are "costly," but they may also exclude providers with relatively sicker patient populations (Jones, 1978). The equilibrium in Model IV occurs with large PGP enrollments composed of people who desire relatively little medical care and a series of IPAs or similar organizations that provide more and more services at increasing premiums. In essence, Model IV describes a relatively extreme form of experience rating in which the healthy pay less and the sick pay more, a rather undesirable outcome of HMO competition.

Despite the potential importance of the competition issue, there has been relatively little research on the subject. Ramsay and Wright (1978) present a simulation model of market responses to HMO growth, but there is no empirical base for their results. Furthermore the available evidence is consistent with a wide range of interpretations. A 1977 Federal Trade Commission study contends that HMOs are responsible for lowering utilization in conventional plans, supporting Model I (Goldberg and Greenberg, 1977). They rest their case on two types of analysis: (1) regressions of hospital utilization by Blue Cross members as a function of HMO market share and other variables; and (2) interviews in various HMO market areas. The regressions, using a cross-section of data from states, show: (1) nonmaternity hospital days per 1000 federal employees and their families in Blue Cross; (2) maternity length of stay for those enrollees; and (3) total hospital days per 1000 for Blue Cross nonfederal enrollees. All have statistically significant negative relationships to HMO market share. The regressions are dominated by four Western states: California, Washington, Oregon, and Hawaii, all of which have both high HMO market shares and low utilization rates. If these four states are omitted, the negative relationship is no longer significant (Enthoven, 1978a, p. 336). The interviews indicate clear competitive reactions by Blue Cross of Northern California to Kaiser's growth. Blue Cross substantially increased coverage of ambulatory services and encouraged direct comparisons with Kaiser. But there is little similar supporting evidence in other areas.

A historical perspective confirms the notion of a competitive response in Northern California. The San Joaquin Foundation for Medical Care was founded to prevent Kaiser from expanding into the Stockton area (Sasuly and Hopkins, 1967). Reactions by FFS physicians to Kaiser in the early 1950s included picketing and leafleting (Garbarino, 1960). Numerous articles appeared in local medical society journals decrying rising hospital utilization and predicting the demise of voluntary Blue Cross and Blue Shield plans. Calls for shorter stays, more outpatient care, and the like, appear with clear references to the dangers that increasing premiums posed to the continued existence of such health insurance programs (Sherrick, 1951, 1952; Thomas, 1951; Moffitt, 1951; Cheney, 1951). Thus the historical situation was consistent with the hypothesis that conventional providers saw the threat posed by HMOs and began to change their practice patterns in order to prevent further competitive losses.

The data presented in Table 14-3 are consistent with Model I in their demonstration that various measures of hospital utilization are lower in SMSAs with early HMO presence. In contrast to the sociodemographic factors in Table 14-1, this pattern seems to be more a *result* of HMO presence than a *cause* of HMO development. Chiswick (1976) also found significantly lower admission rates in SMSAs located in states with HMOs.

Long-term trends in hospital utilization also lend support to Model I. A major weakness in the Goldberg-Greenberg study is that the regressions primarily reflect the lower utilization rates on the West Coast and in Hawaii. These geographic patterns appear in all population groups— Medicare beneficiaries, Blue Cross members, federal employees, those interviewed in the National Health Survey, and the total national hospitalized population (Gornick, 1977; Blue Cross Association, 1974; U.S. Civil Service Commission, 1961–75; U.S. National Center for Health Statistics, "Persons Hospitalized by Number Episodes," 1977; American Hospital Association, 1975b). But, as Figure 14-1 indicates, this well-known pattern first appears between 1950 and 1955, precisely the period of substantial HMO growth on the West Coast and in Hawaii. While this evidence supports Model I, it could also be attributable to a wide variety of other factors, such as a rapidly growing and youthful population, pressure on medical resources, or high levels of employment.

Enthoven provides two sets of empirical support for Model II. One relates to a number of studies of FFS physicians. He shows that where demand is lower, fees are higher and physicians work less. There is also some evidence that physicians can directly influence demand, perhaps by treating problems of minor importance when there is a higher ratio of physicians per capita (Fuchs, 1978; Evans, 1974). Thus FFS physicians might react in the way that Model II predicts. The second set of evidence concerns HMO premiums relative to those of BC-BS for federal employees. Over a ten-year period, HMO premiums stayed within a range of $10 above to $5 below the BC-BS rates (ICF, 1976). This supports the concept that HMOs do not aggressively constrain the growth in costs over time. Much of the evidence in Chapter 8 also supports this idea.

The evidence for Model III is also rather sketchy. The clearest example is Hawaii, where there is low utilization in both Kaiser and the Hawaii Medical Service Association (HMSA). Although HMSA is nominally a Blue Shield plan, it exercises stringent controls over utilization and thus acts in some ways like an IPA or health care alliance (Christianson, 1978). HMSA was founded by local social workers. This legacy, combined with the Hawaiian heritage of plantation-provided medical care, suggests that the HMSA behavior may have more to do with its special history than with a competitive relationship to Kaiser (Bailey, 1971). The ICF study offers

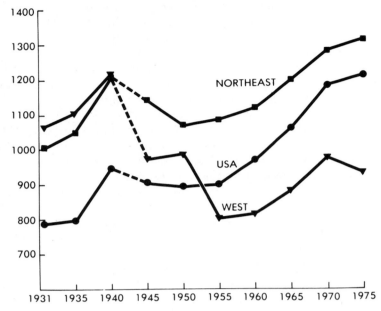

Figure 14-1 Hospital days per 1000 population. Northeast region is composed of Maine, New Hampshire, Vermont, Massachusetts, Rhode Island, Connecticut, New York, New Jersey, and Pennsylvania. West Region is composed of California, Oregon, Washington, Montana, Idaho, Wyoming, Colorado, New Mexico, Arizona, Utah, Nevada, and, from 1960 on, Alaska and Hawaii. *Sources:* 1931–1949: Annual Presentation of Hospital Data by the Council on Medical Education and Hospitals of the American Medical Association in the *Journal of the American Medical Association.* These data refer to the utilization of general; maternity; eye, ear, nose, and throat; children's; orthopedic; and isolation hospitals. 1945–1975: *American Hospital Directory,* 1946, and annual guide issues of *Hospitals,* Journal of the American Hospital Association. These data refer to nonfederal short-term general and other special hospitals. Civilian resident population of each state is presented in U.S. Bureau of the Census, Current Population Reports, Series P-25. The civilian population figures are used instead of the more common total resident figures, because the hospital statistics exclude military hospitals.

support for the argument by showing slower premium growth in markets with competing HMOs than in those with a single HMO (ICF, 1976). But there are only eight market areas, and alternative explanations exist for much of the observed behavior (Enthoven, 1978a, p. 346). Christianson (1978) offers a detailed description of competition among seven HMOs in Minneapolis-St. Paul. Six of these organizations were formed within the past five years, however, and Christianson focuses primarily on HMO behavior, rather than on the long-term responses of conventional providers. Similarly, IPAs have often been formed in response to PGPs, but the long-term outcome of such competition is still unknown (Lavin, 1978; Meier and Tillotson, 1978; Christianson and McClure, 1978; Dietz, 1978a,b; Knox, 1978; Enright, 1979). Zelten (1977) reports that conventional insurers dropped their rates in response to the entry of a new HMO in Tucson. Similar actions may explain an unusual rate freeze by Nebraska BC-BS after the opening of an HMO in Lincoln (Miller, 1979).

At first glance, additional support for the competitive model comes from Rochester, New York where there has been intense competition between several HMOs and the local BC-BS plan. The inpatient medical-surgical utilization rate for members under sixty-five years of age was relatively constant from 1974 to 1977 at about 625 days. It had dropped precipitously to 547 by mid-1979, a decline much larger than any other Eastern Blue Cross Plan. Much of this decline has been attributed to a competitive effect (Finger Lakes Health Systems Agency, 1980). There are a number of alternative explanations, however. Rochester has had aggressive health planning since the late 1940s and traditionally has had a low ratio of beds per capita. It also has an actively interested group of large employers who encourage innovation and cost control (VonBerg, 1972). In addition, a unique regional budgeting strategy is being implemented (Sorensen and Saward, 1978). And changes in New York state policies toward nursing home reimbursement have made it more difficult to transfer Medicare and Medicaid recipients out of hospitals. Given the tight bed supply, this could force down the BC-BS utilization rate (Wersinger, 1979).

The Minneapolis situation has been highly publicized as an example of vigorous competition and rapid HMO growth (Christianson, 1978). It therefore warrants further examination. The market share of HMOs grew from 2 percent in 1972, to 4 percent in 1975, to 10 percent in 1978. This phenomenon occurred through the establishment of six HMOs, widespread dual choice among major employers, and much visibility. The potential for savings is also present: the HMOs average about 550 hospital days per 1000 enrollees, 38 percent below the Blue Cross group average of 885. Yet between 1975 and 1977, while HMO enrollment doubled, overall hospital utilization in the Minneapolis-St. Paul metropolitan area stayed constant or increased slightly (American Hospital Association, 1976, 1977, 1978). Even ignoring a competitive effect, if the new HMO enrollees actually experienced a 38 percent reduction in hospital use, there should have been an area-wide decline of fourteen days per 1000. Obviously, many factors could explain this result, but it is consistent with both the notions of no major competitive response and the selective enrollment of low utilizers in HMOs. New data for 1978 indicate a downturn in hospital use in the Twin Cities (Ellwein, 1979). However, it is noteworthy that large declines occur for Medicare beneficiaries, who are served by conventional FFS practitioners. This may reflect a very effective competitive response carrying over into general modes of practice, or it may indicate the importance of unrelated factors, such as effective PSROs.

The previous discussion noted the generally low hospital utilization in the western states and suggested that this might provide support for the competitive model. A contrary approach would examine total expenditures on health care, because even if conventional providers constrained hospitalization in the face of HMO competition, they might maintain their incomes by increasing charges and providing more physician services (Models II or IV). Dyckman (1978) finds that after adjusting for the cost of living, surgical fees are highest in Los Angeles and were also high in New York, San Francisco, and Sacramento, all areas with high HMO market penetration. In fact, one response by Blue Cross of Northern California to Kaiser competition was to increase its coverage of ambulatory services and encourage efforts to reduce hospitalization.

If competition between HMOs and conventional providers had an impact on overall costs, one might expect it to appear in California, with its massive Kaiser plan, competing HMOs in Southern California, and a documented history of Blue Cross concern. While the most recently available figures on per capita health expenditures by state are for 1969, they provide little support for the competitive model (Cooper, Worthington, and Piro, 1975). (More recent data for the Medicare population yield similar results.) California ranked third among the fifty states. But how could this happen when hospitalization in California is so low? The answer is that, while hospitalization is the largest single type of medical expenditure and is easily measurable, there are other pieces of the pie. Perhaps as a result of the improved ambulatory care coverage by conventional insurers, California ranked second in the share of per capita expenditures for physicians' services. (Washington state, also with high HMO penetration, was first.) Consequently, California ranked forty-sixth in the share of expenditures for hospital care. Thus, while by some standards the mix of medical services bought by Californians may be more efficient, there is no evidence that even massive HMO enrollment has resulted in overall cost containment.

While most interest in the competitive enrollment has been focused on the impact of HMOs on conventional providers, it is also important to underscore the importance of the precise nature of the market environment on HMO performance. The previously mentioned study of University of California employees demonstrates clear price sensitivity in enrollment choice (Piontkowski and Butler, 1979). In response to consistently higher Blue Cross premiums, Kaiser enrollment has more than doubled, from 7500 in 1967 to 15,500 in 1978, while Blue Cross enrollment remained stable at about 9200. But the more interesting issue is on the cost side. Between 1971 and 1978 the Kaiser premium rose 78 percent, while the increase for Blue Cross was nearly twice that—146 percent. By 1978 the additional employee cost for choosing Blue Cross over Kaiser was $246 for single and $551 for family coverage.

One cannot translate Kaiser premiums into expenditures, because they are based on a community rate that represents the experience of all Northern California Kaiser members. The Blue Cross premium, however, reflects the University of California experience, and suggests that the stable group of enrollees was increasingly composed of high utilizers. This conjecture is supported by what has occurred at Stanford during the same period. There Kaiser and Blue Cross enrollments grew at about the same rate, as did their premiums, suggesting that the widening differential at the University of California reflects a shifting enrollment mix, rather than general cost increases faced by all Blue Cross enrollees (Stanford University Personnel Office, 1979). The reason for the different patterns at the two universities is not yet clear, but they probably relate to different patterns of employer contributions and their effects on net premium cost to the enrollee. This conjecture is supported by the enrollment data presented in Figure 14-2. The 1974 change in employer contribution at the University of California increased the net premium differential for Blue Cross families from about 15 percent to 50 percent. In the subsequent two years the net Kaiser enrollment increased markedly. Then, beginning in 1976, total Blue Cross premiums began increasing rapidly relative to Kaiser, perhaps reflecting an increasingly more costly enrollee mix. Moreover, while the Blue Cross gross premiums are only 56 percent higher, the

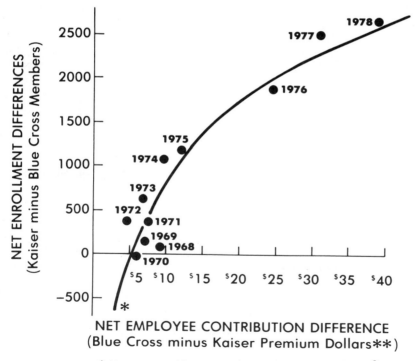

* Line computed from regression $y = -2094 + 1280\, \ell nX$ ($R^2 = .89$)

** 1976 constant dollars

Figure 14-2   Family plan enrollment trends: 1968–1978. (*Source:* Piontkowski and Butler, 1980.)

structure of the employer contribution magnifies this to almost a fourfold difference. People involved in the marketing of HMOs understand the importance of premium structures and employer contributions in influencing not only total enrollment, but the potential for self-selection (Zelten, 1977; Meier and Tillotson, 1978).

In summary, the question of the external effects of HMOs has barely been researched. In part, this is because HMO enrollments have been limited to a small number of areas. The nature of HMOs suggests that they can be valuable resources for teaching and research. While some steps have been taken along these lines, most teaching efforts have been along traditional lines, and most research is a straightforward, in-house type of evaluation. This is not to criticize these efforts. Teaching programs must meet accreditation standards, and an institution must have a strong base to undertake major innovations. In-house researchers find it difficult to do critical and comparative studies, while outside researchers rarely have the time or access to truly understand an organization (Weiss, 1972).

Perhaps the most significant area of externalities is the competitive influence of HMOs. If the enrollment of 10 to 20 percent of the population in HMOs had an impact on the remaining 80 to 90 percent, be it positive or negative, then the policy implications would be enormous. Several models of such competitive impacts have been outlined, ranging from increased cost and utilization controls by conventional providers to increased fees and utilization. Bits and snatches of evidence are available to support each of the alternatives, and it is possible that the true situation is a combination of several models.

SUMMARY

In comparison with previous chapters, this one exhibits a relative dearth of data and an apparent difficulty in presenting conclusive findings. To a substantial degree, this reflects the issues at hand, the nature of the medical care market, and the availability of data. The independent variables, such as sponsorship, goals, consumer involvement, organizational structure, legal constraints, and even the method of physician payment, are difficult to define and impossible to quantify accurately. Moreover, the potential combinations among the factors in just this chapter far exceed the number of HMOs, let alone the number of research studies. Of course, not all combinations exist, but for almost any distinction one wishes to make, a closer look at the data will reveal potentially confounding variables that may vitiate the conclusions.

This inconclusive situation results partly from the relative lack of competition in the medical care market; this allows "inefficient" organizations to survive. The basic tools of economics are designed to study equilibrium situations and, within that context, behavior of firms and individuals at the margin. In a perfectly competitive environment all firms are identical, because any firm less efficient than the others will fall by the wayside. If the market environment is expanded to allow heterogeneous consumers, then different firms may each find a comfortable niche. But if one recognizes that the observed situation is a snapshot during a dynamic sorting-out process, rather than a stable equilibrium, then it becomes impossible to generalize from the snapshot to what is likely to occur in the long run. In spite of these caveats, one can draw some impressions from the data.

The goals of an HMO seem to have a substantial influence on its performance, but clear and objective measures of goals are difficult to develop. Various proxies, such as who has sponsored the organization, the profit-nonprofit status, and the extent of consumer control, have only limited value in predicting performance. There are some clear relationships in extreme cases. For instance, a great many of the Southern California prepaid health plans cited for fraud and poor quality of care were obviously de facto for-profit plans, even though they had been incorporated as nonprofit entities. On the other hand, some clearly for-profit physician-sponsored plans have an excellent history of providing quality care. There is also evidence that consumer cooperatives provide more special services and options for their members, although at somewhat higher cost. But of the two best known cooperatives, one (Washington, D.C.) has experienced major difficulties, while the other (Puget Sound) has been highly successful.

The organizational structure and incentives within an HMO also exert a major influence on performance. Given the previous discussion about the lack of competition, it is to be expected that a great deal of variation exists. Most studies deal with operating HMOs, but for every operating HMO there are several that failed while trying to get off the ground. Such failures are expensive individually, and collectively they can jeopardize support for HMO initiation. One common denominator of early failure is a lack of managerial expertise and a clear sense of what an HMO can and cannot be.

Within operating HMOs important issues arise concerning the structuring of incentives for and control of hospital and physician services. There may be an inherent conflict between the organization's interests and those of the providers within the organization, but some arrangements can exacerbate while others mute this tension. The HMO would like its physicians to work hard and care for its enrollees as efficiently as possible without severely compromising quality and consumer satisfaction. Physicians generally prefer less effort, more income, and interesting cases—all of which are expensive to the HMO. Conflicts seem to be exacerbated by FFS payments to providers without counterbalancing risk-sharing that is meaningful to the individual practitioner. "Meaningful" in this case depends on the size of the risk-sharing pool; if a physician's costs or savings are shared by only five physicians, they will be more meaningful than if they are shared by 500. Risk-sharing should also be on the same basis for the HMO and its physicians. Since hospitalization is controlled by physicians, they should be financially sensitive to their decisions concerning hospital use. In a similar fashion, some HMOs seem to be able to control the use of expensive specialty services by putting primary care physicians in charge of such use and making them sensitive to the costs of specialty care. Conflicts of interest also occur when physicians work only part-time for an HMO. Although small HMOs may have no choice, both theory and evidence support the argument that full-time practitioners are better for the HMO.

The issue of hospital control is more ambiguous. While some of the most successful HMOs have had their own hospitals, it must be remembered that they developed in eras of tight bed supply and opposition by local providers. This made hospital control a necessity. Given the current bed surplus, the high capital expense of new facilities, and restrictions by health planning agencies, it is unlikely that many HMOs will have the opportunity to own hospitals. Moreover, if they can use their bargaining power effectively, they may even do better by contracting with existing facilities.

External or environmental factors are likely to have a substantial influence on the development and long-term success of HMOs. While historically, legal factors have been important in restricting the spread of HMOs and constraining the types of organizational structure, such restrictions seem to be of less importance today. The market environment is likely to continue to be important, particularly for the development of large prepaid group practices requiring a substantial population base. HMOs definitely compete with conventional insurers and also pose a potential threat to physicians and hospitals in conventional practice. The response of such providers can influence both whether an HMO develops and how rapidly it grows. More importantly, the entry of HMOs may lead conventional providers to change their behavior in ways that affect the overall utilization and cost of medical care. Whether such changes are beneficial or detrimental remains to be determined. While they are perhaps the least understood impact of HMOs, they may be the most important.

FIFTEEN

What We Know, Don't Know, and Need to Know

This book was designed to provide a critical and comprehensive analysis of the state of knowledge about HMO performance. In carrying out this task, I have attempted to be led by the available data and then to offer interpretations that flow from the evidence. Complete objectivity, of course, is impossible to attain, so the reader has been invited to examine the data and to draw his or her own conclusions.

Each stage of analysis increases the author's influence—through the selection of one table rather than another, the subtle juxtaposition of figures, the interpretation of results, and the specific choice of words. Thus I recommend that the reader begin with the most detailed level of presentation in the preceding chapters, then consult the original works, and add new studies to the analysis. Few people, however, have the time and inclination to carry out such a task, so there are always demands for brief summaries of the crucial findings. Such summaries become further and further abbreviated, losing their qualifications, uncertainties, and rigor at each step.

This chapter is a compromise between the rigorous position that readers should not be given summaries because many important qualifications are thereby omitted, and the other position that important results buried in the midst of detailed data analysis are useless to nonacademic readers. The compromise takes the form of an extensive summary of specific points that have been identified as being supported by some evidence, along with a summary of questions for which answers are not readily available. References to specific chapters are provided. Further summarization will not be attempted, but a discussion is included that outlines the patterns that appear in our knowledge and ignorance. In particular, the first section highlights the dimensions of HMO performance that seem most clearly understood. The second section may be interpreted as a summary agenda for further research. The third section provides an extensive summary of what is known and not known about HMO performance.

WHAT WE KNOW ABOUT HMO PERFORMANCE

The detailed analyses in the preceding chapters demonstrated that some conclusions about HMO performance can be stated forcefully, while others are necessarily surrounded by qualifications. As indicated in the preface to this volume, this project was begun with some preconceived notions concerning how HMOs work and what the available evidence might show. As the study progressed and the evidence accumulated, some notions were strongly supported, others were moved into the realm of uncertainty, and still others were reversed. If, for a specific issue, one begins without any strong beliefs, then a small amount of data can substantially shift one's "best guess." If one begins with a strong belief in a specific outcome, then a great many contradicting bits of evidence are necessary to shift that opinion.*

This framework is an interactive one. The beliefs or conclusions that result from one round of analysis become the expectations of the next round. It is appropriate, therefore, that the conclusions or statements in this chapter concerning what we know about HMOs include some sense of my level of confidence or certainty. As in all such cases, the estimates are subjective. Numerical probability estimates would convey a false appearance of precision. Instead three levels of certainty are indicated by stars. One star means that there is some evidence or justification for making the statement, but my confidence level is low, and new data could easily alter the conclusion. Two stars mean that there is more substantial evidence, but the results should still be considered too uncertain to rely upon for important decisions, without further investigation. For instance, one or two carefully designed studies providing contrary evidence would raise serious questions about a two-star conclusion. Thus actions based upon such conclusions should be monitored carefully, and policies should be easily reversible. Three stars mean that the conclusion is based on convincing evidence from a substantial number of studies. Contrary evidence would be met initially with skepticism, and a large number of studies would be necessary to reverse a three-star conclusion.

About 10 percent of the conclusions in this chapter can be stated with substantial confidence, and another 40 percent are reasonably firm. Some areas are more likely than others to have firm conclusions. The results with respect to total cost, hospital utilization, and consumer satisfaction with access, coverage, and humaneness are areas of substantial certainty. Findings with respect to technical efficiency, trends in cost, quality of care, physician satisfaction, delivery of care to the poor, and the influence of organizational and environmental factors are all subject to qualification. Many of the conclusions in these latter groups are likely to be supported by further research, but some will probably be reversed.

*The reader familiar with Bayesian analysis will recognize the analogy. The Bayesian approach is used only in a general sense, however; no probabilities have actually been computed.

WHAT WE DO NOT KNOW ABOUT HMO PERFORMANCE: A PRELIMINARY RESEARCH AGENDA

Any issue about which there is a great deal of uncertainty requires more research. On another level, there are issues about which it is impossible to venture even a tentative conclusion. In both cases the evaluation must be subjective, but a crucial aspect of assigning importance to research questions is the potential use of the information. A policy-maker concerned with hospital production efficiencies will develop a research agenda entirely different from that of a consultant advising physicians on whether to join PGPs. Beyond such special-interest research questions are issues that (1) play a crucial methodological role and thus can affect a broad range of more specific results, or (2) are so broadly based as to have an impact on almost any policy concerning HMOs. The remainder of this section will highlight those research questions that appear to be of major importance.

The most crucial question for further research is the importance of self-selection on estimates of utilization, cost, and satisfaction. As described in Chapter 3, the only way to approach the question of HMO performance in a comprehensive manner is to rely on observational studies that compare enrollees in different plans. People are able to choose the plans they prefer, and statistical adjustments for age-sex-health status differences cannot guarantee that enrollees in two different types of plans are identical. In particular, such adjustments cannot guarantee that HMO enrollees do not prefer, for one reason or another, the style of pracice and lower utilization rates offered by that organization, and they may have been low utilizers regardless of plan. Two randomized, controlled trials have been undertaken, which are expensive and will provide data only on two HMOs (Perkoff, Kahn, and Haas, 1976; Newhouse, 1974). Furthermore, no realistic policy would include the random assignment of people to health plans or the elimination, by fiat, of the FFS option. This means that we need to know how people selectively enroll and disenroll in health plans and what impact this has on the overall evaluation of the various systems.

In similar fashion, nothing is known about the potential impact of self-selection by providers on HMO performance. It may be the case that 20 percent of the physician population prefers a style of practice that involves relatively low use of medical resources. If these physicians differentially choose to practice in HMOs (or differentially choose to stay in an HMO after a trial period), then the potential for generalizing from the existing HMO experience will be seriously limited.

Both selection cases involve serious methodological issues, because if HMOs differentially attract or retain people who are naturally inclined to be low utilizers of care, then not only are the HMO rates artificially depressed, but the rates for the comparison group are artificially inflated. The medical care system may or may not work better with self-selection, but it is important that its influence be determined.

Turning to more specific issues, if self-selection is important, as is suggested by the evidence in Chapter 3, we have little understanding of why and how it occurs. For instance, how important are nonmedical factors such as waiting time, continuity, and friendliness in a person's choice of provider? How does this influence the decision to join an HMO? How important is disenrollment behavior in shaping the long-term mix of HMO enrollees? To what extent can and do organizations or groups of providers choose to influence the type of enrollees they will attract and thus "select" their patients? Similar questions occur with respect to the physician's choice of the setting in which to work.

In a number of instances, clear differences in HMO performance have been identified, but the causes of these differences remain a mystery. One of the most consistent observations is the lower hospitalization rates in PGPs. Yet there is little understanding of either the micro or macro aspects of hospital utilization. At a micro level, what determines whether a patient with specific symptoms will be admitted to or discharged from the hospital? At a macro level, why do admission rates vary so much among HMOs? Between HMOs and conventional providers? Across seasons and geographic regions? Or why have utilization rates for both Blue Cross and HMO enrollees shown a substantial downward trend since the late 1960s (well before the advent of PSROs)? Without a better understanding of how the medical care system operates in general, it is difficult to understand how HMOs operate.

Just as decisions to admit and prolong hospitalization remain largely a mystery, so too do decisions about ambulatory care. For instance, even the best statistical models explain less than a quarter of the variation in individual use of ambulatory services. But, without such background information, how can one determine the role that out-of-plan use plays for HMO enrollees? Is it part of common doctor-shopping or second opinion behavior? Does it serve as a special safety valve for dissatisfied patients? Or do people expect to use some out-of-plan services when they join an HMO? Similarly, without a better understanding of what determines the content of an ambulatory care visit, that is, what is done to and for the patient, it is impossible to evaluate ambulatory visits in HMOs.

Although this book has documented a number of important differences in medical care delivery between HMOs as a group and the conventional system, little is known about *how* these differences occur. The initial assumption is that the altered financial arrangements of the HMO change the economic incentives facing the provider, so that fewer rather than more services are offered. Yet physicians claim to be unaware of financial constraints within the HMO, and they often point to the complete coverage for enrollees as giving them a free hand in practicing good medicine. Economics is built on the assumption that incentives often act as an "invisible hand," and one need only observe behavior in order to see the incentives at work. The economic model rarely addresses how incentives lead to long-term changes. In a competitive environment, inefficient producers may recognize impending disaster, change their ways, and become efficient. It is more likely, however, that the inefficient firm simply goes bankrupt and is replaced by another. The latter, if it is efficient, prospers and grows. If it is inefficient, it too will fail, and the cycle repeats itself. This free market model may be an appropriate description of how the economy works in the long run, but it seems grossly inadequate for describing the forces shaping the short-term behavior of medical providers. An understanding of *how* financial and other incentives influence physician behavior must rely upon detailed analyses of the role of specific organizational factors within both HMOs and the conventional sector. Very little is known about the influence of peer pressure, physician selection, size of practice group, goals of the organization, direct involvement of consumers, type of administrative structure, or control over referral patterns. Yet many policies and regulations directed specifically toward HMOs address these issues with little empirical underpinning.

One may argue that it is unnecessary to know how HMOs do what they do; instead, we should merely foster a competitive environment and let the "invisible hand" determine the optimal set of providers. There are two important drawbacks to such a strategy. The first is that the market is likely to work slowly, more slowly than will be politically acceptable, so that some "friendly encouragement" in the right direction may be necessary. For example, competition may eventually lead to a geographic redistribution of providers, but the Congress might use relocation subsidies and National Health Service Corps placements to hasten the process. The second drawback is that the implications of a competitive market environment are largely unknown. Research is needed to unveil the factors that induce and inhibit HMO birth and development. Almost nothing is known about the dynamics of enrollment, utilization, and premiums in multiple choice situations. For instance, competition leading to greater efficiency is desirable, but competition leading to experience rating and a quest for low-risk enrollees is undesirable. Similarly, little is known about the competitive influence of HMOs on conventional providers. It may, in fact, be the most important aspect of HMO performance, yet the evidence is far from conclusive.

Setting a research agenda requires an understanding of three major areas: (1) the state of knowledge and ignorance; (2) the policy relevance of the potential answers to specific questions; and (3) the feasibility of carrying out research in each area. This book has attempted to address the first area. Policymakers in and out of government will be outlining the second area through discussions about the future shape of the medical care system. It is the researchers' task to create innovative approaches to the more crucial questions on the agenda.

A SUMMARY OF WHAT WE KNOW AND DO NOT KNOW ABOUT HMOS

Feasible Types of HMOs

What We Know. The generic definition allows a very wide range of organizational forms. Over time, new variations appear and diversity seems to have increased (Chapters 2, 14).**

What We Do Not Know. The limits of feasible variants are not yet known, that is, will the next ten years show an increase or decrease in the number of *different kinds* of HMO-type organizations (Chapter 14)?

Reasons for Consumer Enrollment in HMOs

What We Know. Within dual choice situations HMO enrollees sometimes differ with respect to age and other sociodemographic factors. Selection seems to depend at least partially on subtle differences among alternative plans in coverage and cost (Chapter 3).* People having good ongoing relationships with physicians are unlikely to sever those ties for moderate cost savings (Chapter 3).***

What We Do Not Know. Do selection patterns change over time as the same group of consumers is repeatedly offered an enrollment choice? For instance, is the mix of enrollees in two or more plans different five years after dual choice is made available (Chapter 3)? Little is known about preferences for the quantity and style of medical care and whether this influences enrollment (Chapter 3).

Impact of Consumer Self-Selection on Measures of Performance

What We Know. There is some evidence that in a newly offered dual choice situation, people joining PGPs were lower than average utilizers of hospital care when they had conventional coverage (Chapter 3).* Preenrollment use of ambulatory services was sometimes higher, sometimes lower. The difference appears related to specific aspects of the dual choice situation (Chapter 3).* Adverse selection seems more likely to occur consistently in IPA options (Chapter 3).*

What We Do Not Know. To what extent does self-selection account for differences in cost and utilization (Chapters 3, 4, 5, 6)? To what extent does self-selection determine observed levels of satisfaction (Chapters 3, 11)? Can and should self-selection be encouraged or discouraged (Chapters 3, 14)? Do people self-select differently with respect to expected needs for ambulatory versus inpatient care (Chapters 3, 5, 6, 14)?

*Some evidence to support, but could be easily reversed by new data.
**More substantial evidence, but should still be considered tentative (one or more well designed studies to the contrary would raise serious questions).
***Very consistent evidence; contrary results would be a surprise and a large number of contrary data points would be required to reverse.

Impact of Disenrollment by Consumers

What We Do Not Know.   How important is voluntary disenrollment relative to enrollment in determining the mix of enrollees? Does voluntary disenrollment have an important impact on quality and performance—Hirschman's exit, voice, and loyalty argument (Chapters 3, 10, 11, 14)?

Total Cost of Medical Care: Premium plus Out-of-Pocket

What We Know.   Enrollees in prepaid group practices (PGPs) experience 10 to 40 percent lower costs than people in conventional plans. These results, however, are based on a small number of points and largely reflect Kaiser's experience (Chapter 4).** There is no evidence that enrollees in individual practice associations experience lower costs (Chapter 4).*

What We Do Not Know.   The total expenditure results are sensitive to a number of methodological issues such as age-sex composition, selection, and regional factors; how sensitive they are is not known (Chapter 4).

Split in Total Cost between Premium and Out-of-Pocket

What We Know.   HMOs typically offer more comprehensive coverage for about the same premium as conventional insurance plans. Although HMO premiums used to be somewhat higher, in many instances they are now even lower than conventional plans (Chapter 4).*** Out-of-pocket costs (including out-of-plan use) for HMO enrollees tend to show less variability than the same costs for enrollees in conventional plans. Thus there is a much lower probability of incurring large expenses. This seems to be true for both PGP and IPA enrollees (Chapter 4).**

What We Do Not Know.   What is the appropriate unit for measuring consumer welfare, the individual or the family? What is the appropriate unit of time to evaluate costs, one, two, or more years? How sensitive or risk averse are consumers to fluctuations in medical expenditures (Chapter 4)?

  To what extent do out-of-pocket costs for HMO enrollees represent supplementary charges for covered services, or the costs of uncovered services, or consumer preference for out-of-plan services, even though they would be covered if obtained within the plan (Chapter 4)?

Number and Mix of Services

What We Know.   Using a fixed set of weights, or prices, PGPs seem to deliver fewer units of medical care per enrollee per year, largely because of lower hospitalization (Chapter 4).**

What We Do Not Know. Are weights based on prices or relative value studies derived from the conventional FFS sector appropriate measures of services in HMOs? Would the results be different if more weight were given to ambulatory services and less given to hospital services, tests, and procedures (Chapter 4)?

Hospital Utilization Rates

What We Know. PGPs demonstrate substantially lower rates of hospital use (days per 1000 enrollees) (Chapter 5).*** These utilization rates are 35 percent lower than for people in comparison groups.** IPAs also demonstrate somewhat lower utilization rates, but the results are less clear. On the average their utilization rates are 5 to 25 percent lower (Chapter 5).**

Length of Stay

What We Know. Length of stay does not consistently differ between HMOs and their comparison populations (Chapter 5).** The comparability in length of stay seems to result from complicated changes in case mix and diagnosis-specific length of stay (Chapter 5).*

What We Do Not Know. What are the determinants of diagnosis-specific lengths of stay in various regions and settings (Chapter 5)?

Admission Rates

What We Know. PGPs seem to have lower admission rates for diagnosis and for X-rays and laboratory tests (Chapter 5).* Some PGPs perform a large fraction of their surgery on a do-not-admit basis (Chapters 5, 7).* The overall utilization rate difference is largely attributable to lower admission rates among HMO enrollees rather than to shorter stays (Chapter 5).***

What We Do Not Know. How important is do-not-admit surgery in conventional practice (Chapters 5, 7)?

Reasons for Differences in Admission Rates

What We Know. In general HMOs do not have a consistently higher or lower proportion of surgical admissions than do comparison groups (Chapter 5).** IPAs, however, have a consistently lower proportion of surgical admissions (Chapter 5).* PGPs do not seem to have achieved a disproportionately greater "reduction" in "discretionary procedures" than in any other procedures. There is no evidence for IPAs (Chapter 5).**

What We Do Not Know.   What accounts for the lower admission rates in HMOs? Do they (1) identify "discretionary" admissions in all diagnostic categories; (2) underhospitalize across the board; (3) hospitalize appropriately while conventional providers overhospitalize; (4) have a mix of patients who, for various subtle reasons, need or prefer less hospitalization; or (5) achieve the differences in some other way (Chapter 5)?

How do HMOs obtain the above results? Is it through financial incentives, nonfinancial incentives, selection of physicians or patients, referral procedures, or some other variable (Chapter 5)?

Ambulatory Care

What We Know.   On the average, PGP enrollees have somewhat more ambulatory visits per year than people in comparison groups, but the difference is less than 10 percent, and nearly as many PGPs show fewer visits per year as show more (Chapter 6).** IPA enrollees had nearly 20 percent more visits than their comparison groups, and six of seven IPA studies showed higher visit rates (Chapter 6).** HMO enrollees seem more likely to have at least one physician visit per year, suggesting that access barriers are less of a problem for them than for people with conventional insurance (Chapter 6).** HMOs seem to reduce both the proportion of people without any visits and those with very large numbers of visits within a year (Chapter 6).*

These differences in ambulatory use seem to reflect differences in coverage. When HMO coverage is much better than conventional coverage, ambulatory use is higher; when coverages are comparable, HMO enrollees are as likely to use fewer services as they are to use more (Chapter 6).**

What We Do Not Know.   How important are the lower financial barriers to ambulatory care use, relative to changes in the physical and organizational setting (Chapters 6, 14)? What explains the large variation in PGP performance (Chapter 6)? Is ambulatory care a substitute or a complement for hospital use (Chapter 6)?

What is the relative importance of solo practice versus FFS payment to the practitioners in explaining the higher ambulatory visit rates in IPAs (Chapters 6, 14)? How important are the financial costs of ambulatory care relative to nonprice factors, such as travel and waiting time, and the organization's policies with respect to encouraging or discouraging initial and follow-up visits (Chapter 6)?

Efficiencies in Providing Inpatient Care

What We Know.   Expenses per patient day in hospitals controlled by PGPs are not consistently higher or lower than in nearby community hospitals of the same size (Chapter 7).* Shorter lengths of stay in the same PGP hospitals result in lower costs per case (Chapter 7).* There is substantial variation in hospitalization rates, length of stay, and the use of do-not-admit surgery across hospitals within a single Kaiser region (Chapter 7).*

What We Do Not Know.   What are differences in diagnosis-specific treatment costs between HMOs and conventional providers (Chapter 7)?

Regionalization of Inpatient Facilities

What We Know.   There is some evidence that the formal system of Kaiser hospitals has fewer specialized facilities of various types than does the informal system of all other hospitals in the region. That is, Kaiser hospitals have fewer specialized facilities than would be expected, given their size and distance from one another (Chapter 7).*

What We Do Not Know.   Does regionalization save the medical care system substantial amounts of money (Chapter 7)?
    Does regionalization impose substantial nonmonetary travel costs on the patient, and the patient's family (Chapter 7)?

Differences in the Mix of Ambulatory Services

What We Know.   PGPs seem to provide somewhat more laboratory tests and X-rays than do conventional providers. Part of this difference may be attributable to a lack of coverage under conventional insurance (Chapters 7, 9).* There is substantial variation in the use of tests, procedures, referrals, and telephone calls among physicians within specific practice settings and this may even exceed differences across settings (Chapter 7).*

What We Do Not Know.   Do the differences in measured content of the ambulatory visit have any effect on outcome (Chapters 7, 10)? Do PGP physicians substitute tests or prescriptions for time spent with the patient (Chapters 7, 10, 12)? What is the relative importance of financial incentives versus organizational and physician-selection factors in the style of ambulatory practice (Chapters 7, 14)?

Economies of Scale in Ambulatory Practice

What We Know.   It appears that economies of scale in providing ambulatory visits do exist, but they are achieved by relatively small groups of about three to five physicians, and that diseconomies of scale may predominate in larger groups (Chapter 7).*** Most prepaid group practices have relatively large clinical groups, and therefore show physician productivity levels comparable to those of large FFS group practices (Chapter 7).**

What We Do Not Know.   To what extent does the lower physician productivity in large groups represent problems of coordination and inefficiency, rather than self-selection by physicians who prefer relatively lower incomes and more leisure (Chapters 7, 12)? What are the roles of financial and organizational incentives in physician productivity (Chapters 7, 14)?

Intensive Use of Specialists

What We Know.   The productivity of specialists, and surgeons in particular, may be substantially higher in HMOs, because their staffing patterns are designed to keep such specialists fully occupied with specialty care (Chapters 7, 10).*

What We Do Not Know.   Do specialists who concentrate in certain areas have substantially better outcomes (Chapters 7, 10)?

Use of Allied Health Personnel

What We Know.   There is no evidence that HMOs differ consistently or substantially from FFS groups in their use of allied health personnel (Chapter 7).**

What We Do Not Know.   Is the use of allied health personnel governed by efficiency considerations or by issues such as power, status, professional turf, and concepts of teamwork (Chapter 7)?

Trends in Total Medical Care Costs over Time

What We Know.   Only one pair of studies provides comparable data on premium and out-of-pocket costs over a substantial period for enrollees in various plans. These indicate the lowest rates of growth in costs for enrollees in indemnity plans, IPAs, and Kaiser; another PGP and BC-BS had substantially higher increases. Part of the slower IPA increase can be traced to an increased reliance on out-of-pocket costs (Chapter 8).*

What We Do Not Know.   How reproducible are these time trend results (Chapter 8)? What factors lie behind changes in costs over time: Enrollment mix? Local cost inflation? Changes in utilization rates (Chapters 8, 14)?

Trends in Premiums

What We Know.   For federal government enrollees, premiums have grown at annual rates of 10.4 percent for those with conventional coverage, 9.5 percent for PGP enrollees, and 6.9 percent for IPA enrollees. The initial

premium levels, however, were in reverse order, with IPA enrollees
starting with the highest costs (Chapter 8).**

What We Do Not Know.   What factors account for changes in premiums,
enrollment patterns, benefit coverage, and so on (Chapter 8)? Does
enrollment respond to premiums? How does this simultaneity affect the
results (Chapters 8, 14)?

Trends in Hospitalization

What We Know.   Utilization rates for several HMOs have been falling for
the past twenty to thirty years. In the last decade, however, utilization rates
for BC-BS enrollees in general have been falling at a similar rate (Chapter
8).** The overall rate of hospital days per 1000 enrollees in the Kaiser
Oregon plan has fallen by more than 50 percent since 1951. Reductions in
length of stay and admissions per 1000 are about equally responsible for
this decline (Chapter 8).** It appears that a substantial fraction of the fall in
admissions is attributable to changes in the enrollee mix (Chapter 8).*
There is some evidence that Kaiser Oregon was unable to constrain
utilization while it had a substantial bed surplus (Chapter 8).*

What We Do Not Know.   What accounts for long-term changes in hospital
utilization rates (Chapter 8)? How have such dramatic changes been
achieved (Chapter 8)?

Trends in Ambulatory Visits and Ancillary Services

What We Know.   The rate of ambulatory visits per enrollee shows little
trend over the long term, but this is based on limited evidence (Chapter 8).*
There have been substantial increases in the use of X-rays and laboratory
procedures. These increases seem to reflect both national technological
changes and short-run enrollment cycles within the HMO (Chapter 8).*

What We Do Not Know.   What are the trends in ambulatory visit rates in
other HMOs? How do they compare with national trends, adjusting for
population differences (Chapter 8)?

Trends in the Costs of Providing Inpatient Services

What We Know.   There seems to be little difference in long-run trends in
cost per patient day for HMOs and conventional hospitals. The falling
length of stay for HMO members resulted in a slower rise in cost per case
(Chapter 8).*

What We Do Not Know.   Are these cost patterns observable in other
HMO-controlled hospitals (Chapter 8)?

Trends in Physician Productivity

What We Know.   The average panel size (enrollees per physician) and visits per physician have been falling over time, much as has been the case for physician productivity nationally (Chapter 8).*

What We Do Not Know.   Are these patterns observable in other PGPs? In FFS groups? (Chapter 8)

Preventive Services

What We Know.   If preventive services are defined as checkups, periodic exams, immunizations, pre- and postnatal care, and diagnostic screenings, then some HMOs clearly provide more of such services than does the FFS sector, while for other HMOs there is no difference between HMO enrollees and people in comparison groups. The explanation lies with the better coverage of such services in HMOs. Conventional systems with coverage for preventive services have as many visits as or more visits than HMOs (Chapter 9).** There is some evidence that Kaiser, at least, is deemphasizing annual physical exams (Chapter 9).* When given the option to modify their benefit package, a majority of enrollees are unwilling to add certain preventive services to a conventional insurance package for a modest premium increase (Chapter 9).* The average HMO offers much better coverage for preventive services and much higher utilization rates for its enrollees than the average conventional plan (Chapter 9).***

What We Do Not Know.   Why do physicians offer and patients demand various types of medical care? Are preventive visits really for prevention, or do they meet other needs? Do preventive visits make any difference in health outcomes? Does the content of a preventive visit vary across settings? (Chapter 9)
   Do HMOs provide a more cost-effective mix of preventive services, emphasizing those proven to work well and deemphasizing those with little proven efficacy (Chapter 9)? Are differences in the use of preventive services across settings attributable to self-selection of patients or physicians (Chapter 9)?

Quality of Medical Care

What We Know.   Structure, process, and outcome measures often bear little relationship to one another, and some measures may be biased in favor of or against HMOs. For example, HMOs tend to be composed of younger, more recently trained physicians, who are more likely to be board eligible. PGPs and FFS groups are likely to have better written records than solo practitioners, who provide more personal continuity of care. FFS reimbursement may encourage clinically unnecessary tests that increase scores on process measures (Chapter 10).**

What We Do Not Know.   How should quality in medical care be measured (Chapter 10)?

Quality: Structural Measures

What We Know.   HMOs have more control over types and quality of physicians than does the open FFS system (Chapter 10).** Many of the better-known HMOs have higher proportions of board-certified specialists and are more likely to use qualified surgeons. However, some HMOs with demonstrably good quality using other measures emphasize generalists rather than specialists for the bulk of their services. Some of the California PHPs for Medicaid enrollees had markedly lower measures of structural quality. Thus the potential for quality control exists in HMOs, but it may not always be exercised (Chapter 10).**

Informal consultations with peers occur no more frequently in group practices than among solo providers (Chapter 10).* Groups seem to offer more opportunities for continuing education (Chapter 10).*

What We Do Not Know.   Do HMOs exercise more effective control over the quality of their medical staffs than do comparable groups of FFS providers (Chapter 10)? If generic HMO incentives do not guarantee high quality levels, what factors determine good or poor HMO performance (Chapters 10, 14)?

Quality: Process Measures

What We Know.   Process measures based on complete, legible records are biased in favor of PGPs and IPAs and against solo FFS practitioners, that is, they measure the records rather than the process itself (Chapter 10).** Early evaluations of specific group practices within HIP show substantial variation in quality. These reviews were then used to implement corrective actions (Chapter 10).*

PGPs provide more tests and more complete examinations, but these may reflect differences in coverage, not inherent quality. One carefully executed study does indicate the more appropriate use of services in a PGP, even when complete coverage was available for FFS providers (Chapter 10).*

PGP enrollees are more likely to be treated by an "appropriate" specialist in a large hospital than are FFS patients in general. There are few differences, however, between PGPs and the larger FFS multispecialty groups (Chapter 10).** PGP enrollees are more likely to continue to receive care within the same organization, but are less likely to be seen by the same practitioner (Chapter 10).*

What We Do Not Know.   What is the evidence that quality review systems in FFS settings, for example, PSROs, lead to improvements in quality (Chapter 10)? Are these results reproducible? What is the relative importance of prepayment versus group practice (Chapter 6)?

Prescribing Patterns

What We Know.   In one HMO prescribing patterns seem to be no different from those in FFS settings and even include similar proportions of brand name versus generic drugs and drugs of questionable efficacy. In another setting, prescription drugs were used much more appropriately in the HMO (Chapter 10).* It appears that prescribing patterns in the FFS sector can be changed if sufficient effort and incentives are applied (Chapter 10).*

What We Do Not Know.   Are prescribing patterns useful measures of quality (Chapter 10)?

Quality: Outcome Measures

What We Know.   Comparisons of HMO outcomes with respect to explicit outcome criteria, such as hypertension control, show substantial gaps between performance and what the investigators thought results should be. Similar gaps appear in FFS settings, and these gaps may be the result of unrealistic expectations (Chapter 10).* Early studies at HIP showed significantly lower mortality and prematurity rates. More recent studies suggest that HMO enrollees may have no better outcomes than FFS patients, and in some cases their outcomes may be somewhat worse (Chapter 10).* HMO members seem to have somewhat better measures of health status, particularly as indicated by disability days per episode of illness (Chapter 10).**

What We Do Not Know.   Are these tentative outcome findings reproducible in large, methodologically sound studies (Chapter 10)? Does patient self-selection play any role in these outcome differences across settings (Chapter 10)?

Consumer Satisfaction

What We Know.   There are few methodologically sound or comprehensive studies (Chapter 11).* HMO enrollees seem more knowledgeable about their medical care options and seem to have more opinions about almost everything (Chapter 11).**

What We Do Not Know.   Is there a bias in questionnaires given to PGP and solo FFS patients resulting from the PGP enrollees answering questions about their prepaid group *in general,* while the FFS patient focuses on his or her particular physician (Chapter 11)?

Access to Care

What We Know.   PGP enrollees spend less time waiting in the physician's office when they have an appointment than do FFS patients (Chapter 11).*** IPA and PGP enrollees are more satisfied with their office waiting times than are FFS patients (Chapter 11).** PGP enrollees have to schedule appointments further in advance and are more dissatisfied with this (Chapter 11).*** Few consistent differences appear with respect to telephone access, house calls, time allocated for appointment and availability of physicians (Chapter 11).* Physical access seems somewhat more difficult for PGP enrollees (Chapter 11).**

What We Do Not Know.   Do differences in appointment scheduling and office waiting times reflect prepayment incentives or group practice performance (Chapters 11, 14)? Do differences in appointment scheduling and office waiting times lead to patient self-selection, with those having nonurgent, schedulable visits, but a high value of time, preferring PGPs (Chapters 3, 11)? Do PGPs tend to enroll only people who live or work relatively close to the clinic (Chapter 3, 7, 11)?

Financial Coverage

What We Know.   PGP enrollees are much more satisfied with their financial coverage than are enrollees in conventional plans (Chapter 11).*** IPA enrollees seem only somewhat more satisfied with their coverage than conventional enrollees (Chapter 11).*

Continuity of Care

What We Know.   PGP enrollees are somewhat less likely to report having a personal physician or seeing the same physician. They are, however, more likely to seek care from the same place in urgent situations (Chapter 11).*

What We Do Not Know.   Is continuous care from one setting with different providers sharing the same records better or worse than care that is more likely to be with a single physician, recognizing that in the latter instance, a larger proportion of visits will be to emergency rooms or other sources with no sharing of records (Chapter 11)?

One major reason for not joining a PGP is a prior strong attachment to a physician. Does this mean that people who join PGPs are less interested in continuity of care (Chapters 3, 11)?

Information Transfer

What We Know. PGP enrollees are less satisfied with the willingness of plan physicians to listen and to explain. There is more dissatisfaction with their willingness to explain than to listen (Chapter 11).** IPA enrollees are about as satisfied as people in conventional plans (Chapter 11).*

Humaneness

What We Know. PGP enrollees seem consistently less satisfied about their interactions with physicians (Chapter 11).*** Results concerning interactions with the staff are mixed. Some PGP enrollees are more satisfied with their interactions with ancillary personnel than are FFS patients (Chapter 11).**

What We Do Not Know. Are some of these results a reflection of large, bureaucratic group practices, rather than prepaid groups per se? There is some evidence that small PGPs are evaluated more favorably than large ones (Chapters 11, 14). Are the different evaluations by PGP enrollees with respect to physicians and staff a reflection of different approaches to the use of appointments and scheduling (Chapter 11)?

Perceptions of Quality

What We Know. PGP enrollees are slightly more dissatisfied with the quality of their care, but there are studies showing both more and less dissatisfaction (Chapter 11).* IPA enrollees seem at least as satisfied or more satisfied with their quality of care than are people in other plans (Chapter 11).*

What We Do Not Know. To what extent do perceptions of quality reflect the ability of the patient to find a physician willing to do what he or she wants done (Chapters 3, 11)?

Overall Attitudinal Measures

What We Know. Results regarding attitudinal measures are mixed for both PGP and IPA enrollees, with a slight leaning toward less satisfaction among HMO members (Chapter 11).*

What We Do Not Know. How sensitive are these overall results to specific questionnaires, and in particular, are the Hulka scales valid measures for comparing HMO and FFS enrollees (Chapter 11)?

Out-of-Plan Use as a Measure of Satisfaction

What We Know.   About 5 to 10 percent of PGP members are regular users of outside services, and these people are likely to be the same ones who report substantial dissatisfaction in surveys (Chapter 11).**

What We Do Not Know.   Why do people belong to an HMO and continue to use outside services on a regular basis without then switching to a conventional plan (Chapter 11)?

Disenrollment as a Measure of Satisfaction

What We Know.   There appears to be a great deal of inertia in choice of plan, so disenrollment behavior must be measured over a long period of time (Chapter 11).** In a number of PGPs there is a low voluntary disenrollment rate despite greater expressed dissatisfaction. To a substantial degree this suggests that PGPs' financial advantages outweigh their negative aspects (Chapter 11).**

What We Do Not Know.   Do disenrollment rates vary with individuals' experience in the plan (Chapters 3, 11)? In one situation, enrollees in both a PGP and BC-BS had identical and complete financial coverage at no cost. The PGP enrollees were more dissatisfied, yet their disenrollment rate was no greater than that observed in dual choice situations with substantial financial advantages to the HMO enrollees. What explains this behavior (Chapter 11)?

Long-Term Changes in Enrollment Patterns

What We Know.   Over periods of more than a decade, both PGPs and IPAs have tended to substantially increase their enrollment shares within employee groups having multiple choice options (Chapter 11).***

What We Do Not Know.   What are the long-term dynamics of enrollment in multiple choice situations? How sensitive are people to financial and other differences (Chapters 3, 11, 14)?

Role of the Physician in HMOs

What We Know.   The decision of a physician to participate in an HMO has often involved behavior seen by the rest of the profession as aberrant. Thus switching back and forth is difficult for both financial and psychological reasons, and this may influence the willingness of HMO physicians to voice complaints (see Hirschman). (Chapters 3, 12)*

What We Do Not Know.   What determines physician choice of the setting in which to work (Chapter 12)?

Physician Workload and Income

What We Know.   PGP physicians have shorter work weeks and earn correspondingly less than those in FFS groups. They also have more fixed schedules (Chapter 12).** PGP physicians are more satisfied with their work weeks and earnings than physicians are in other settings even though both are lower (Chapter 12).** Income distribution within a group is often a major point of contention and is the primary reason given for leaving a group (Chapters 12, 14).*

What We Do Not Know.   Do physicians who join PGPs have a greater preference for more stable work weeks, fringe benefits, and more moderate incomes, than do those who prefer FFS practice? Do these preferences develop after joining (Chapters 3, 12)?

Physician Satisfaction with Patient Interactions

What We Know.   There is evidence that PGP physicians feel they are faced with "demanding patients" who do not accept the traditional patient role and, instead, demand certain services guaranteed in the contract (Chapter 12).* There is also evidence that PGP physicians find themselves with rigid appointment schedules and not enough time to deal adequately with the difficult problems posed by the psychosomatic or "worried well" patient. Instead, they label the complaints as trivial and blame the system for lowering access costs (Chapter 12).*

What We Do Not Know.   Is the content and style of physician-patient interactions really different across settings (Chapters 11, 12)? How important are differences between prepayment and group practice settings in influencing physician-patient interactions (Chapters 11, 12)?

Physician Satisfaction with Autonomy

What We Know.   Physician autonomy in PGPs appears to be less of a problem than might be expected, because the physician group can generally set its own rules, and the health plan is generally supportive and nonintrusive. The health plan provides a buffer and frees the physician from having to deal with a wide variety of separate insurers, government agencies, and the like (Chapter 12).**

Physician Satisfaction with Ability to Practice "Good Medicine"

What We Know.   Some HMO physicians are attracted by the fact that complete coverage allows them to deliver care without worrying about the patient's ability to pay (Chapter 12).* PGP and FFS group physicians sometimes feel constrained to refer patients within the system. They also feel an incongruity between their largely ambulatory practice and their hospital-oriented training (Chapter 12).* Reports of low self-esteem by PGP practitioners seem related to early battles with organized medicine, and this is no longer an issue (Chapter 12).*

What We Do Not Know.   If the HMO physician practices as if cost were not a constraint, what accounts for the lower utilization rates (Chapters 12, 14)? How do physicians in conventional practice deal with the contrast between their hospital-based training and the realities of practice (Chapter 12)?

Recruitment and Turnover of Physicians

What We Know.   PGPs do not seem to face major problems in recruiting new physicians, except in the cases of certain subspecialties where market incomes far exceed what the average physician earns (Chapter 12).** Turnover rates appear to be moderate for well established HMOs (Chapter 12).**

What We Do Not Know.   What factors determine the selection of physicians into and out of HMOs? Does this selection influence how the organization performs (Chapters 12, 14)?

HMOs Serving the Poor

What We Know.   Enrollment of Medicaid eligibles in HMOs is usually difficult because the proposed coverage is often no better than Medicaid coverage while it restricts choice; and frequent changes in enrollment eligibility create a substantial administrative burden for the HMO (Chapter 13).**

HMOs serving the poor (generally Medicaid eligibles) fall into two major categories: (1) demonstration projects in which special incentives made HMO enrollment attractive for the beneficiaries and the administrative problems worthwhile for the HMO; and (2) situations in which Medicaid contracts were attractive to the HMO as its major business, and the HMO seemed to the Medicaid eligibles to be a better source of care than the conventional system (Chapter 13).**

It often appears that when few other medical care alternatives are available, the poor are willing to join HMOs regardless of their quality (Chapter 13).*

What We Do Not Know. Under what circumstances is the enrollment of Medicaid eligibles attractive to both the poor and the HMOs?

Prepaid Health Plans in California

What We Know. Many marketing abuses can be traced to state guidelines that did not provide for start-up costs, authorized many plans in each service area, and refused to allow access to mailing lists of eligibles (Chapter 13).** Some plans undoubtedly reaped excessive profits through subsidiaries of de jure nonprofit health plans, while others paid apparently excessive administrative costs to their subsidiaries (Chapters 13, 14).** In some cases quality of care was clearly inferior to what it should have been, but comparisons of PHPs and Medicaid mills reveal both extremely large differences in utilization rates and poor quality in both settings (Chapters 10, 13, 14).*

What We Do Not Know. What guidelines would allow HMOs to market to the poor without encouraging such abuses (Chapter 13)? How does one design a payment scheme for HMOs that allows for a reasonable return on investment while maintaining cost control incentives (Chapters 13, 14)? How did the profits, providers' incomes, and quality of care in the PHPs compare with those of FFS providers treating predominantly Medicaid populations (Chapter 13)?

Utilization Rates of the Poor

What We Know. Overall, rates of ambulatory care utilization of the poor in HMOs are comparable to that of both the nonpoor in HMOs and the poor in conventional systems. Differences appear, however, in the use of specific services. The poor are less likely to use the telephone and more likely to use the emergency room within the HMO (Chapter 13).*

Patient perceptions of ease of access, waiting, and appointment times show a wide variety among HMOs. Many of the differences appear related to variations in the structure and performance of the local FFS system rather than the HMOs (Chapters 13, 14).*

What We Do Not Know. What levels of utilization *should* the poor have within an HMO, that is, what should be the standard for comparison and how do various providers measure up (Chapter 10)?

Feasibility of HMO Care for the Poor

What We Know. New federal regulations limiting Medicare and Medicaid enrollments in HMOs to a maximum of 50 percent may render it impossible for PGPs to locate themselves so as to serve both the poor and the middle class. Providing coverage for the working poor, as well as eliminating employer-based insurance coverage, may be necessary. Some mainstream HMOs have provided high-quality care for the poor at reasonable cost, but the number of such enrollees has always been relatively small (Chapter 13).*

What We Do Not Know. What types of environmental, and in particular, financing arrangements are most conducive to the appropriate enrollment of the poor in HMOs (Chapters 13, 14)?

Influence of Sponsorship on Performance

What We Know. The reason behind establishment of an HMO seems to have an important impact on its chances for success and subsequent performance. Simple categories of sponsors, such as provider and consumer, however, are not reliable guides to the organization's goals (Chapter 14).*

Profit-Nonprofit Status

What We Know. Similarly, profit or nonprofit structure is an unreliable indicator. There have been both good and bad organizations of each type (Chapter 14).**

What We Do Not Know. How can one distinguish *ex ante* organizations seeking to provide quality services over the long term from the "fast buck" operators (Chapter 14)?

Consumer Involvement

What We Know. Substantive and effective consumer involvement may lead to better HMOs, but the evidence is scanty. It probably is true that effective involvement is incompatible with extremely poor HMOs (Chapter 14).*

What We Do Not Know. Is there an optimal level of consumer control that achieves an appropriate balance between consumer and provider satisfaction (Chapters 11, 12, 14)?

Administrative Factors

What We Know. The management of an HMO is much more complex than that of a conventional FFS medical practice. Particularly in the start-up phase, it seems important to have substantial expertise (Chapter 14).*

What We Do Not Know.   Is a centralized or decentralized form of management best for an HMO, or does the choice of administrative structure depend on other variables (Chapter 14)?

Methods of Paying the Physicians

What We Know.   A wide range of schemes exists within HMOs, ranging from fixed salaries based on tenure to FFS payments to capitation schemes (Chapter 14).** Problems seem to occur when (1) primary physicians are only partly involved in the HMO, (2) physicians share in the financial implications of some of their actions but not others, and (3) physicians are paid on an FFS basis by the organization without having effective countervailing incentives to constrain costs (Chapter 14).*

What We Do Not Know.   Are there consistent differences in HMO performance and provider satisfaction associated with the different payment schemes? Are certain schemes clearly better than others (Chapters 13, 14)?

Hospital Control by the HMO

What We Know.   Advantages of direct control relate to proximity (physician time, reducing duplicate equipment for inpatient and outpatient use, and so on) and hospital technology and efficiency. HMO hospitals do not seem to be run particularly more efficiently, but they may be able to restrain the excessive purchase of new equipment to compete for physicians (Chapters 7, 8, 14).* Major disadvantages include the cost of capital and potential further duplication of hospital facilities that may then lead to conflicts with health planning agencies (Chapter 14).*

What We Do Not Know.   How large are the differences, if any, between the costs of inpatient care in hospitals directly controlled by HMOs and in those for which the HMO is a major customer (Chapters 7, 14)?

Access to Specialists

What We Know.   Some HMOs have made special attempts to use the primary care physician as a gatekeeper to specialty care. This may reduce costs, but little is known about its true impact on cost, quality, and satisfaction (Chapter 14).*

What We Do Not Know.   Is giving the primary-care physician responsibility for all medical care a feasible and effective means of organization? Will it work only with selected physicians and patients (Chapter 14)?

Legal Constraints on HMO Development

What We Know.   Although restrictive state laws had been a problem in HMO development and have shaped the particular organizational structures taken by many HMOs, they do not now seem to be a major stumbling block (Chapter 14).* The ways in which laws have been interpreted and enforced at local levels seem more important than the letter of the law (Chapter 14).*

What We Do Not Know.   Exactly what impact have the legal constraints had on HMO development and the ability of people in various areas to even begin plans for HMOs, that is, do certain requirements make HMOs legal, but infeasible (Chapter 14)? What is the impact of various regulatory reporting and staffing requirements on HMO development and growth (Chapter 14)? How effective are local HMO backers in changing the legal setting (Chapter 14)?

Sociodemographic Factors and HMO Development

What We Know.   HMOs seem to have developed first in areas that were relatively wealthy, liberal, unionized, and had extensive health insurance coverage, rapid population growth, high density, and large total populations (Chapter 14).*

What We Do Not Know.   What factors are necessary or sufficient for HMO development? Are these factors different for starting an HMO than for promoting rapid growth? Are these factors different for PGPs and IPAs (Chapter 14)?

HMOs in the Health Insurance Market

What We Know.   HMOs seem to have kept their premiums within a narrow range set by competing conventional insurance premiums. In recent years, however, some conventional premiums have grown much more rapidly than those of the HMOs (Chapters 8, 14).** Dual choice options have traditionally been available to only a limited segment of the population (Chapter 14).**

What We Do Not Know.   What are the dynamics of the competitive effects of HMOs, if in fact they exist (Chapter 14)? What determined the availability of dual choice options? How will the mandatory dual choice provisions change this? And what are the likely implications for HMOs and conventional insurers (Chapter 14)?

Teaching and Research in HMOs

What We Know.   Although HMOs could serve as important settings for integrating training in patient care, there is little evidence that this has taken place (Chapter 14).* Some HMOs have used their extensive medical records to provide large-scale and long-term epidemiological studies. Few HMOs have experimented with major innovations in medical care delivery (Chapter 14).*

What We Do Not Know.   What incentives and structural changes are necessary in order to better utilize the potential of HMOs for medical education and research (Chapter 14)?

Impact of HMOs on the Conventional System

What We Know.   There is some evidence that the presence of HMOs may lead the conventional system to respond by constraining its utilization rates and costs. Hospital utilization rates are lower in areas with substantial HMO enrollments, and in some cases the lower utilization occurred contemporaneously with HMO growth. Other data, however, indicate no measurable effect of HMOs on the hospitalization of non-HMO enrollees (Chapter 14).*

There is also the possibility that HMOs achieve some of their utilization advantage through a subtle form of selection by which they attract and retain a population that prefers less hospitalization. This would have major implications for both the analysis of cost and utilization and for the desirability of various types of market competition (Chapters 3, 4, 5, 6, 14).*

Areas with substantial HMO enrollment have no lower overall medical care costs. HMO competition may have led to a substitution of ambulatory services and higher physician fees (Chapter 14).*

What We Do Not Know.   How important is the competitive influence of HMO enrollment, that is, will a 10 percent market penetration by HMOs have a noticeable impact on conventional providers (Chapter 14)? Is there a selection effect, and how important is it in explaining utilization differences between HMOs and conventional plans (Chapters 3, 14)?

CONCLUSION

This book represents an effort to gather, analyze, and synthesize what is known about HMO performance at the beginning of the 1980s. As this chapter illustrates, research findings on some questions are consistent; however, there are substantial areas about which little is known or the evidence is contradictory. For some of these it is possible to design the necessary research projects, and sufficient time and research support will fill in the gaps in our knowledge. In other areas, however, the questions are far more intractable, and clear answers will be difficult to develop.

Policy-making does not necessarily wait for solid research conclusions. Pressing human problems cannot be ignored, and policy-makers frequently must rely on logic, intuition, and limited evidence to frame their decisions. One message of this book is that things are not always what they seem at first glance. A second message is that well-intentioned plans often have unintentioned adverse consequences. These cautions, however, should not lead to policy paralysis. It has been demonstrated that HMOs can provide good quality medical care to substantial numbers of enrollees at lower cost than the conventional system, while maintaining reasonable levels of consumer and provider satisfaction. We also know that HMOs do not offer an answer to everyone, and further experimentation with other types of medical care delivery systems is necessary.

Recognizing the uncertainties about various aspects of HMO performance, experimentation should be encouraged, but with careful monitoring and built-in flexibility. As we experiment in designing an improved health care delivery system some failures will inevitably occur, but the existing evidence on HMO performance suggests that prepaid systems will be among the successful policy options of the future.

Reference List

Abrams, Herbert L. "The Overutilization of X-Rays," *New England Journal of Medicine,* **300**:21 (May 24, 1979: 1213–1216.

Abt Associates. *A Study of Administrative Costs in Physicians Offices and Medicaid Participation.* Cambridge: Abt Associates Inc., 1977.

Acton, Jan Paul. "Demand for Health Care Among the Urban Poor, with Special Emphasis on the Role of Time," in Richard N. Rosett (ed.), *The Role of Health Insurance in the Health Services Sector.* New York: National Bureau of Economic Research, 1976

———. "Nonmonetary Factors in the Demand for Medical Services: Some Empirical Evidence," *Journal of Political Economy,* **83**:3 (June 1975): 595–614.

Aday, Lu Ann. "Economic and Non-Economic Barriers to the Use of Needed Medical Services," *Medical Care,* **13**:6 (June 1975): 447–456.

———. "Response to Critique of 'Economic and Non-Economic Barriers to the Use of Needed Medical Services,'" *Medical Care,* **14**:8 (August 1976): 717–720.

———, Andersen, R., and Anderson, O. "Social Surveys and Health Policy: Implications for National Health Insurance," *Public Health Reports,* **92**:6 (November-December 1977): 508–517.

Aiken, Linda H., et al. "The Contribution of Specialists to the Delivery of Primary Care: A New Perspective," *New England Journal of Medicine,* **300**:24 (June 14, 1979): 1363–1370.

American Association of Medical Clinics, AMA, Medical Group Management Association. *Group Practice: Guidelines to Joining or Forming a Medical Group.* Chicago: American Medical Association, 1970.

American Association of Professional Standards Review Organizations. Letter to Members of National Council re Screening Criteria. Stockton, Ca.: AAPSRO, January 8, 1978.

American Heart Association. *Recommendations for Human Blood Pressure Determination by Sphygmomanometers.* New York: American Heart Association, 1967.

American Hospital Association. *American Hospital Directory.* Chicago: American Hospital Association, 1946.

———. *Financial Relationships between Hospitals and Comprehensive Health Care Delivery Organizations.* Chicago: AHA, 1975.

———. *Guide to the Health Care Field, 1975 Edition.* Chicago: AHA, 1975.

———. *Hospital Statistics, 1975 Edition.* Chicago: AHA, 1975.

———. *Hospital Statistics, 1976 Edition.* Chicago: AHA, 1976.

————. *Hospital Statistics, 1977 Edition.* Chicago: AHA, 1977.

————. *Hospital Statistics, 1978 Edition.* Chicago: AHA, 1978.

————. "The Nation's Hospitals: A Statistical Profile," *Hospitals, JAHA,* **36,** part 2 (August 1, 1962): 414.

American Medical Association. "Annual Presentation of Hospital Data by the Council on Medical Education and Hospitals," *Journal of the American Medical Association,* 1931–1940.

————. "Minutes of the 85th Annual Session, June 11–15, 1934," *Journal of the American Medical Association,* **102** (1934): 2200.

————. *Opinions of AMA Members 1973.* Chicago: AMA, 1973.

————. *Profile of Medical Practice '74.* Chicago: AMA, 1974.

————, Commission on Medical Care Plans. "Report of the Commission—Findings, Conclusions and Recommendations," *Journal of the American Medical Association,* Special Edition (January 17, 1959).

————, Commission on Medical Care Plans (Larson). *Report on the Commission . . . Part II. Statistical Appendices and Background Materials.* Chicago: AMA, 1958.

American Medical News. "Are Physicians Overworked?" *American Medical News Impact* (August 23, 1976).

Andersen, Ronald. *A Behavioral Model of Families' Use of Health Services.* Chicago: Center for Health Administration Studies, Research Series #25, 1968.

————, Kravits, Joanna, and Anderson, Odin W. "The Public's View of the Crisis in Medical Care: An Impetus for Changing Delivery Systems?" *Economic and Business Bulletin,* **24:**1 (Fall 1971): 44–52.

————, Lion, Joanna, and Anderson, Odin W. *Two Decades of Health Services: Social Survey Trends in Use and Expenditures.* Cambridge: Ballinger Publishing Co., 1976.

Anderson, James G. "Health Services Utilization: Framework and Review," *Health Services Research,* **8:**3 (Fall 1973): 184–199.

Anderson, Odin W., and Sheatsley, Paul B. *Comprehensive Medical Insurance: A Study of Costs, Use, and Attitudes under Two Plans.* New York: Health Insurance Foundation: Research Series No. 9, 1959.

————. *Hospital Use: A Survey of Patient and Physician Decisions.* Chicago: Center for Health Administration Studies, University of Chicago, 1967.

Andrus, Len Hughes, and Mitchell, Ferd H. *Health Care for the American People: Unfinished Agenda; Group Practice.* Prepared for Conference on Medical Care for the American People: Unfinished Agenda, Georgetown University School of Medicine, Virginia, May 18–20, 1977.

Angermeier, Ingo. "Impact of Community Rating and Open Enrollment on a Prepaid Group Practice," *Inquiry,* **13:**1 (March 1976): 48–53.

Anonymous. "HEW's Dual Option Regulations, Impact," *Medical World News,* **17:**23 (February 9, 1976).

Anonymous. "HMOs' Stormy Tryout in Los Angeles Area," *Medical World News* (June 15, 1973): 17–19.

Anonymous. "Some Management Firms Make Studies of Prepaid Health Plans," *Federation of American Hospitals Review,* **11:**4 (June 1978): 36–38.

Anonymous. "The Two Barriers to HMO Success: The Doctors and the Patients," *Modern Healthcare,* **1:**2 (May 1974).

Arnstein, Sherry R. "A Ladder of Citizen Participation," *AIP Journal* (July 1969).

Arrow, Kenneth J. "Uncertainty and the Welfare Economics of Medical Care," *American Economic Review*, **53**:5 (December 1963): 941–973.

Ashcraft, Marie, et al. "Expectations and Experience of HMO Enrollees after One Year: An Analysis of Satisfaction, Utilization and Costs," *Medical Care*, **16**:1 (January 1978): 14–32.

Auger, Richard, and Goldberg, Victor. "Prepaid Health Plans and Moral Hazard," *Public Policy*, **22** (1974): 353–393.

Bacon, Donald C. "Medicaid Abuse: Even Worse Than Feared," *US News and World Report* (June 4, 1979).

Bahn, Robert. "Where Doctors Stand on Prepaid Group Medicine," *Hospital Physician* (November 1970): 66–67, 122.

Bailar, John C. "Mammography: A Contrary View," *Annals of Internal Medicine*, **84**:1 (January 1976): 77–84.

Bailey, Richard M. "Economies of Scale in Medical Practice," in Herbert Klarman (ed.), *Empirical Studies in Health Economics*. Baltimore: Johns Hopkins Press, 1970, pp. 255–273, 274–277.

———. "Philosophy, Faith, Fact, and Fiction in the Production of Medical Services," *Inquiry*, **7**:1 (March 1970).

———. *Medical Care in Hawaii: 1970*. Berkeley: University of California, Institute of Business and Economic Research, February 1971.

Baker, A. Sherwood. "What Do Family Physicians in a Prepaid Group Do in Their Offices?" *The Journal of Family Practice*, **6**:2 (1978): 335–340.

Banta, David, and Bosch, Samuel J. "Organized Labor and the Prepaid Group Practice Movement," *Archives of Environmental Health*, **29**:1 (July 1974): 43–51.

Barker, Karlyn. "Yeklell, Antonelli Seen Pressuring Hospital, GHA Link," *Washington Post*, **100** (December 16, 1976). Reprinted in *Medical Care Review*, **34**:1 (January 1977): 42–47.

Barr, Richard. "The New Mexico Health Care Corporation: One Hospital's Involvement in an HMO," in Robert A. Zelten and Susan Bray (eds.), *Health Maintenance Organizations*. Presentations from the 1976 Guest Lecture Series Training Program in HMO Management, Leonard Davis Institute of Health Economics, University of Pennsylvania, pp. 93–103.

Bashshur, Rashid L., and Metzner, Charles A. "Patterns of Social Differentiation Between Community Health Association and Blue Cross-Blue Shield," *Inquiry*, **4** (1967): 23–44.

———. "Vulnerability to Risk and Awareness of Dual Choice of Health Insurance Plan," *Health Services Research* (Summer 1970): 106–113.

———, and Worden, C. "Consumer Satisfaction with Group Practice: The CHA Case," *American Journal of Public Health*, **57**:11 (November 1967): 1991–1994.

Bator, Francis M. "The Anatomy of Market Failure," *Quarterly Journal of Economics*, **72**:3 (August 1958): 351–379.

Bear, Michael R. "Downward Trend in the Incidence of Tonsillectomy with Adenoidectomy," *PAS Reporter*, **15** (May 16, 1977): 1–8.

Beck, Leif C., and Kalogredis, Vasilios J. "Dividing the Group Income Pie," *Pennsylvania Medicine* (September 1977): 31–33.

Becker, Gary S. "A Theory of the Allocation of Time," *Economic Journal*, **75** (September 1965): 493–517.

Becker, Marshall H., Drachman, Robert H., and Kirscht, John P. "A Field Experiment to Evaluate Various Outcomes of Continuity of Physician Care," *American Journal of Public Health*, **64**:11 (November 1974), 1062–1070.

Becker, Marshall H., et al. "Selected Psychosocial Models and Correlates of Individual Health-Related Behaviors," *Medical Care*, **15:**5 (Supplement) (May 1977): 27–46.

Berkanovic, Emil, and Reeder, Leo G. "Can Money Buy the Appropriate Use of Services? Some Notes on the Meaning of Utilization Data," *Journal of Health and Social Behavior*, **15** (June 1974): 93–99.

Berkanovic, Emil, et al. *Perceptions of Medical Care: The Impact of Prepayment.* Lexington, Ma.: D.C. Heath, 1974.

Berki, Sylvester E. "Economic Effects of National Health Insurance," *Inquiry*, **8:**2 (June 1971): 37–55.

——— and Ashcraft, Marie L. "On the Analysis of Ambulatory Utilization: An Investigation of the Roles of Need, Access and Price as Predictors of Illness and Preventive Visits." Forthcoming in *Medical Care*.

Berki, Sylvester E., et al. "Enrollment Choice in a Multi-HMO Setting: The Roles of Health Risk, Financial Vulnerability, and Access to Care," *Medical Care*, **15:**2 (February 1977): 95–114.

———. "Enrollment Choices in Different Types of HMOs: A Multivariate Analysis," *Medical Care*, **16:**8 (August 1978): 682–697.

———. "Health Concern, HMO Enrollment, and Preventive Care Use," *Journal of Community Health*, **3:**1 (Fall 1977): 3–31.

Biblo, Robert L. "Marketing and Enrollment Strategies for Prepaid Group Practice Plans," in U.S. Office for Health Maintenance Organizations, *Marketing Prepaid Health Care Plans*, U.S. Department of Health, Education and Welfare Publication No. HSM 73-6207, 1972, pp. 5–38.

Bice, Thomas W. "Risk Vulnerability and Enrollment in a Prepaid Group Practice," *Medical Care*, **13:**8 (August 1975): 698–703.

———, Eichhorn, Robert L., and Fox, Peter D. "Socioeconomic Status and Use of Physician Services: A Reconsideration," *Medical Care*, **10:**3 (May-June 1972): 261–271.

Bird, David. "Public Can't View City H.I.P. Reports," *New York Times*, **124:**29 (April 20, 1975). Reprinted in *Medical Care Review*, **32:**5 (May 1975): 534–535.

Birnbaum, Roger W. "Appendix B: Selected HMO Planning Data," in Birnbaum, *Prepayment and Neighborhood Health Centers: Guidelines for the Planning of or Conversion to a Health Maintenance Organization.* Washington, D.C.: Office of Health Affairs, OEO, 1972, pp. 69–81.

———. "The Harvard Community Health Plan: To Provide Broad Access to Quality, Comprehensive Health Care," *Public Welfare*, **29:**1 (January 1971): 42–46.

———. *Health Maintenance Organizations: A Guide to Planning and Development.* New York: Spectrum, 1976.

Blanchard, Leland B. "Why We're Losing Family Doctors," *Prism* (March 1975): 57–59.

Blue Cross Association. *The Use of Hospitals by Blue Cross Members in 1972.* Research Series 12, March 1974.

Blue Cross Association. "The Use of Hospitals by Blue Cross Members in 1965," *Blue Cross Reports*, **4:**4 (October-December 1966).

Blue Cross Association. *The Use of Hospitals by Members of Blue Cross Plans in 1973.* Research Series 13, April 1975.

Blue Cross Association, Research and Development, Health Economics Center. Personal communications. Chicago, April 12, 1977; July 28, 1978.

Blue Cross and Blue Shield. *Fact Book 1976.* Chicago: Blue Cross Association and National Association of Blue Shield Plans, 1976.

————. "Press Release: Blue Cross-Blue Shield HMOs," *Medical Care Review,* **35:**8 (August 1978): 799–800.

Blue Cross and Blue Shield Association. "Reserves, Expenses, and Revenues," *Financial Outlook,* **10** (May 1978): 6.

Blue Cross and Blue Shield of Michigan. "Surgical Patient Study: Press Release," *Medical Care Review,* **34:**4 (April 1977): 412–413.

Blumberg, Mark S. *Problems in Access to Health Care; Data from the 1974 U.S. Health Interview Survey.* Unpublished paper, January 12, 1978.

————. *The Relative Merits of Prepaid Group Practice: A Brief History of HMO Precursors.* Oakland, Ca.: Kaiser Foundation Health Plan, December 1977.

————, and Gentry, Douglas W. "Routine Hospital Charges and Intensity of Care: A Cross-Section Analysis of Fifty States," *Inquiry,* **15:**1 (March 1978): 58–73.

Boan, J. A. *Group Practice.* Monograph for Royal Commission on Health Services. Ottawa, Canada: Queen's Printer, 1966.

Bombardier, Claire. *Variations in the Utilization of Medical Care: Economic Considerations.* Unpublished paper, 1976.

Borsody, Robert P. "HMO's and the Neighborhood Health Centers," *Clearinghouse Review,* **6:**3 (July 1972): 123–129.

Bosch, Samuel J., et al. "Medical Student Roles in Prepaid Group Practice," *Journal of Medical Education,* **48:**4 (April 1973), Part 2: 142–153.

————. "A Proposed Network to Improve Access to High-Quality Health Care for Medicaid-Eligible Families," *Journal of Community Health,* **4:**4 (Summer 1979): 302–311.

Bothwell, James L., and Cooley, Thomas F. *Efficiency in the Provision of Health Care: An Economic Analysis of Health Maintenance Organizations.* Unpublished draft, 1978.

Bovbjerg, Randall. "Medical Malpractice Standard of Care: HMO's and Customary Practice," *Duke Law Journal* (1975): 1375–1414.

Bradwell, A. R., Carmatt, M. H. B., and Whitehead, T. P. "Explaining the Unexpected Abnormal Results of Biochemical Profile Investigations," *Lancet,* **7888** (November 2, 1974): 1071–1074.

Breo, Dennis. "HMO Skirmish Heats Up in Rochester, N.Y.—and the Doctors' Plan May Be First Casualty," *American Medical News,* **18:**11 (October 27, 1975). Reprinted in *Medical Care Review,* **33:**1 (January 1976): 27–32.

————. "In Florida, Testing Centers Are Big Business—But MDs Are Questioning Their Value," *American Medical News,* **19:**15 (November 22, 1976). Reprinted in *Medical Care Review,* **34:**1 (January 1977): 48–52.

Breslow, Lester. *Do HMO's Provide Health Maintenance?* Paper presented to Delta Omega, San Francisco, November 7, 1973.

————. "Statement Prepared for Senate Permanent Subcommittee on Investigations of the Committee on Government Operations, March 12, 1975," in U.S. Senate, Committee on Government Operations, Permanent Subcommittee on Investigations. *Prepaid Health Plans,* Washington D.C.: USGPO, 1975, pp 52–63.

————, and Hochstim, Joseph R. "Sociocultural Aspects of Cervical Cytology in Alameda County, California," *Public Health Reports,* **79:**2, (February 1964): 107–112.

Brewster, Agnes W., and Seldowitz, Estelle. "Medical Society Relative Value Scales and the Medical Market," *Public Health Reports,* **80:**6 (June 1965): 501–509.

Brewster, Agnes W., Allen, Scott I., and Holen, Arlene. "Patterns of Drug Use by Type in a Prepaid Medical Plan," *Public Health Reports,* **79:**5 (May 1964): 403–409.

Broida, Joel H. "Macro and Micro Assessment of an Alternative Delivery System: The HMO: Methodology and Output." Presented at APHA, Chicago, November 16–20, 1975.

Broida, Joel and Lerner, Monroe. "Knowledge of Patient's Method of Payment by Physicians in a Group Practice," *Public Health Reports*, **90**:2 (March-April 1975): 113–118.

Broida, Joel, et al. "Impact of Membership in an Enrolled Prepaid Population on Utilization of Health Services in a Group Practice," *New England Journal of Medicine*, **292**:15 (April 10, 1975): 780–783.

Brook, Robert H. "Critical Issues in the Assessment of Quality of Care and Their Relationship to HMO's," *Journal of Medical Education*, **48**:4 (April 1973), Part 2: 114–134.

———. *Quality of Care Assessment: Comparison of Five Methods of Peer Review*. National Center for Health Services Research and Development. Washington, D.C.: USGPO, 1973.

———, and Stevenson, Robert L. "Effectiveness of Patient Care in an Emergency Room," *New England Journal of Medicine*, **283**:17 (October 22, 1970): 904–907.

Brook, Robert H. and Williams, Kathleen N. "Effect of Medical Care Review on the Use of Injections: A Study of the New Mexico Experimental Medical Care Review Organization," *Annals of Internal Medicine*, **85**:4 (October 1976): 509–515.

Brook, Robert H., Berg, Morris H., and Schechter, Philip A. "Effectiveness of Non-Emergency Room Care Via Emergency: A Study of 116 Patients with Gastro-intestinal Symptoms," *Annals of Internal Medicine*, **78**:3 (March 1973): 333–339.

Bruzelius, Nils. "Dukakis Signs Bill, Lauds Health Plans," *Boston Globe*, October 22, 1976. Reprinted in *Medical Care Review*, **33**:10 (November 1976): 1143–1144.

Bunker, John P. "A Comparison of Operations and Surgeons in the United States and in England and Wales," *New England Journal of Medicine*, **282**:3 (January 15, 1970): 135–144.

Burch, George E., and Shewey, Lana. "Sphygmomanometric Cuff Size and Blood Pressure Recordings," *Journal of the American Medical Association*, **225**:10 (September 3, 1973): 1215-1218.

Burke, Richard T. *Guidelines for HMO Marketing*. Minneapolis: InterStudy, 1973.

———, with George Strumpf. *Sharing the Risk: A Guide for the Young HMO*. Minneapolis: InterStudy, 1973.

Burkett, Gary L., et al. "A Comparative Study of Physicians' and Nurses' Conceptions of the Role of the Nurse Practitioner," *American Journal of Public Health*, **68**:11 (November 1978): 1090–1096.

Burney, Ira L., et al. "Geographic Variation in Physicians' Fees: Payments to Physicians Under Medicare and Medicaid," *Journal of the American Medical Association*, **240**:13 (September 22, 1978): 1368–1371.

California Department of Health. "Prepaid Health Plans: The California Experience," in U.S. Senate, Committee on Government Operations, Permanent Subcommittee on Investigations, *Prepaid Health Plans*, Hearings, March 13–14, 1975, 94th Congress, 1st Session. Washington, D.C.: USGPO, 1975.

California Medical Association, Bureau of Research and Planning. "Physician Participation in the Medi-Cal Program: Highlights of Findings From a 1977 Survey, Part 1," *Socioeconomic Report: Division of Research and Socioeconomics*, **17**:3 (April-May 1977).
———. "A Survey of Physician Participation in the Medi-Cal Program," *Socioeconomic Report*, **15**:2 (February-March 1975).

California Office of the Auditor General. *Department of Health Prepaid Health Plans: Report to the Joint Legislative Audit Committee*. Sacramento: April 1974.

California State Legislative Analyst. "A Review of the Regulation of Prepaid Health Plans by the California Department of Health." Sacramento: November 15, 1973. Reprinted in U.S.

Senate, Committee on Government Operations, *Prepaid Health Plans Hearings,* March 13–14, 1975. Washington, D.C.: USGPO, 1975.

Campbell, Donald T. "Reforms as Experiments," *American Psychologist,* **24**:4 (April 1969): 409–429.

Carnoy, Judith, and Koo, Linda. "Kaiser-Permanente: A Model American Health Maintenance Organization," *International Journal of Health Services,* **4**:4 (1974): 599–615.

Carnoy, Judy, Coffee, Lee, and Koo, Linda. "The Kaiser Plan," *Health/Pac Bulletin,* **55** (November 1973).

Carter, Katherine K., and Allison, Thaine H., Jr. *A Comparison of Utilization and Costs in Kaiser and Non-Kaiser Hospitals in California.* California Health Facilities Commission Research Report 78-2, November 1978.

Cauffman, Joy G., Roemer, Milton I., and Shultz, Carl S. "The Impact of Health Insurance Coverage on Health Care of School Children," *Public Health Reports,* **82**:4 (April 1967): 323–328.

Center for Research in Ambulatory Health Care Administration. *The Organization and Development of a Medical Group Practice,* Cambridge: Ballinger Publishing Company, 1976.

Chamberlain, Jocelyn. "Screening for the Early Detection of Diseases in Great Britain," *Preventive Medicine,* **4** (1975): 268.

———. "Selected Data on Group Practice Prepayment Plan Services," *Group Health and Welfare News,* Special Supplement (June 1967).

Chamberlin, R. W., and Radebaugh, J. F. "Delivery of Primary Health Care-Union Style: A Critical Review of the Robert F. Kennedy Plan for the United Farm Workers of America," *New England Journal of Medicine,* **294**:12 (March 18, 1976): 641–645.

Chambers, Mark, and Russell, Richard. "Two Hospitals Consolidate Services to Save $375,000 Annually," *Forum,* **2**:3 (1978): 14–15.

Chavkin, David F., and Treseder, Anne. "California's Prepaid Health Plan Program: Can the Patient Be Saved?" *Hastings Law Journal,* **28** (January 1977): 685–760.

Chicago Daily News. "State Cancels Two Health Plans From Medicaid," *Chicago Daily News* (May 18, 1976). Reprinted in *Medical Care Review,* **33**:6 (June 1976): 636–637.

Chen, Milton M., Bush, J. W., and Patrick, Donald L. "Social Indicators for Health Planning and Policy Analysis," *Policy Sciences,* **6**:1 (March 1975): 71–89.

Cheney, Garnett. "President's Page: Physician Responsibility in Medical Welfare Plans," *San Francisco Medical Society Bulletin,* **24**:11 (December 1951): 17 and 42.

Chiswick, Barry R. "Hospital Utilization: An Analysis of SMSA Differences in Occupancy Rates, Admission Rates and Bed Rates," *Explorations in Economic Research,* **3**:3 (Summer 1976): 326–378.

Christianson, Jon B. *The Competitive Impact of Health Maintenance Organizations: Minneapolis-St. Paul.* Excelsior, Minn.: InterStudy, 1978.

———, and McClure, Walter. *Competition in the Delivery of Medical Care.* Excelsior, Minn.: InterStudy, 1978.

Cobb, Beatrix. "Why Do People Detour to Quacks?" *The Psychiatric Bulletin* (Summer 1954): 66–69.

Cochrane, Archibald L. *Effectiveness and Efficiency: Random Reflections on Health Services.* London: Nuffield Provincial Hospitals Trust, 1972.

———, and Elwood, P. C. "Screening: The Case Against It," *Medical Officer,* **121**:5 (January 31, 1969): 53–57.

Coffey, Rosanna M., and Hornbrook, Mark C. "National Health Insurance: Research

Findings on Selected Issues," in U.S. National Center for Health Statistics and National Center for Health Services Research, *Health: United States, 1976-77,* Washington, D.C.: USGPO, 1977, DHEW Pub. No. (HRA) 77-1232.

Cohen, Harold. Testimony in *Technology and the Cost of Health Care.* Hearings before the U.S. House, Committee on Science and Technology, September 26, 27, October 6, 1978. Washington, D.C.: USGPO, 1978, pp. 121–150.

Cohn, Victor. "Doctors in GHA Want Own Firm," *Washington Post,* **99** (March 17, 1976): Reprinted in Medical Care Review, **33:**4 (April 1976): 406–407.

––––––. "Hospital Shift Set by GHA," *Washington Post,* **99** (February 1, 1976): 1. Reprinted in *Medical Care Review,* **33:**3 (March 1976): 278–280.

Collen, Morris F. *A Ten-Year Program Report: Medical Methods Research.* Oakland, Ca.: The Permanente Medical Group, December 1970.

––––––. "Research with a Defined Population," in Anne R. Somers (ed.), *The Kaiser-Permanente Medical Care Program: A Symposium.* New York: The Commonwealth Fund, 1971, pp. 129–137.

––––––, et al. "Dollar Cost per Positive Test for Automated Multiphasic Screening," *New England Journal of Medicine,* **283:**9 (August 27, 1970): 459–463.

––––––, et al. "Multiphasic Checkup Evaluation Study. 4. Preliminary Cost Benefit Analysis for Middle-Aged Men," *Preventive Medicine,* **2:**2 (June 1973): 236–246.

Collins, Jean E. "Maintaining an HMO by Marketing to Members," *Medical Group Management* (September-October 1977): 40–44.

Colombo, Theodore J., Saward, Ernest W., and Greenlick, Merwyn R. "The Integration of an OEO Health Program into a Prepaid Comprehensive Group Practice Plan," *American Journal of Public Health,* **59:**4 (April 1969): 641–650.

Coltin, Kathy, Neisuler, Ross, and Lurie, Robert S. *Utilization of Preventive Services by Poor, Near-Poor, and Non-Poor Members of an HMO.* Presented at 106th Annual Meeting of the American Public Health Association, October 16, 1978.

Columbia University School of Public Health and Administrative Medicine. *Family Medical Care under Three Types of Health Insurance.* New York: Foundation on Employee Health, Medical Care and Welfare, Inc., 1962.

––––––. *Prepayment for Medical and Dental Care in New York State.* New York: Commissioner of Health and the Superintendent of Insurance, 1962.

Comanor, William S. "Competition in Health Care and the Impact of Federal Tax Policy." Testimony before a Joint Session of the Oversight Subcommittee of the Ways and Means Committee and the Tax Expenditure Task Force of the Budget Committee, U.S. House of Representatives, July 9, 1979.

Committee for the Special Research Project in the Health Insurance Plan for Greater New York. *Health and Medical Care in New York City.* Cambridge: Harvard University Press, 1957.

Condie, Spencer, and Lyon, J. Lynn. "Private and HMO Patient Reactions Toward Limited Access to Physicians." Paper presented at Pacific Sociological Association meeting, Victoria, B.C., April 1975.

Connelly, Shirley V., and Connelly, Patricia A. "Physicians' Patient Referrals to a Nurse Practitioner in a Primary Medical Care Clinic," *American Journal of Public Health,* **69:**1 (January 1979): 73–75.

Consumers Union of U.S., Inc. "Health Maintenance Organizations: Are HMO's the Answer to Your Medical Needs?" *Consumer Reports* (October 1974).

Cook, Wallace H. "Profile of the Permanente Physician," in Ann R. Somers (ed.), *The Kaiser-Permanente Medical Care Program: A Symposium.* New York: Commonwealth Fund, 1971.

Cooper, Barbara S., and Worthington, Nancy L. "Medical Care Spending for Three Age Groups," *Social Security Bulletin,* **35**:5 (May 1972): 3−16.

————, and Piro, Paula A. *Personal Health Care Expenditures by State.* U.S. Department of Health, Education and Welfare Publication No. (SSA) 75-11906. Washington, D.C.: USGPO, 1975.

Cooper, Barbara, et al. *Medical Care Expenditures, Prices and Costs: Background Book.* Social Security Administration, Office of Research and Statistics, September 1975. U.S. Department of Health, Education and Welfare Publication No. (SSA) 75-11909. Washington, D.C.: USGPO.

Corbin, Mildred, and Krute, Aaron. "Some Aspects of Medicare Experience with Group Practice Prepayment Plans," *Social Security Bulletin,* **38**:3 (March 1975): 3−11.

Covell, Ruth. *Delivery of Health Services for the Poor.* Program Analysis, U.S. Department of Health, Education and Welfare, Office of the Assistant Secretary (Planning and Evaluation), 1967.

Cowan, Edward. "U.S. Suit Says Prepaid Health Plan in Florida Was Illegally Opposed," *New York Times,* **128** (November 28, 1978): 3b. Reprinted in *Medical Care Review,* **36**:1 (January 1979): 38−39.

Coyne, Joseph S. *A Comparative Study of the Performance and Characteristics of Multihospital Systems.* Dissertation, School of Public Health, University of California, Berkeley, 1978.

Crane, Steven. *The Effect of Formal Control on the Provision and Distribution of Hospital Facilities.* Stanford University, Health Services Research Program, Research Workshop in Health Economics, May 1978.

Crawford, Ronald L., and McCormack, Regina C. "Reasons Physicians Leave Primary Practice," *Journal of Medical Education,* **46**:4 (April 1971): 263−268.

Curran, William J. "The Questionable Virtues of Genetic Screening Laws," *American Journal of Public Health,* **64**:10 (October 1974): 1003−1004.

————, and Moseley, George B. "The Malpractice Experience of HMOs," *Northwestern University Law Review,* **70**:1 (1975): 69−89.

Cutler, John L., et al. "Multiphasic Checkup Evaluation Study: I. Methods and Population," *Preventive Medicine,* **2**:2 (June 1973): 197−206.

Daniels, Marcia, and Schroeder, Steven A. "Variation among Physicians in Use of Laboratory Tests: II. Relation to Clinical Productivity and Outcomes of Care," *Medical Care,* **15**:6 (June 1977): 482−487.

Darsky, Benjamin J., Sinai, Nathan, and Axelrod, Solomon J. *Comprehensive Medical Services under Voluntary Health Insurance: A Study of Windsor Medical Services.* Cambridge: Harvard University Press, 1958.

Davis, Karen. "Medicaid Payments and Utilization of Medical Services by the Poor," *Inquiry,* **13**:2 (June 1976): 122−135.

————, and Reynolds, Roger. "The Impact of Medicare and Medicaid on Access to Medical Care," in Richard N. Rosett (ed.), *The Role of Health Insurance in the Health Services Sector.* New York: National Bureau of Economic Research, 1976.

DeFriese, Gordon H. "On Paying the Fiddler to Change the Tune: Further Evidence from Ontario Regarding the Impact of Universal Health Insurance on the Organization and Patterns of Medical Practice," *Milbank Memorial Fund Quarterly/Health and Society,* **53**:2 (Spring 1975): 117−148.

Densen, Paul M. "Design of Reporting Systems for Health Care Programs," *Medical Care,* **11**:2 (March-April 1973, Supplement): 145−157.

————, Balamuth, Eve, and Shapiro, Sam. *Prepaid Medical Care and Hospital Utilization.* Chicago: American Hospital Association, 1958.

Densen, Paul M., Deardorff, Neva R., and Balamuth, Eve. "Longitudinal Analyses of Four Years of Experience of a Prepaid Comprehensive Medical Care Plan," *Milbank Memorial Fund Quarterly,* **36:**1 (January 1958): 5–45.

Densen, Paul M., Shapiro, Sam, and Einhorn, Marilyn. "Concerning High and Low Utilizers of Service in a Medical Care Plan, and the Persistence of Utilization Levels Over a Three Year Period," *Milbank Memorial Fund Quarterly,* **37:**3 (July 1959): 217–250.

Densen, Paul M., et al. "Prepaid Medical Care and Hospital Utilization: Comparison of a Group Practice and a Self-Insurance Situation," *Hospitals,* **36** (November 16, 1962): 62–68, 138.

————. "Prepaid Medical Care and Hospital Utilization in a Dual Choice Situation," *American Journal of Public Health,* **50:**11 (November 1960): 1710–1726.

deVise, Pierre. *Misused and Misplaced Hospitals and Doctors: A Locational Analysis of the Urban Health Care Crisis.* Washington, D.C.: Association of American Geographers, Commission on College Geography, Resource Paper 22, 1973.

Dewey, Donald. *Where Have the Doctors Gone: The Changing Distribution of Private Practice Physicians in the Chicago Metropolitan Area, 1950-1970.* Chicago: Illinois Regional Medical Program, Chicago Regional Hospital Study, 1973.

Diehr, Paula, Jackson, Kathleen O., and Boscha, M. Vicki. "Access to Medical Care: The Impact of Outreach Services on Enrollees of a Prepaid Health Insurance Program," *Journal of Health and Social Behavior,* **16:**3 (September 1975): 326–340.

Diehr, P. K., et al. in William C. Richardson (ed.), *The Seattle Prepaid Health Care Project: Comparison of Health Services Delivery.* "Chapter II, Utilization: Ambulatory and Hospital," National Technical Information Service, PB 267488-SET, 1976.

Dietz, Jean. "Harvard Plan Growth Vexes the Competition," *Boston Globe* (October 9, 1978). Reprinted in *Medical Care Review,* **35:**10 (November 1978): 1050–1051.

————. "Stone OK's New Health Insurance," *Boston Globe* (September 15, 1978). Reprinted in *Medical Care Review,* **35:**10 (November 1978): 1049–1050.

Di Paolo, Vince. "Bills Are Lower in Contracted Units," *Modern Healthcare,* **8:**1 (January 1978): 13–14.

Donabedian, Avedis. "An Evaluation of Prepaid Group Practice," *Inquiry,* **6:**3 (September 1969): 3–27.

————. "Evaluating the Quality of Medical Care," *Milbank Memorial Fund Quarterly,* **44:**3 (July 1966), Part 2: 166–203.

————. *Medical Care Appraisal: Quality and Appraisal.* New York: American Public Health Association, 1968.

————. *Needed Research in the Assessment and Monitoring of the Quality of Medical Care.* Hyattsville, Md.: National Center for Health Services Research, July 1978. U.S. Department of Health, Education and Welfare Publication No. (PHS) 78-3219.

————. "The Numerology of Utilization Control," *Inquiry,* **11:**3 (September 1974): 229–232.

————. "The Quality of Medical Care," *Science,* **200** (May 26, 1978): 856–858.

D'Onofrio, Carol N., and Mullen, Patricia Dolan. "Consumer Problems with Prepaid Health Plans in California," *Public Health Reports,* **92:**2 (March-April 1977): 121–134.

Dorrity, Thomas G. "HMOs versus Ethical Medicine," April 20, 1972. Reprinted in U.S. House of Representatives, Committee on Interstate and Foreign Commerce, Hearings on HR

51 and HR 4871, *Health Maintenance Organizations-1973,* March 6 and 7, 1973. Serial 93-26. Washington, D.C.: USGPO.

Dorsey, Joseph. "The HMO Act of 1973 (P.L. 93-222) and Prepaid Group Practice Plans," *Medical Care,* **13:**1 (January 1975).

———— (ed). *How a Group Practice Maintains Its Own Health in a Troubled Economy: A Discussion of Hospital Utilization and Physician Productivity.* Proceedings of the Medical Directors Educational Conference, Vol. 1, No. 1, Medical Directors Division, Group Health Association of America, Inc. Held as an Advance Joint Session of the Group Health Institute, Denver, Colorado, June 13, 1976.

————. "The Prepaid Group Practice Plan in the Education of Future Physicians: Initial Efforts at the Harvard Community Health Plan," *Medical Care,* **11:**1 (January-February 1973): 12–20.

Dowling, William L. "Prospective Reimbursement of Hospitals," *Inquiry,* **11:**3 (September 1974): 163–180.

Downey, Gregg W. "A Haven for HMOs in New Haven," *Modern Healthcare,* **2:**5 (November 1974): 21–27.

Dozier, Dave, et al. *Final Report on the Survey of Consumer Experience under the State of California's Employees' Hospital and Medical Care Act.* Sacramento: State of California, 1968.

————. *1970-71 Survey of Consumer Experience Report of the State of California Employees' Medical and Hospital Care Program Prepared under the Policy Direction of the Medical Advisory Council to the Board of Administration of the Public Employees' Retirement System.* Sacramento: State of California, 1973.

————. *Report of the Medical and Hospital Advisory Council to the Board of Administration of the California State Employees' Retirement System.* Sacramento: June 1964.

DuBois, Donald M. "Organizational Viability of Group Practice," *Group Practice* (April 1967): 261–270.

Dun and Bradstreet. *The Business Failure Record.* New York: Dun and Bradstreet, Inc., 1978.

Durenberger, David. *Health Incentives Reform Act of 1979,* Senate Bill 1485, 96th Congress, First Session, July 12, 1979.

Dutton, Diana Barbara. *A Causal Model of the Use of Health Services: The Role of the Delivery System.* Unpublished doctoral dissertation, Massachusetts Institute of Technology, February 1976.

————. *Explaining Low Use of Health Services by the Poor: Costs, Attitudes, or Systems?* Paper presented at the Pacific Sociological Association 48th Annual Meeting, April 20-23, 1977. Sacramento, Ca.

————. *Patterns of Ambulatory Use in Five Health Care Delivery Systems.* Health Services Research, Discussion paper, Stanford University, 1976.

————. *Patterns of Physician Satisfaction in Five Different Delivery Systems,* draft, August 1978.

————, and Silber, Ralph S. *Children's Health Outcomes In Six Different Ambulatory Care Delivery Systems.* Stanford, Ca.: Stanford University School of Medicine, Health Services Research Division, March 1979.

Dyckman, Zachary Y. *A Study of Physicians' Fees.* Staff Report prepared by the Council on Wage and Price Stability. Washington, D.C.: USGPO, 1978.

Eamer, Richard K. "For-Profits Are Measurably More Efficient: Corporation Executive," *Modern Hospital,* **116:**4 (April 1971): 116.

Egdahl, Richard H. "Foundations for Medical Care," *New England Journal of Medicine,* **288:**10 (March 8, 1973): 491–498.

———, and Walsh, Diana Chapman. "Industry-Sponsored Health Programs: Basis for a New Hybrid Prepaid Plan," *New England Journal of Medicine,* **296** (1977): 1350–1353.

Egdahl, Richard H., Taft, Cynthia H., and Linde, Kenneth J. "Method of Physician Payment and Hospital Length of Stay," *New England Journal of Medicine,* **296:**6 (February 10, 1977): 339–340.

Egdahl, R. H., et al. "The Potential of Organizations of Fee-For-Service Physicians for Achieving Significant Decreases in Hospitalization," *Annals of Surgery,* **186:**3 (September 1977): 388–399.

Egger, Ross L. "The 5 Doctors Who Made Me Leave Group Practice," *Medical Economics,* **54:**5 (March 7, 1977): 231–236.

Ehrenberg, A. S. C. *Data Reduction: Analyzing and Interpreting Statistical Data.* London: John Wiley and Sons, 1975.

Eisenberg, Barry S. "Income Distribution Policies in Group Practices," *Medical Group Management* (November-December 1977): 42–44.

Eisenberg, Howard. "The New Boom in Prepaid Groups," *Medical Economics* (September 28, 1970): 29ff.

Eisenberg, John M., and Rosoff, Arnold J. "Physician Responsibility for the Cost of Unnecessary Medical Services," *New England Journal of Medicine,* **299:**2 (July 13, 1978): 76–80.

Eisenberg, John, et al. "Patterns of Pediatric Practice by the Same Physicians in a Prepaid and Fee-For Service Setting," *Clinical Pediatrics,* **13:**4 (April 1974): 352–359.

Ellwein, Linda Krane. *Health Care Trends: Minneapolis/St. Paul: Summary Highlights* Excelsior, Minn.: InterStudy. August 1979.

Ellwood, Paul. "The Biggest HMO Advocate Backs Off on Prepayment," *Medical Economics* (August 1976): 29–40.

———, et al. "Health Maintenance Organizations: Concept and Strategy," *Hospitals,* **45** (March 16, 1971): 53.

Engel, George L. "The Need for a New Medical Model: A Challenge for Biomedicine," *Science,* **196:**4286 (April 8, 1977): 129–134.

Engel, Gloria. "The Effect of Bureaucracy on the Professional Autonomy of the Physician," *Journal of Health and Social Behavior,* **10:**1 (March 1969): 30–41.

Engelland, Ann L., Alderman, Michael H., and Powell, Hugh B. "Blood Pressure Control in Private Practice: A Case Report," *American Journal of Public Health,* **69:**1 (January 1979): 25–29.

Enright, Steven B. "I.P.A.: The Initials That May Mean Your Future," *Medical Economics* (February 19, 1979): 124–137.

Enthoven, Alain. "Competition of Alternative Health Care Delivery Systems," in *Competition in the Health Care Sector: Past, Present, and Future.* Proceedings of U.S. Federal Trade Commission Conference, Bureau of Economics, Washington, D.C., June 1-2, 1977, edited by Warren Greenberg, March 1978, pp. 322–351.

———. "Consumer-Centered vs. Job-Centered Health Insurance," *Harvard Business Review* (January-February 1979): 141–152.

———. "Consumer-Choice Health Plan," *New England Journal of Medicine,* **298:**12-13 (March 23 and March 30, 1978): 650-658 and 709-720.

Epstein, Steven B., and Kopit, William G. "Legal Considerations in the Organization and Operation of HMOs," in Robert A. Zelten and Susan Bray (eds.), *Health Maintenance Organizations.* Presentations from the 1976 Guest Lecture Series Training Program in HMO

Management, Leonard Davis Institute of Health Economics, University of Pennsylvania, pp. 45–54.

Etzioni, Amitai, and Doty, Pamela. "Profit in Not-For-Profit Corporations: The Example of Health Care," *Political Science Quarterly*, **91** (Fall 1976): 433–453.

Evans, Robert G. "Supplier-Induced Demand: Some Empirical Evidence and Implications," in Mark Perlman (ed.), *The Economics of Health and Medical Care*. London: MacMillan, 1974, pp. 162–173.

Evashwick, Connie J. "The Role of Group Practice in the Distribution of Physicians in Nonmetropolitan Areas," *Medical Care*, **14**:10 (October 1976): 808–823.

Falk, I. S. "A Community Group Practice Prepayment Plan Linked with the Medical School Center in New Haven, Connecticut." Proceedings 19th Annual Group Health Institute, New York, June 4-6, 1969.

——, and Senturia, J. *Medical Care Program for Steelworkers and Their Families.* Pittsburgh: United Steelworkers of America, 1960.

Federa, R. Danielle. *Cost Consciousness and Ancillary Diagnostic Test Utilization: Evaluation of an Educational Program in an HMO Setting.* Boston: Ernst and Ernst, 1978.

Fein, Rashi. *The Doctor Shortage: An Economic Diagnosis.* Washington: Brookings Institution, 1967, pp. 62–89.

——, and Weber, Gerald I. *Financing Medical Education: An Analysis of Alternative Policies and Mechanisms.* New York: Carnegie Commission on Higher Education and the Commonwealth Fund, 1971.

Feldstein, Martin S. "Hospital Cost Inflation: A Study of Nonprofit Price Dynamics," *American Economic Review*, **61**:5 (December 1971): 853–872.

——. "Econometric Studies of Health Economics," in M. Intriligator and D. Kendrick, *Frontiers of Quantitative Economics.* Amsterdam: North-Holland, 1974.

——, and Allison, Elizabeth. *Tax Subsidies of Private Health Insurance: Distribution, Revenue Loss and Effects.* Cambridge: Harvard Center for Community Health, Health Care Policy Discussion Paper Series No. 2, October 1972.

Feldstein, Paul J. *Prepaid Group Practice: An Analysis and Review.* Bureau of Hospital Administration, School of Public Health, University of Michigan, Ann Arbor, Michigan, June 1971.

Ferber, Bernard. "An Analysis of Chain-Operated for Profit Hospitals," *Health Services Research*, **16**:1 (Spring 1971): 53.

Fessel, W. J., and Van Brunt, E. E. "Assessing the Quality of Care from the Medical Record," *New England Journal of Medicine*, **286**:3 (January 20, 1972): 134–138.

Fetter, Robert B., and Thompson, John D. "Patients' Waiting Time and Doctors' Idle Time in the Outpatient Setting," *Health Services Research* (Summer 1966): 66–90.

Fielding, Jonathan E. "Successes of Prevention," *Milbank Memorial Fund Quarterly/Health and Society*, **56**:3 (Summer 1978): 274–302.

Fineberg, Harvey V. *Clinical Chemistries: The High Cost of Low-Cost Diagnostic Tests.* Prepared for the Sun Valley Forum, August 1977.

Finger Lakes Health Systems Agency. *Health Maintenance Organizations in Rochester, New York: History, Current Performance, and Future Prospects.* Rochester: Finger Lakes Health Systems Agency. Task Force on Prepaid Health Care, 1980.

Finkler, Steven A. *The Cost-Effectiveness of Health Care Regionalization.* Research Paper #436, Graduate School of Business, Stanford University, March 1978.

Foltz, Anne-Marie, and Kelsey, Jennifer L. "The Annual Pap Test: A Dubious Policy Success," *Milbank Memorial Fund Quarterly/Health and Society*, **56**:4 (1978): 426–462.

Fortune. *How Major Industrial Corporations View Employee Benefit Programs*. New York: Time, Inc., 1975.

Fottler, Myron D., Gibson, Geoffrey, and Pinchoff, Diane M. "Physician Attitudes Toward the Nurse Practitioner," *Journal of Health and Social Behavior*, **19** (September 1978): 303–311.

Fox, Maurice. "Why People Are Mad at Doctors," *Newsweek* (January 10, 1977): 4.

Fox, Peter D., and Bice, Thomas W. "Socioeconomic Status and the Use of Physician Services Revisited," *Medical Care*, **14**:8 (August 1976): 714–717.

Fox, Renee C. "Is There a 'New' Medical Student?" in Laurence R. Tancredi (ed.), *Ethics of Health Care*. Washington, D.C.: National Academy of Sciences, 1974, 197–220.

Francis, V., Korsch, B. M., and Morris, M. J. "Gaps in Doctor-Patient Communication: Patient's Response to Medical Advice," *New England Journal of Medicine*, **280**:10 (March 6, 1969): 535–540.

Franklin, B., and McLemore, S. "Attitudes Toward and Reported Utilization of a Student Health Center," *Journal of the American College Health Association*, **17** (October 1970): 54–59.

––––––. "Factors Affecting the Choice of Medical Care among University Students," *Journal of Health and Social Behavior*, **11** (December 1970): 311–319.

Freeborn, Donald K., et al. "Determinants of Medical Care Utilization: Physicians' Use of Laboratory Services," *American Journal of Public Health*, **62**:6 (June 1972): 846–853.

––––––. "Health Status, Socioeconomic Status, and Utilization of Outpatient Services for Members of a Prepaid Group Practice," *Medical Care*, **15**:2 (February 1977): 115–128.

Freeland, Mark, Calaf, George, and Schendler, Carol Ellen. "Projections of National Health Expenditures, 1980, 1985, and 1990," *Health Care Financing Review*, **1**:3 (Winter 1980): 1–28.

Freidson, Eliot. "Client Control & Medical Practice," *American Journal of Sociology*, **65**:4 (January 1960): 374–382.

––––––. *Doctoring Together: A Study of Professional Social Control*. New York: Elsevier, 1975.

––––––. *Patients' Views of Medical Practice: A Study of Subscribers to a Prepaid Medical Plan in the Bronx*. New York: Russell Sage Foundation, 1961.

––––––. "Prepaid Group Practice and the New Demanding Patient," *Milbank Memorial Fund Quarterly*, **51**:4 (Fall 1973): 473–488.

––––––, and Mann, John H. "Organizational Dimensions of Large Scale Medical Practice," *American Journal of Public Health*, **61**:4 (April 1971): 786–795.

Freidson, Eliot, and Rhea, Buford. "Physicians in Large Medical Groups," *Journal of Chronic Diseases*, **17**:9 (September 1964): 827–836.

––––––. "Processes of Control in a Company of Equals," *Social Problems*, **11**:2 (Fall 1963): 119–131.

Friedman, Gary D., Dales, Loring G., and Ury, Hans K. "Mortality in Middle-Aged Smokers and Non-smokers," *New England Journal of Medicine*, **300**:5 (February 1, 1979): 213–217.

Friedman, Gary D., et al. "Kaiser-Permanente Epidemiologic Study of Myocardial Infarction. Study Design and Results for Standard Risk Factors," *American Journal of Epidemiology*, **99** (1974): 101–116.

Fuchs, Victor R. "The Supply of Surgeons and the Demand for Operations," *Journal of Human Resources*, **13** (1978 Supplement): 35–56.

––––––. *Who Shall Live? Health, Economics, and Social Choice*. New York: Basic Books, 1974.

————, and Kramer, Marcia J. *Determinants of Expenditures for Physicians Services in the United States 1948-1968*. New York: NBER Occasional Paper 117, December 1972. Washington: National Center for Health Services Research and Development.

Fuller, Norman, and Patera, Margaret. *Report on a Study of Medicaid Utilization of Services in a Prepaid Group Practice Health Plan*. U.S. Department of Health, Education and Welfare, Public Health Service, Bureau of Medical Services, January 1976.

————, and Koziol, Krista. "Medicaid Utilization of Services in a Prepaid Group Practice Health Plan," *Medical Care,* **15:**9 (September 1977): 705–737.

Gaffney, John C. (ed.), *Profile of Medical Practice, 1978*. Chicago: American Medical Association, Center for Health Services Research and Development, 1979.

Galiher, Claudia B., and Costa, Marjorie A. "Consumer Acceptance of HMOs," *Public Health Reports,* **90:**2 (March-April 1975): 106–112.

Garbarino, Joseph W. *Health Plans and Collective Bargaining*. Berkeley: University of California Press, 1960.

Garfield, Sidney R. "The Delivery of Medical Care," *Scientific American,* **222:**4 (April 1970): 15–23.

————. "Multiphasic Health Testing and Medical Care as a Right," *New England Journal of Medicine,* **283:**20 (November 12, 1970): 1087–1089.

————, et al. "Evaluation of an Ambulatory Medical-Care Delivery System," *New England Journal of Medicine,* **294:**8 (February 19, 1976): 426–431.

Garner, Dewey D., Liao, Winston C., and Sharpe, Thomas R. "Factors Affecting Physician Participation in a State Medicaid Program," *Medical Care,* **17:**1 (January 1979): 43–58.

Gaus, Clifton. "Who Enrolls in a Prepaid Group Practice: The Columbia Experience," *Johns Hopkins Medical Journal,* **128:**1 (January 1971): 9–14.

————, Cooper, Barbara S., and Hirschman, Constance G. "Contrasts in HMO and Fee-For-Service Performance," *Social Security Bulletin,* **39:**5 (May 1976): 3–14.

Gerst, Arthur, Rogson, Lorraine, and Hetherington, Robert. "Patterns of Satisfaction with Health Plan Coverage: A Conceptual Approach," *Inquiry,* **6:**3 (September 1969): 37–51.

Gertman, Paul M. "Physicians as Guiders of Health Services Use," in Selma J. Mushkin (ed.), *Consumer Incentives for Health Care*. New York: Prodist, 1974, 362–382.

Gibbens, Stephen F. *Hospitalization Savings under Prepayment: California Medi-Cal* (An Analysis of Consolidated Medical Systems Ltds. Operations), February 1973.

Gibson, Robert M., and Fisher, Charles R. "National Health Expenditures, Fiscal Year 1977," *HCFA Health Notes* (May 1978).

Gintzig, Leon and Shouldice, Robert T. *Prepaid Group Practices: An Analysis of a Delivery System: The Reports and Comparisons of Selected Aspects of Several Prepaid Group Practice Plans*. George Washington University: Department of Health Care Administration, School of Government and Business Administration, 1971.

Glaser, William A. *Paying the Doctor: Systems of Remuneration and Their Effects*. Baltimore: Johns Hopkins Press, 1970.

Goldbeck, Willis B. *Health Care Costs: A Dilemma for all Americans*. Statement made before the Select Committee on Small Business, U.S. Senate, August 21, 1978. Washington, D.C.: Washington Business Group on Health, 1978.

Goldberg, Lawrence G., and Greenberg, Warren. "The Emergence of Physician-Sponsored Health Insurance: A Historical Perspective," in Warren Greenberg, (ed.), *Competition in the Health Care Sector: Past, Present, and Future*. Washington, D.C.: USGPO, 1978.

————. *The HMO and Its Effects on Competition.* Washington, D.C.: Federal Trade Commission, Bureau of Economics, 1977.

Goldberg, Theodore. *The Effects of Collectively Bargained New Benefits on Prepaid Group Practice Plans.* Proceedings 19th Annual Group Health Institute, New York, June 4-6, 1969.

Goldberg, Victor P. "Some Emerging Problems of Prepaid Health Plans in the Medi-Cal System," *Policy Analysis,* **1:**1 (Winter 1975).

Goldstein, George S. *Consumer Participation in UMWA-Related Health Clinics.* Paper presented at the Panel on Consumer Participation in a National Health Service, 106th Annual Meeting of the American Public Health Association, Los Angeles, California, October 17, 1978.

Golladay, Frederick L., Manser, Marilyn E., and Smith, Kenneth R. "Scale Economies in the Delivery of Medical Care: A Mixed Integer Programming Analysis of Efficient Manpower Utilization," *Journal of Human Resources,* **9:**1 (Winter 1974): 50−62.

Golladay, Frederick L., Miller, Marianne, and Smith, Kenneth R. "Allied Health Manpower Strategies: Estimates of Potential Gains from Efficient Task-Delegation," *Medical Care,* **11:**6 (November-December 1973): 457−469.

Goodman, L. J., Bennett, T. H., and Odem, R. J. *Group Medical Practice in the United States, 1975.* Chicago: Center for Health Services Research and Development, American Medical Association, 1976.

Gordis, Leon, and Markowitz, Milton. "Evaluation of the Effectiveness of Comprehensive and Continuous Pediatric Care," *Pediatrics,* **48:**5 (November 1971): 766−776.

Gornick, Marian. "Medicare Patients: Geographic Differences in Hospital Discharge Rates and Multiple Stays," *Social Security Bulletin,* **40:**6 (June 1977): 1−20.

Goss, Steve. "Retrospective Application of the HMO Risk Sharing Savings Formula for Six Group Practice Prepayment Plans for 1969, 1970," *Actuarial Note,* No. 88 U.S. Department of Health, Education and Welfare, Social Security Administration 76-11500 (11-75).

Gossett, Jay W. "Medicine's Capital City Faces an Influx of HMOs," *Medical Economics,* **48:**25 (1972): 200.

Gould, William. *Hospitals: Occupancy Too Low or Stays Too Long?* Palo Alto, Ca.: National Bureau of Economic Research, mimeo, 1979.

Grady, George F., and Wetterlow, Leslie H. "Pertussis Vaccine: Reasonable Doubt?" *The New England Journal of Medicine,* **298:**17 (April 27, 1978): 966−967.

Graham, Fred E., II. "Group vs. Solo Practice: Arguments and Evidence," *Inquiry,* **9:**2 (June 1972): 49−60.

Greenberg, Ira G., and Rodburg, Michael L. "The Role of Prepaid Group Practice in Relieving the Medical Care Crisis," *Harvard Law Review,* **84:**4 (February 1971): 887-1001.

Greenfield, Carol A., et al. "Use of Out-of-Plan Services by Medicare Members of HIP," *Health Services Research* (Fall 1978): 243−260.

Greenfield, Sheldon, et al. "Protocol Management of Dysuria, Urinary Frequency and Vaginal Discharge," *Annals of Internal Medicine,* **81** (1974): 452−457.

Greenlick, Merwyn R., and Darsky, Benjamin J. "A Comparison of General Drug Utilization in a Metropolitan Community with Utilization under a Drug Prepayment Plan," *American Journal of Public Health,* **58:**11 (November 1968): 2121−2136.

Greenlick, Merwyn, and Saward, Ernest. "Impact of a Reduced-Charge Drug Benefit in a Prepaid Group Practice Plan," *Public Health Reports,* **81:**10 (October 1966): 938−940.

Greenlick, Merwyn R., et al. *Characteristics of Men Most Likely to Respond to an Invitation to Be*

Screened. Presented at 105th Annual Meeting of American Public Health Association, November 1, 1977, Washington, D.C.

―――. "Comparing the Use of Medical Care Services by a Medically Indigent and a General Membership Population in a Comprehensive Prepaid Group Practice," *Medical Care,* **10**:3 (May-June 1972): 187–200.

―――. "Determinants of Medical Care Utilization: The Role of Telephone in Total Medical Care," *Medical Care,* **11**:3 (April 1973).

―――. *Do Not Admit Surgery.* Interim Report, HCFA Contract No. 600-77-0040. Portland, Oregon: Kaiser Health Services Research Center, Circa 1978.

Gregory, Robert. *Northwest Healthcare: An Insurance Company-Physician Alliance for More Cost-Effective Healthcare.* Presented at the Health Staff Seminar, Washington, D.C., January 25, 1978. Seattle, Wash.: Northwest Healthcare.

Group Health Association of America. *Sample Operating Prepaid Group Practice Medical Care Programs: Organizational and Financial Relationships,* mimeo, June 22, 1972.

Group Health and Welfare News. "HIP Completes First Major Reorganization in 25 Years," *Group Health and Welfare News,* **12**:2 (January 1972). Reprinted in *Medical Care Review,* **29**:3 (March 1972): 251–252.

Group Health Foundation. "National HMO Rate Would Stifle Competition," *Group Health News,* **20**:1 (January 1979). Reprinted in *Medical Care Review,* **36**:2 (February 1979): 151–153.

Group Health News. "Quality Assurance and Utilization Review Studied in Prepaid Group Practice," *Group Health News,* **18**:7 (January 1977). Reprinted in *Medical Care Review,* **34**:2 (February 1977): 170–171.

Gumbiner, Robert. *HMO: Putting It All Together.* St. Louis: C.V. Mosby, 1975.

Gupte, Pranay. "New York's Medicaid 'Mills': A Growing Number of Inquiries, With Patients Caught in the Middle," *New York Times,* **126** (November 23, 1976): 42c. Reprinted in *Medical Care Review,* **33**:11 (December 1976): 1318–1320.

Guptill, Paul B., and Graham, Fred E., II. "Continuing Education Activities of Physicians in Solo and Group Practice: Report on a Pilot Study," *Medical Care,* **14**:2 (February 1976): 173–180.

Guze, Samuel B. "Can the Practice of Medicine Be Fun For a Lifetime?" *Journal of the American Medical Association,* **241**:19 (May 22, 1979): 2021–2023.

Guzick, David S., and Jahiel, Rene I. "Distribution of Private Practice Offices of Physicians with Specified Characteristics Among Urban Neighborhoods," *Medical Care,* **14**:6 (June 1976): 469–488.

Haggerty, Robert J. "Teaching Ambulatory Care in an HMO," *Journal of Medical Education,* **48**:4 (April 1973), Part 2: 154–157.

Halenar, John F. "Big Business Turns Up the Heat on Doctors," *Medical Economics* (July 9, 1979): 111 ff.

Haley, T. W. "Physicians Association of Clackamas County," *Hospitals,* **45**:6 (March 16, 1971).

Hall, Robert P. "Experience With Medicaid HMO Contract," in *Rural Health Care Delivery: Proceedings of a National Conference on Rural Health Maintenance Organizations,* Louisville, Ky., July 8-10, 1974. U.S. Senate Committee on Agriculture and Forestry, 93rd Congress, 2nd Session. Washington, D.C.: USGPO, 1974.

Handschin, Richard. "Group Health Cooperative of Puget Sound," in Arizona Regional Medical Program, *Workshop on Alternative Methods for Delivery of Health Services Casa Grande* (September 23-24, 1971), 43–55.

Harrelson, E. Frank, and Donovan, Kirk M. "Consumer Responsibility in a Prepaid Group Health Plan," *American Journal of Public Health,* **65:**10 (October 1975): 1077–1086.

Harrington, Donald C. "San Joaquin Foundation for Medical Care," *Hospitals,* **45:**6 (March 1971): 67–68.

Harrington, R. L., Burnell, George M., and Koreneff, C. *Systems Approach to Mental Health Care in a HMO Model: Project Brief . . . As Of August 31, 1974.* Unpublished paper.

Harris, Jeffrey E. "The Internal Organization of Hospitals: Some Economic Implications," *Bell Journal of Economics,* **8:**2 (Autumn 1977): 467–482.

Harvard Business School. *The Kaiser-Permanente Medical Care Program.* President and Fellows of Harvard College, 1972.

Hastings, J. E. F., et al. "Prepaid Group Practice in Sault Ste. Marie, Ontario—Part I: Analysis of Utilization Records," *Medical Care,* **11:**2 (March-April 1973): 91–103.

————. "An Interim Report on the Sault Ste. Marie Study: A Comparison of Personal Health Services Utilization," *Canadian Journal of Public Health,* **61** (July-August 1970), 289–296.

Havighurst, Clark C. "Health Maintenance Organizations and the Market for Health Services," *Law and Contemporary Problems,* **35:**4 (1970): 716–795.

————. "Professional Restraints on Innovation in Health Care Financing," *Duke Law Journal,* 1978:2 (May 1978): 303–387.

————. "Regulation of Health Facilities and Services by 'Certificate of Need'," *Virginia Law Review,* **59:**7 (October 1973): 1143–1232.

————. "State Regulation of HMOs: Arranging for a 'Fair Market Test'," in *Rural Health Care Delivery: Proceedings of a National Conference on Rural Health Maintenance Organizations,* Louisville, Ky., July 8-10, 1974, Subcommittee on Rural Development of the Senate Committee on Agriculture and Forestry, 93rd Congress, 2nd Session (Committee Print 1974), pp. 90–96.

Heagarty, Margaret C., and Robertson, Leon S. "Slave Doctors and Free Doctors. A Participant Observer Study of Physician Patient Relations in a Low Income Comprehensive Care Program," *New England Journal of Medicine,* **284:**12 (March 25, 1971): 636–641.

Health Insurance Plan of Greater New York. *Information for Physicians.* Unpublished paper (circa 1970).

Health Law Newsletter. "Prepaid Health Plans," *Health Law Newsletter* (June 1976). Reprinted in *Medical Care Review,* **33:**8 (August 1976): 886–888.

Health Maintenance Organization of Pennsylvania. *The HMO of Private Physicians' Offices.* Willow Grove, Pa., May 1978.

Health/PAC (eds.). *Feelings About the Kaiser Foundation Health Plan on the Part of Northern California Carpenters and Their Families.* San Francisco: Health/PAC, April 5, 1973.

————. *Materials on Pre-Paid Health Plans.* San Francisco: Health/PAC, April 1974.

Hedrick, W. L. "Mass Screening: Preventive Medicine or Public Sedative?" *Medical Economics,* **54:**4 (February 21, 1977): 127.

Herbert, Michael E. *A Financial Guide for HMO Planners.* Minneapolis: Interstudy, September 1972.

Hershey, John C., Abernathy, W. J., and Baloff, N. "Comparison of Nurse Allocation Policies—A Monte Carlo Model," *Decision Sciences,* **5** (January 1974): 58–72.

Hershey, John C., and Kropp, Dean H. "A Re-Appraisal of the Productivity Potential and Economic Benefits of Physician's Assistants," *Medical Care,* **17:**6 (June 1979): 592–606.

————, and Kuhn, Ingeborg M. *Physicians' Assistants in Ambulatory Health Care Settings: Need for Improved Analysis.* Health Services Administration Program, Stanford University, Research Paper, October 1975.

————. "The Productivity Potential of Physician's Assistants: An Integrated Approach to Analysis," *Journal of Medical Systems,* **2** (1978): 123.

Hershey, John C., Luft, Harold S. and Gianaris, Joan M. "Making Sense Out of Utilization Data," *Medical Care,* **13:**10 (October 1975): 838–854.

Hessler, R. M., and Walters, M. J. "Consumer Evaluation of Health Services: Implications for Methodology and Health Care Policy," *Medical Care,* **13:**8 (August 1975): 683–693.

Hester, James, and Sussman, E. "Medicaid Prepayment: Concept and Implementation," *Milbank Memorial Fund Quarterly/Health and Society,* **52:**4 (Fall 1974): 415–444.

Hetherington, Robert W., Hopkins, Carl E., and Roemer, Milton I. *Health Insurance Plans: Promise and Performance.* New York: Wiley-Interscience, 1975.

Heyssel, Robert M., and Seidel, Henry M. "The Johns Hopkins Experience in Columbia, MD," *New England Journal of Medicine,* **295:**22 (November 25, 1976): 1225–1231.

Hicks, Nancy. "Future of H.I.P. Still in Dispute," *New York Times* (September 11, 1972): 33.

————. "H.I.P. Considers Two Merger Plans," *New York Times,* **121:**61 (August 20, 1972). Reprinted in *Medical Care Review,* **29:**9 (October 1972): 1006–1007.

Hildebrand, Polly K. *Environmental Conduciveness to Health Maintenance Organizations: A Population Ecology Explanation.* Unpublished dissertation proposal, Sociology of Education, Stanford University, February 1978. *See* Keller, Polly.

Hirsch, Gary B., and Bergan, Thomas B. *Simulating Ambulatory Care Systems, Part Four: Final Report,* Contract HSM-110-70-356. Newton, Mass.: Organization for Social and Technical Innovation, Inc., January 1973.

Hirschman, Albert O. *Exit, Voice, and Loyalty: Responses to Decline in Firms, Organizations and States.* Cambridge: Harvard University Press, 1970.

Holahan, John. "Foundations for Medical Care: An Empirical Investigation of the Delivery of Health Services to a Medicaid Population," *Inquiry,* **14:**4 (December 1977): 352–368.

————. *Physician Reimbursement under National Health Insurance.* Washington, D.C.: The Urban Institute, August, 1977.

————, et al. *Physician Pricing In California: Executive Summary.* Working Paper 998–10. Washington, D.C.: The Urban Institute, April 1978.

Holland, W. "Screening for Disease: Taking Stock," *Lancet,* **1** (December 21, 1974): 1494–1497.

Hudes, Jack, et al. *Are HMO Enrollees Being Attracted by a Liberal Maternity Benefit?* Presented at the Joint National Meeting of the Institute of Management Sciences/Operations Research Society of America, May 1, 1979.

Hulka, Barbara S., et al. "Scale for the Measurement of Attitudes Toward Physicians and Primary Health Care," *Medical Care,* **8:**5 (September-October 1970): 429–436.

————. "Satisfaction with Medical Care in a Low Income Population," *Journal of Chronic Diseases,* **24:**10 (November 1971): 661–673.

Huntley, Robert R., and Howell, Julianne R. *Program Project in Evaluative Research in HMO's: Final Report, Year I.* Washington, D.C.: Georgetown University School of Medicine, Department of Community Medicine and International Health, June 28, 1974.

Hurtado, Arnold V. "Utilization Control and Quality Assurance at the Kaiser-Permanente

Medical Care System," in Michael A. Newman (ed.), *The Medical Director in Prepaid Group Practice Health Maintenance Organizations.* Proceedings of a Conference, Denver (1973), Health Maintenance Organization Service, U.S. Department of Health, Education and Welfare.

————, Greenlick, Merwyn R., and Colombo, Theodore J. "Determinants of Medical Care Utilization: Failure to Keep Appointments," *Medical Care,* **10:**3 (May-June 1973): 189–198.

Hurtado, Arnold V., Marks, Sylvia D., and Greenlick, Merwyn R. *Hospital Utilization Study II.* Portland, Ore.: Kaiser Foundation Hospitals Health Services Research Center, 1977. Research Report Series, Report No. 4.

Hurtado, Arnold V., et al. "Unscheduled Use of Ambulatory Care Services," *Medical Care,* **12:**6 (June 1974): 498–511.

Hustead, Edwin, Chief Actuary, U.S. Civil Service Commission. Personal communication, June 5, 1978.

ICF Inc. *Analysis of HMO Markets.* Washington, D.C.: ICF, September 1976.

Illich, Ivan. *Medical Nemesis: The Expropriation of Health.* New York: Pantheon-Random House, 1976.

Jackson, Jeffrey O., and Greenlick, Merwyn R. "The Worried-Well Revisited," *Medical Care,* **12:**8 (August 1974): 659–667.

Jaggar, Franz M., et al. *Comparative Evaluation of the Costs, Quality, and System Effects of Ambulatory Surgery Performed in Alternative Settings.* Prepared for presentation at the Annual Meeting of the American Public Health Association, Los Angeles, October 18, 1978.

Jensen, David A., Warren, J. William, and Seigal, Barbara. *Implementation of Utilization Controls in a Prepaid Health Plan Sponsored by Hospitals and Their Medical Staff: The New Mexico Health Care Corporation.* Presented to the American Public Health Association, November 18, 1975.

Johnson, Richard E., et al. "Studying the Impact of Patient Drug Profiles in an HMO," *Medical Care,* **14:**10 (October 1976): 799–807.

Johnson, Richard L. "Data Show for Profit Hospitals Don't Provide Comparable Service: Consultant," *Modern Hospital,* **116:**4 (April 1971): 117.

Jones, Ellen, et al. "HIP Incentive Reimbursement Experiment: Utilization and Costs of Medical Care, 1969 and 1970," *Social Security Bulletin,* **37:**12 (December 1974): 3–34.

Jones, Stanley B. "Regulation Under a Consumer Choice Approach to National Health Insurance: The Domino Theory of NHI," in William R. Roy (ed.), *Effects of the Payment Mechanism on the Health Care Delivery System.* Hyattsville, Md.: U.S. Department of Health, Education and Welfare, National Center for Health Services Research, 1978. DHEW Pub. No. (PHS) 78-3227.

Julius, Stevo, et al. "Home Blood Pressure Determination: Value in Borderline (Labile) Hypertension," *Journal of the American Medical Association,* **229:**6 (August 5, 1974): 663–666.

Jurgovan and Blair, Inc. *Health Maintenance Organization Viability.* Rockville, Md.: Jurgovan and Blair, Inc., March 1979.

Kaiser Foundation Health Plan. "Arbitration Proves to be a Quicker, Equitable Way to Settle Malpractice," *Planning for Health,* **22:**2 (Spring 1979): 2.

————. "Health Examinations: An Important Message," *Planning for Health,* **19:**1 (Spring 1976): 2–3.

Kaiser Foundation Health Plan Inc. Department of Medical Economics, Central Office personal communications, Oakland, Ca., April 18, 1977, July 27, 1978.

Kaiser Foundation Hospital. *Internship Training Program.* Oakland, Ca., 1969.

Kaiser Foundation Hospitals. *Educational Programs 1975-76.*

Kaiser Foundation Medical Care Program. *1963 Annual Report: The Role of the Independent Medical Groups,* Oakland, Ca., 1964.

———. *1966 Annual Report: The Medical Center: A Product of This Century.* Oakland, Ca.: Kaiser Foundation Health Plan, 1967.

———. *1968 Annual Report: The Doctor and the Machine; Computer in Medicine.* Oakland, Ca.: Kaiser Foundation Health Plan, 1969.

———. *1973 Annual Report: Measuring Quality and Accessibility.* Oakland, Ca.: Kaiser Foundation Health Plan, 1974.

———. *1975 Annual Report: Changing Patterns of Health Care.* Oakland, Ca.: Kaiser Foundation Health Plan, 1976.

Kaiser-Permanente Medical Care Program. *Facts, 1973.* Oakland, Ca.: Kaiser-Permanente Medical Care Program, 1973.

———. *Facts, 1976.* Oakland, Ca., 1976.

———, Oregon Region. *Statistical Data Reports, 1971-1975.* Portland, Ore.: Kaiser-Permanente Medical Care Program.

Kasl, Stanislav V., and Cobb, Sidney. "Health Behavior, Illness Behavior and Sick Role Behavior," *Archives of Environmental Health,* **12**:2 (February 1966): 246−266.

Kasteler, Josephine, et al. "Issues Underlying Prevalence of 'Doctor Shopping' Behavior," *Journal Health and Social Behavior,* **17**:4 (December 1976): 328−339.

Katz, Dolores. "Big Three, UAW Plan Health Plan to Rival Blues," *Detroit Free Press,* **148** (May 10, 1978): 3a. Reprinted in *Medical Care Review,* **35**:6 (June 1978): 588−589.

Keeler, Emmett B., Relles, Daniel A., and Rolph, John E. "An Empirical Study of the Differences Between Family and Individual Deductibles in Health Insurance," *Inquiry,* **14**:3 (September 1977): 269−277.

Kehrer, Barbara H., and Intriligator, Michael D. "Malpractice and Employment of Allied Health Personnel," *Medical Care,* **13**:10 (October 1975): 876−883.

Keller, Polly E. *Environmental Conduciveness to Health Maintenance Organizations: A Population Ecology Explanation.* Unpublished Ph.D. Dissertation, School of Education, Stanford University, August 1979.

Kelman, H. R. "Evaluation of Health Care Quality By Consumers," *International Journal of Health Services,* **6**:3 (1976): 431−442.

Kerr, Lorin E. "Desire, Expectation and Reality in a Union Health Program," *New England Journal of Medicine,* **178**:21 (May 23, 1968): 1149.

Kessel, Reuben A. "Price Discrimination in Medicine," *Journal of Law and Economics,* **1**:1 (October 1958): 20−53.

Kimbell, Larry J., and Lorant, John H. *Physician Productivity and Returns to Scale.* Paper presented at the Health Economics Research Organization Meeting, New York, December 1973.

———. *Production Functions for Physicians' Services.* Paper presented at the Econometric Society meeting, Toronto, December 1972.

Kirchner, Merian. "The Real World of Hospital Finance 5: Can Doctors Truly Do Much About Hospital Costs?" *Medical Economics,* **55**:9 (May 1, 1978): 79−102.

Kirkman, Don. " 'Surgicenters' Eyed To Trim Health Costs," *Rocky Mountain News* (December 3, 1978). Reprinted in *The Green Sheet,* **25**:263 (December 13, 1978): R3.

Kisch, Arnold I., and Reeder, Leo G. "Client Evaluation of Physician Performance," *Journal of Health and Social Behavior,* **10**:1 (March 1969): 51−58.

————, and Viseltear, Arthur J. *The Ross-Loos Medical Group.* U.S. Public Health Service, Medical Care Administration, Case Study No. 3, 1967.

Kissam, Philip C. "Health Maintenance Organizations and the Role of Antitrust Law," *Duke Law Journal,* **1978:**2 (May 1978): 487–541.

————. *Health Maintenance Organizations, Anticompetitive Behavior and the Role of Antitrust Law and Policy.* Presented at The Antitrust Laws and the Health Services Industry, American Enterprise Institute, Washington, D.C., December 19–20, 1977.

Klarman, Herbert E. "Analysis of the HMO Proposal—Its Assumptions, Implications and Prospects," in *Health Maintenance Organizations: A Reconfiguration of the Health Services System.* Proceedings of the Thirteenth Annual Symposium on Hospital Affairs, University of Chicago, Center for Health Administration Studies, May 1971, pp. 24–38.

————. "Economic Research in Group Medicine," in *New Horizons in Health Care.* Proceedings of the First International Congress on Group Medicine, Winnipeg, Manitoba, April 26–30, 1970, 178–193.

————. "Effect of Prepaid Group Practice on Hospital Use," *Public Health Reports,* **78:**11 (November 1963): 955–965.

Klitsner, Irving N. "Affecting Hospital Utilization Patterns," in Joseph L. Dorsey (ed.), *How A Group Practice Maintains Its Own Health in a Troubled Economy.* Washington, D.C.: Group Health Association of America, Inc., 1976.

Knox, Richard A. "New Health Plan 'Fighting for Life'," *Boston Globe* (March 15, 1978). Reprinted in *Medical Care Review,* **35:**4 (April 1978): 367–368.

Koepsell, Thomas D., Soroko, Sharon, and Riedel, Donald C. *"Appropriateness of Hospital Admission under a Prepaid Group Practice and a Fee-For-Service Health Plan."* Presented at the APHA Annual Meeting (Medical Care Section), Los Angeles, Ca., October 15–19, 1978.

Korsch, Barbara M., and Negrete, Vida Francis. "Doctor-Patient Communication," *Scientific American* (August, 1972): 66.

Korsch, Barbara, Gozzi, Ethel, and Francis, Vida. "Gaps in Doctor-Patient Communication, 1. Doctor-Patient Interaction and Patient Satisfaction," *Pediatrics,* **42:**5 (November 1968): 855–971.

Kosa, John, Antonovsky, Aaron, and Zola, Irving Kenneth (eds.). *Poverty and Health: A Sociological Analysis.* Cambridge: Harvard University Press, 1969.

Koutsopoulos, K. C., Meyer, R. J., and Henley, D. "Psychometric Modeling of Consumer Decisions in Primary Health Care," *Health Services Research,* **12:**4 (Winter 1977): 427–437.

Kravits, Joanna, and Schneider, John. "Health Care Need and Actual Use by Age, Race and Income," in Ronald Andersen, Joanna Kravits, and Odin W. Anderson (eds.), *Equity in Health Services: Empirical Analyses in Social Policy.* Cambridge: Ballinger Publishing, 1975, pp. 169–187.

Kress, John R., and Singer, James. *HMO Handbook.* Rockville, Md.: Aspen Systems Corp., 1975.

Krizay, John, and Wilson, Andrew. *The Patient as Consumer: Health Care Financing in the United States.* Lexington, Mass.: The Twentieth Century Fund, Lexington Books, 1974.

Kushman, John Everett, and Nuckton, Carole Frank. "Further Evidence on the Relative Performance of Proprietary and Nonprofit Hospitals," *Medical Care,* **15:**3 (March 1977): 189–204.

Ladimer, Irving. *Consumer Impact on Policy Development: Implications for Prepaid Group Health Agencies.* Paper presented at 105th Annual Meeting of the American Public Health Association, November 1, 1977, Washington, D.C.

Lairson, Paul D., Record, Jane C., and James, Julia C. "Physician Assistants at Kaiser: Distinctive Patterns of Practice," *Inquiry,* **11**:3 (September 1974): 207–219.

Lancaster, Kelvin. "A New Approach to Consumer Theory," *Journal of Political Economy,* **74**:2 (April 1966): 132–157.

Lane, Millicent. "HMO Health Improving: Growth Stops," (Michigan) *State Journal* (May 20, 1979). Reprinted in *DHEW Green Sheet,* **26**:111 (June 6, 1979): R19.

Lathem, Willoughby. "Community Medicine: Success or Failure?" *New England Journal of Medicine,* **295**:1 (July 1, 1976): 18–23.

Lavin, John H. "The Town That's Squeezing Out Private Practice," *Medical Economics,* **55**:15 (July 24, 1978) 27–44.

Lawrence, David. Personal communication. September 26, 1979.

Lebow, Jay L. "Consumer Assessments of Quality of Medical Care," *Medical Care,* **12**:4 (April 1974): 328–337.

Lee, Maw-Lin. "A Conspicuous Production Theory of Hospital Behavior," *Southern Economic Journal,* **38**:1 (July 1971): 48–58.

———. "Interdependent Behavior and Resource Misallocation in Hospital Care Production," *Review of Social Economy,* **30**:1 (March 1972): 84–95.

Lee, Sidney S., and Butler, Lawrence M. "The Three-Layered Cake: A Plan for Physician Compensation," *New England Journal Of Medicine,* **291**:5 (August 1, 1974): 253–256.

Leff, Arnold M., et al. "Private Practice in the Public Sector: A Unique Relationship Among Local Government Physicians, and Health Care Consumers in Cincinnati," *Medical Care,* **15**:10 (October 1977): 838–848.

Levin, Peter J. "Encouraging Group Practice: With Gun and Net Through the Health Establishment," *American Journal of Public Health,* **61**:5 (May 1971): 941–956.

Levine, Daniel M., et al. "The Role of New Health Practitioners in a Prepaid Group Practice: Provider Differences in Process and Outcomes of Medical Care," *Medical Care,* **14**:4 (April 1976): 326–347.

Levy, Howard, and Fein, Oliver. "Crippled H.I.P.," *Health/PAC Bulletin,* **45** (October 1972): 15–22.

Lewis, Charles E. "Does Comprehensive Care Make a Difference: What Is The Evidence?" *American Journal of Diseases of Children,* **122** (December 1971): 469–474.

———. "The State of the Art of Quality Assessment—1973," *Medical Care,* **12**:10 (October 1974): 799–806.

Lewis, Howard L. "A Togetherness Spirit in Connecticut," *Modern Healthcare,* **2**:1 (July 1974): 25–29.

Lewis, Oscar. "The Culture of Poverty," *Scientific American,* **215** (October 1966): 19–25.

Lewis, Richard. "Oregon County Buying Prepaid Care for the Needy," *American Medical News* (July 27, 1979): 1, 14, 15.

Lewis, Russell F. "The Greater Marshfield Community Health Plan—A Community Experiment," *Wisconsin Medical Journal,* **72**:6 (June 1973): 17–23.

Light, Harold, and Match, Robert. "The Potential of the Teaching Hospital for the Development of Prepaid Group Practices," *Medical Care,* **14**:8 (August 1976): 643–653.

Lindsay, Cotton M. "Real Returns to Medical Education," *Journal of Human Resources,* **8**:3 (Summer 1973): 331–348.

———. "More Real Returns to Medical Education," *Journal of Human Resources,* **11**:1 (Winter 1976): 127–130.

Lipton, Helene L. *Regulatory Climate for HMOs in California: The Knox-Keene Health Care Service Plan Act.* San Francisco: UCSF Health Policy Program, mimeo, June 1978.

LoGerfo, James P. "Hypertension: Management in a Prepaid Health Care Project," *Journal of the American Medical Association,* **233**:3 (July 21, 1975): 245–248.

———, Larson, Eric, and Richardson, William C. "Assessing the Quality of Care for Urinary Tract Infection in Office Practice: A Comparative Organizational Study," *Medical Care,* **16**:6 (June 1978): 488–495.

Logerfo, James P., et al. "Quality of Care," in William C. Richardson (ed.), *The Seattle Prepaid Health Care Project: Comparison of Health Services Delivery.* National Technical Information Service, PB 267488-SET, 1976.

———. "Rates of Surgical Care in Prepaid Group Practices and the Independent Setting: What Are the Reasons for the Differences?" *Medical Care,* **17**:1 (January 1979): 1–10.

Logsdon, Donald N., Magagna, Jeanne, and Varela, Alice. *Quality Assurance Program of a Prepaid Group Practice Plan.* Presented at 1975 Group Health Institute Conference, June 23–26, 1975.

Lorant, John H., and Kimbell, Larry J. "Determinants of Output in Group and Solo Medical Practice," *Health Services Research,* **11**:1 (Spring 1976): 6–20.

Louis, Daniel Z., and McCord, John J. *Evaluation of California Prepaid Health Plans: Executive Summary.* Santa Barbara, Ca.: General Research Corp., 1974.

Lubalin, James S., et al. *Evaluation of the Accomplishments of Selected HMOs-Funded Projects,* Draft Final Report, Contract HSA 105-74-10, Santa Barbara, Ca.: General Research Corp., May, 1974.

Luft, Harold S. "Benefit-Cost Analysis and Public Policy Implementation: From Normative to Positive Analysis," *Public Policy,* **24**:4 (Fall 1976).

———. *Competition and Regulation: The Selection and Competitive Effects of HMOs,* Grant no. 18-p-97127/9-01 from the Health Care Financing Administration, 1979.

———. "National Health Care Expenditures: Where Do the Dollars Go?" *Inquiry,* **13**:4 (December 1976) 344–363.

———, and Crane, Steven, *Interhospital Resource Allocation in Health Maintenance Organizations and Conventional Systems of Hospitals.* Presented at Joint National Meeting of The Institute for Management Sciences/Operations Research Society of America, May 1, 1979, New Orleans.

Luft, Harold S., Judith Feder, Holahan, John, and Lennox, D. Karen. "Health Maintenance Organizations," in Judith Feder, John Holahan, and Theodore Marmor (eds.), *National Health Insurance: Conflicting Goals and Policy Choices,* Washington, D.C.: Urban Institute, 1980.

Lum, Doman. *Comparison of Organizational Sponsorship and Service Arrangement Variables among Prepaid Medical Group Practices in the United States.* Unpublished Ph.D. dissertation, School of Applied Social Sciences, Case Western Reserve University, 1974.

———. "The Health Maintenance Organization Delivery System: A National Study of Attitudes of HMO Project Directors on HMO Issues," *American Journal of Public Health,* **65**:11 (November 1975): 1192–1201.

Lyle, Carl B., et al. "Cost of Medical Care in a Practice of Internal Medicine," *Annals of Internal Medicine,* **81**:1 (July 1974): 1–6.

———. "Practice Habits in a Group of Eight Internists," *Annals of Internal Medicine,* **84**:5 (May 1976): 594–601.

Lyons, Thomas F., and Payne, Beverly C. "The Relationship of Physicians' Medical Recording Performance to Their Medical Care Performance," *Medical Care,* **12**:8 (August 1974): 714–720.

McAuliffe, William E. "Measuring the Quality of Medical Care: Process Versus Outcome," *Milbank Memorial Fund Quarterly/Health and Society,* **57:**1 (Winter 1979): 118–152.

―――. "Studies of Process-Outcome Correlations in Medical Care Evaluations: A Critique," *Medical Care,* **16:**11 (November 1978): 907–930.

McCaffree, Kenneth M., and Newman, Harold F. "Prepayment of Drug Costs under a Group Practice Prepayment Plan," *American Journal of Public Health,* **58:**7 (July 1968): 1212–1218.

McCaffree, Kenneth M., et al. "Comparative Costs of Services," in William C. Richardson (ed.), *The Seattle Prepaid Health Care Project: Comparison of Health Services Delivery.* National Technical Information Service, PB # 267488-SET, 1976.

McCarthy, Eugene G., and Finkel, Madelon Lubin. "Second Opinion Elective Surgery Programs: Outcome Status over Time," *Medical Care,* **16:**12 (December 1978): 984–994.

McClure, Walter. "The Medical Care System under National Health Insurance: Four Models," *Journal of Health Politics, Policy and Law,* **1:**1 (Spring 1976): 22–68.

MacColl, William A. *Group Practice and Prepayment of Medical Care.* Washington, D.C.: Public Affairs Press, 1966.

McElrath, Dennis C. "Perspective and Participation in Prepaid Group Practice," *American Sociological Review,* **26** (1961): 596–607.

McFarland, John B., and Odem, Richard J. "Income and Expenses of Group Practices and the Role of the Business Manager," in American Medical Association, *Profile of Medical Practice, 1974 edition,* pp. 66–79.

McGregor, Maurice, and Pelletier, Gerald. "Planning of Specialized Health Facilities: Size vs. Cost and Effectiveness in Heart Surgery," *New England Journal of Medicine,* **299:**4 (July 27, 1978): 179–181.

McKinlay, John B. "Some Approaches and Problems in the Study of the Use of Services—An Overview," *Journal of Health and Social Behavior,* **13:**2 (June 1972): 115–152.

McKinlay, John B., and Dutton, Diana B. "Social-Psychological Factors Affecting Health Service Utilization," in Selma Mushkin (ed.), *Consumer Incentives for Health Care.* New York: Prodist, 1974.

McLaughlin, Loretta. "Housecalls in the Inner City," *Boston Globe* (April 27, 1978). Reprinted in *Medical Care Review,* **35:**6 (June 1978): 617–619.

MacLeod, Gordon K., and Prussin, Jeffrey A. "The Continuing Evolution of Health Maintenance Organizations," *New England Journal of Medicine,* **288:**9 (March 1, 1973): 439–443.

McNeer, J. Frederick, et al. "Hospital Discharge One Week after Acute Myocardial Infarction," *New England Journal of Medicine,* **298:**5 (February 2, 1978): 229–232.

McNeil, Barbara J., Weichselbaum, Ralph, and Pauker, Stephen G. "Fallacy of the Five-Year Survival in Lung Cancer," *New England Journal of Medicine,* **299:**25 (December 21, 1978): 1397–1401.

McNeil, Richard, Jr., and Schlenker, Robert E. "HMOs, Competition and Government," *Milbank Memorial Fund Quarterly/Health and Society,* **53:**2 (Spring 1975): 195–224.

Maccoby, Nathan, et al. "Reducing the Risk of Cardiovascular Disease: Effects of a Community-Based Campaign on Knowledge and Behavior," *Journal of Community Health,* **3:**2 (Winter 1977): 100–114.

Mahony, Michael J. "Experimental Methods and Outcome Evaluation," *Journal of Consulting and Clinical Psychology,* **46:**4 (1978): 600–672.

Makover, Henry B. "The Quality of Medical Care: Methodology of Survey of the Medical

Groups Associated with the Health Insurance Plan of New York," *American Journal of Public Health*, **41:**7 (July 1951): 824–832.

Maloney, James V. "A Report on the Role of Economic Motivation in the Performance of Medical School Faculty," *Surgery*, **68:**1 (July 1970): 1–19.

Marks, Sylvia D., Hurtado, Arnold V., and Greenlick, Merwyn R. *Hospital Utilization Study I.* Portland, Ore.: Kaiser Foundation Health Services Research Center, Research Report Series No. 2, 1976.

Marshall, Tyler. "Kaiser Plan. The Patients' View: What They Like and What They Don't Like," *Modern Hospital*, **116:**2 (February 1971): 86–87.

Martin, Nancy. "I'd Rather Switch Than Fight," *Medical Economics*, **53:**7 (April 5, 1976): 154ff.

Martin, William C. "Death of a Group," *Medical Economics*, (December 1953): 138ff.

Marton, Keith I. *Assessing the Value of a Diagnostic Test.* Stanford University, Health Services Research Seminar, April 24, 1978.

———. *The Diagnostic Significance of Involuntary Weight Loss.* Presented at National Meeting of American Federation for Clinical Research, May 5–7, 1979.

———, Rudd, Peter, and Sox, Harold C., Jr. *The Comparative Value of Certain Laboratory Tests and the Clinical History in Detecting Pancreatic Cancer.* Palo Alto, Ca.: Veterans Administration Medical Center, 1979. (Mimeo).

Mattera, Marianne Dekker. "Would Chain-Store Practice Suit You?" *Medical Economics* (September 18, 1978): 98–108.

Maxwell, Neil. "Hospitals Work to Cut Expenses and Fend Off Government Controls," *The Wall Street Journal* (October 27, 1978).

Mechanic, David. "Factors Affecting Receptivity to Innovations in Health-Care Delivery among Primary-Care Physicians," in Mechanic, David, *Politics, Medicine and Social Disease.* New York: Wiley-Interscience, 1974, pp. 69–87.

———. *The Growth of Bureaucratic Medicine.* New York: Wiley-Interscience, 1976.

———. "The Growth of Bureaucratic Medicine: An Inquiry Into the Dynamics of Patient Behavior and the Organization of Medical Care," *American Journal of Sociology*, **82:**5 (March 1977): 1134–1139.

———. "The Organization of Medical Practice and Practice Orientation among Physicians in Prepaid and Nonprepaid Primary Care Settings," *Medical Care*, **13:**3 (March 1975): 189–204.

———. "Physicians," *Research and Analytic Report Series* 3-76, University of Wisconsin-Madison, Health Economics Research Center, Center for Medical Sociology and Health Services Research, 1976.

Meier, Gerald B., and Tillotson, John. *Physician Reimbursement and Hospital Use in HMOs.* Excelsior, Minn.: InterStudy, September 1978.

Menke, Wayne G. "Professional Values in Medical Practice," *New England Journal of Medicine*, **280:**17 (April 24, 1969): 930–936.

Mennemeyer, Stephen T. "Really Great Returns to Medical Education?" *Journal of Human Resources*, **13:**1 (Winter 1978): 75–90.

Mercer, Lyle. "The Role of the Member in Group Health Cooperative of Puget Sound," in U.S. Health Maintenance Organization Service, *Selected Papers on Consumerism in the HMO Movement.* Washington, D.C., USGPO, Department of Health, Education and Welfare Publication No. HSM 73-13012, July 1973.

Metzner, Charles A., and Bashshur, Rashid L. "Factors Associated with Choice of Health Care Plans," *Journal of Health and Social Behavior*, **8** (December 1967): 291–299.

————, and Shannon, Gary W. "Differential Public Acceptance of Group Medical Practice," *Medical Care*, **10**:4 (July-August 1972): 279–287.

Meyer, Lawrence. "Group Health in Trouble," *Washington Post*, **101**:1 (January 2, 1978). Reprinted in *Medical Care Review*, **35**:2 (February 1978): 163–167.

Meyer, Priscilla S. "Health-Care Deductibles Are Promoted by Insurance Firms in Bid to Pare Costs," *Wall Street Journal*, **58** (November 2, 1977): 11. Reprinted in *Medical Care Review*, **34**:11 (December 1977): 1300–1302.

Meyers, Samuel M., et al. *Ambulatory Medical Use by Federal Employees: Experience of Members in a Service Benefit Plan and in a Prepaid Group Practice Plan*. Presented at the 105th Annual Meeting of the American Public Health Association, November 1, 1977.

Miller, Jana. "Health Central Affecting Blues in Lincoln," *Lincoln Journal* (April 13, 1979). Reprinted in *DHEW Green Sheet*, **26**:88 (May 3, 1979): R17.

Mitchell, Bridger M., and Phelps, Charles E. "National Health Insurance: Some Costs and Effects of Mandated Coverage," *Journal of Political Economy*, **86**:3 (June 1976): 553–571,.

Mitchell, J. H., and Dunn, J. P. "Comparative Absence Experience Among Employees Covered by a Prepaid or a Blue Cross/Blue Shield Health Insurance Plan," *Journal of Occupational Medicine*, **20**:12 (December 1978): 797–800.

Moffitt, Herbert C., Jr. "Use and Abuse of Hospital Insurance: Editorial," *San Francisco Medical Society Bulletin*, **24**:10 (October 1951): 11.

Monsma, George N., Jr. "Marginal Revenue and the Demand for Physicians' Services," in Herbert Klarman (ed.), *Empirical Studies in Health Economics*. Baltimore: Johns Hopkins Press, 1970, pp. 145–160.

Moore, Stephen. "Cost Containment through Risk-Sharing by Primary-Care Physicians," *New England Journal of Medicine*, **300**:24 (June 14, 1979): 1359–1362.

Moore, Thomas G., Jr., and Breslow, Lester. "California Medical Group Evaluation Report," California Council for Health Plan Alternatives, December 6, 1972. Reprinted in U.S. Senate, Permanent Subcommittee on Investigations, 94th Congress First Session, March 12–14, 1975, Hearings on *Prepaid Health Plans*.

Morehead, Mildred A. "Evaluating the Quality of Medical Care in the Neighborhood Health Center Program of the Office of Economic Opportunity," *Medical Care*, **8**:2 (March-April 1970): 118–131.

————. "The Medical Audit as an Operational Tool," *American Journal of Public Health*, **57**:9 (September 1967): 1643–1656.

————, Donaldson, Rose S., and Seravalli, Mary R. "Comparisons Between OEO Neighborhood Health Centers and Other Health Care Providers of Ratings of the Quality of Health Care," *American Journal of Public Health*, **61**:7 (July 1971): 1294–1306.

Moriarty, Mark M., et al. *The HMO as an Innovation: Determinants of Adoption*. Iowa City: Bureau of Business and Economic Research, July 1977.

Morozumi, John I. "San Joaquin Medical Foundation Plan," in Arizona Regional Medical Program, *Workshop on Alternative Methods for Delivery of Health Services, Casa Grande* (September 23–24, 1971), pp. 23–30.

Morris, Lawrence C. "National HMO Census," Memorandum to Chief Plan Executives, All Blue Cross and Blue Shield Plans, Appendix I: Analysis of Hospital and Physician Utilization, April 10, 1978. Chicago: Blue Cross Association/National Association of Blue Shield Plans.

Mott, F. D., Hastings, J. E. F., and Barclay, A. T. "Prepaid Group Practice in Sault Ste. Marie, Ontario: Part II: Evidence From the Household Survey," *Medical Care*, **11**:3 (May-June 1973): 173–188.

Moustafa, A., Hopkins, Carl E., and Klein, Bonnie. "Determinants of Choice and Change of Health Insurance Plan," *Medical Care,* **9:**1 (January-February 1971): 32−41.

Mueller, Marjorie Smith, and Gibson, Robert M. "National Health Expenditures, Calendar Year 1974," *Research and Statistics Note* 1976-5, April 14, 1976. Social Security Administration, Office of Research and Statistics, U.S. Department of Health, Education and Welfare Publication No. (SSA) 76-11701.

———. "National Health Expenditures, Fiscal Year 1975," *Social Security Bulletin,* **39:**2 February 1976).

Mueller, Marjorie Smith, and Piro, Paula A. "Private Health Insurance in 1974: A Review of Coverage, Enrollment, and Financial Experience," *Social Security Bulletin,* **39:**3 (March 1976).

Mullooly, John P., and Freeborn, Donald K. *The Effects of Length of Membership Upon the Utilization of Ambulatory Care Services: A Comparison of Disadvantaged and General Membership Populations in a Prepaid Goup Practice.* Portland, Ore.: Kaiser Foundation Health Services Research Center, no date, circa 1978.

Multnomah County Oregon, Project Health Division. *National Health Insurance Through State/ Regional/Local Government and Private Sector Health Care Brokerage.* Portland, Ore.: Department of Human Services, 1977.

———. *Project Health: An Overview.* Portland, Ore.: Department of Human Services, 1977.

Nathan, Richard W. "Medicaid 'Mill' Defense," *New York Times,* **125** (September 12, 1976): 16e. Reprinted in *Medical Care Review,* **33:**9 (October 1976): 1013−1014.

National Advisory Commission on Health Manpower. "Kaiser Foundation Medical Care Program," in *Report of the National Advisory Commission on Health Manpower,* Vol. II. Washington: USGPO, 1967, pp. 197−228.

National Chamber Foundation. *A National Health Care Strategy: A Series of Five Reports on Business Involvement with Health.* Washington, D.C.: National Chamber Foundation, 1978.

Neil, Merritt B., Goldsteiin, George S., and Birmingham, Daniel J. "The Medical Foundation of Bellaire—The Bellaire Medical Group: A Case Study of the Development of a Consumer-Oriented, Prepaid Group Practice Health Program in a Rural Area," in *Rural Health Care Delivery: Proceedings of a National Conference on Rural Health Maintenance Organizations,* Louisville, Ky., July 8−10, 1974. Prepared for U.S. Senate, Committee on Agriculture and Forestry, October 30, 1974.

Neilsen, Chris. Personal communication, September 26, 1979.

Nesson, H. Richard. "Quality Assurance and Assessment," in Robert A. Zelten and Susan Bray (eds.), *Health Maintenance Organizations.* Philadelphia: University of Pennsylvania Press, 1977, pp. 259−266.

Neumann, Bruce R., et al. "Consolidation of Community Hospitals," *Journal of Community Health,* **4:**1 (Fall 1978): 73−83.

Neutra, Raymond. "Indications for the Surgical Treatment of Suspected Acute Appendicitis: A Cost-Effectiveness Approach," in John P. Bunker, Benjamin A. Barnes, and Frederick Mosteller (eds.), *Costs, Risks and Benefits of Surgery.* Oxford: Oxford University Press, 1977.

Newhouse, Joseph P. "A Design for a Health Insurance Experiment," *Inquiry,* **11:**1 (March 1974): 5−27.

———. "The Economics of Group Practice," *Journal of Human Resources,* **8:**1 (Winter 1973): 37−56.

———, and Phelps, Charles E. "New Estimates of Price and Income Elasticities of Medical Care Services," in Richard N. Rosett (ed.), *The Role of Health Insurance in the Health Services Sector.* New York: National Bureau of Economic Research, 1976.

———, and Schwartz, William B. "Policy Options and the Impact of National Health Insurance," *New England Journal of Medicine*, **290**:24 (June 13, 1974): 1345–1359.

Newman, Harold F. "Testimony before U.S. House of Representatives, Subcommittee on Public Health and Environment of the Committee on Interstate and Foreign Commerce," *Health Maintenance Organizations*, Hearings, April 11–13, 1972, Serial 92–88.

Newman, Michael A. (ed.). *The Medical Director in Prepaid Group Practice Health Maintenance Organizations*. Proceedings of a Conference, Denver, Colorado, April 1973. Sponsored by Health Maintenance Organization Service, U.S. Department of Health, Education and Welfare.

Newport, John, and Roemer, Milton I. "Comparative Perinatal Mortality under Medical Care Foundations and Other Delivery Models," *Inquiry*, **11**:1 (March 1975): 10–17.

Nolan, Robert L., Schwartz, Jerome L., and Simonian, Kenneth. "Social Class Differences in Utilization of Pediatric Services in a Prepaid Direct Service Medical Care Program," *American Journal of Public Health*, **57**:1 (January 1967): 34–47.

Northrup, Bowen, and Bishop, Jerry E. "Whooping-Cough Vaccine Risks Are Weighed against Benefits in a Vigorous British Debate," *Wall Street Journal* (March 31, 1977): 30.

Numbers, Ronald L. "The Third Party: Health Insurance in America," in Judith Walter Leavitt and Ronald L. Numbers (eds.)., *Sickness and Health in America: Readings in the History of Medicine and Public Health*. Madison: University of Wisconsin Press, 1978, pp. 139–153.

Olsen, Donna, Kane, Robert, and Proctor, Paul. "A Controlled Trial of Multiphasic Screening," *New England Journal of Medicine*, **294**:17 (April 22, 1976): 925–930.

Orr, Ralph. "Chrysler Families Give New Group Health Plan High Ratings," *Detroit Free Press*, **148** (April 3, 1979): 8e. Reprinted in *Medical Care Review*, **36**:5 (May 1979): 475–476.

Orso, Camille. "Delivering Ambulatory Health Care: The Successful Experience of an Urban Neighborhood Health Center," *Medical Care*, **17**:2 (February 1979): 111–126.

Owens, Arthur. "Doctors' Productivity: The Trend Is Down," *Medical Economics*, **53**:1 (January 12, 1976): 100–102.

———. "Their First Year of Practice: A Far Cry from Yours," *Medical Economics*, **50**:3 (February 5, 1973): 150–171.

———. "What Doctors Want Most from Their Practices Now," *Medical Economics*, **54**:5 (March 7, 1977): 88–92.

———. "What's Behind the Drop in Doctors' Productivity?" *Medical Economics*, **55**:15 (July 24, 1978): 102–105.

Palley, Howard A. "The 'Health Insurance Plan' Controversy: Ideology and the Organization of Medical Care," *Journal of Health and Human Behavior*, **6**:4 (Winter 1965): 218–225.

Palmer, Walter K. "Financial Planning," in Robert A. Zelten and Susan Bray (eds.), *Health Maintenance Organizations*. Philadelphia: The Wharton School, University of Pennsylvania, 1977, pp. 149–186.

Parker, Gordon, and Tupling, Hilary. "Consumer Evaluation of Natural Therapists and General Practitioners," *Medical Journal of Australia*, **1** (April 23, 1977): 619–622. Reprinted in *Medical Care Review*, **35**:9 (October 1978): 996–997.

Paulson, L. Gregory, Schroeder, Steven A., and Donaldson, Molla S. "Medical Student Instructional Costs In a Primary Care Clerkship," *Journal of Medical Education*, **54** (July 1979): 551–555.

Pauly, Mark V. "The Economics of Moral Hazard," *American Economic Review*, **58**:3 (June 1968): 531–537.

———. "Efficiency, Incentives and Reimbursement for Health Care," *Inquiry,* **7**:1 (March 1970): 114–131.

———. "What Is Unnecessary Surgery?" *Milbank Memorial Fund Quarterly/Health and Society,* **57**:1 (Winter 1979): 95–117.

Payne, Beverly C., and Lyons, Thomas F. *Detailed Statistics and Methodologies for Studies of Personal Medical Care in Hawaii.* Ann Arbor: University of Michigan School of Medicine, 1972.

Payne, Beverly C., et al. *The Quality of Medical Care: Evaluation and Improvement.* Chicago: Hospital Research and Educational Trust, 1976.

Peck, Richard L. "The HMO That Drove Doctors to Strike," *Medical Economics* (September 18, 1978): 142–160.

Peebles, Thomas C. Personal correspondence, June 3, 1977.

Peel, Evelyn, and Scharff, Jack. "Impact of Cost-Sharing on Use of Ambulatory Services under Medicare," *Social Security Bulletin* (October 1973): 3–24.

Penchansky, Roy, and Berki, Sylvester E. *Evaluating HMO Development: Contributions from the Experience of the Community Health Network,* mimeo. Presented at American Public Health Association Annual Meeting. Miami Beach, October 1976.

Perkoff, Gerald T. "An Effect of Organization of Medical Care upon Health Manpower Distributions," *Medical Care,* **16**:8 (August 1978): 628–640.

———. *Lessons from the Creation of a New Medical Care Setting,* Unpublished manuscript, 1977.

———. "The Medical Care Group of Washington University: A Health Care Experiment," *Missouri Medicine,* **68**:6 (June 1971): 392–394.

———. Personal communication, February 24, 1977.

———., Kahn, Lawrence, and Haas, Philip J. "The Effects of an Experimental Prepaid Group Practice on Medical Care Utilization and Cost," *Medical Care,* **14**:5 (May 1976): 432–449.

———., Kahn, Lawrence, and Mackie, Anita. "Medical Care Utilization in an Experimental Prepaid Group Practice Model in a University Medical Center," *Medical Care,* **12**:6 (June 1974): 471–485.

———., et al. "Lack of Effect of an Experimental Prepaid Group Practice on Utilization of Surgical Services," *Surgery,* **77**:5 (May 1975): 619–623.

The Permanente Medical Group. *The Permanente Medical Group-Northern California,* circa 1970.

———. *General Information,* mimeo 1973.

Perrott, George S. *The Federal Employees Health Benefits Program.* Office for Group Practice Development, U.S. Department of Health, Education and Welfare, 1971.

Peterson, Iver. "Automakers and U.A.W. Initiate Low-Cost, Prepaid Health Plan," *New York Times* (February 13, 1979). Reprinted in *The Green Sheet,* **26**:32 (February 14, 1979).

Peterson, Osler L., et al. "An Analytical Study of North Carolina General Practice, 1953–54," *Journal of Medical Education,* **31**:12 (December 1956), Part 2.

Phelan, Jerry, Erickson, Robert, and Fleming, Scott. "Group Practice Prepayment: An Approach to Delivering Organized Health Services," *Health Care: Part II* (Autumn 1970), *Law and Contemporary Problems* (Duke University School of Law).

Phelps, Charles E. "Illness Prevention and Medical Insurance," *Journal of Human Resources,* **13** Supplement (1978): 183–207.

Pineault, Raynald. "The Effect of Prepaid Group Practice on Physicians' Utilization Behavior," *Medical Care,* **14**:2 (February 1976): 121–136.

Piontkowski, Dyan. *Selection of Health Insurance By an Employee Group in Northern California,* San Francisco: University of California San Francisco, Health Policy Program, 1979.

————, and Butler, Lewis. "Selection of Health Insurance by an Employee Group in Northern California," *American Journal of Public Health,* **70:**3 (March 1980): 274–276.

Pirsig, Robert M. *Zen and the Art of Motorcycle Maintenance.* New York: William Morrow and Co., 1974.

Pollack, Jerome. *A Plan for Prepaid Health Care at Harvard.* Proceedings of the 19th Annual Group Health Institute, New York, June 4–6, 1969.

Pope, Clyde R. "Consumer Satisfaction in a Health Maintenance Organization," *Journal of Health and Social Behavior,* **19** (September 1978): 291–303.

————. *Illness with a High Emotional Component and the Use of Medical Services.* Portland, Ore.: Health Services Research Center, Kaiser Foundation Hospitals, 1978.

————, Freeborn, D. K., and Greenlick, M. R. *Use of Outside Physicians by Members of a Group Practice Prepayment Plan.* Presented at American Public Health Association Annual Meeting, November 12–16, 1972.

————. *Members' Evaluation of Their Experience in a Group Practice Prepayment Plan,* Presented at American Public Health Association Annual Meeting, November 1972.

Pope, Clyde R., Yoshioka, Samuel, and Greenlick, Merwyn R. "Determinants of Medical Care Utilization: The Use of Telephone for Reporting Symptoms," *Journal of Health and Social Behavior,* **12** (June 1971): 155–162.

Powles, John. "On the Limitations of Modern Medicine," *Science, Medicine and Man,* **1:**1 (1973): 1–30.

Prussin, Jeffrey A. "HMOs: Organizational and Financial Models," *Hospital Progress,* **55:**4–6 (April-June 1974).

Prybil, Lawrence. "Physician Terminations in Large Multispecialty Groups," *Medical Group Management,* **18:**5,6 (July, September 1971).

Quigley, Dennis F. "Changes in Selected Health Care Plans," *Monthly Labor Review* (December 1975): 22–26.

Rabin, David, Bush, Patricia J., and Fuller, Norman A. "Drug Prescription Rates before and after Enrollment of Medicaid Population in an HMO," *Public Health Reports,* **93:**1 (January-February 1978): 16–23.

Rafferty, John A. "Enfranchisement and Rationing: The Effects of Medicare on Discretionary Hospital Use," *Health Services Research,* **10:**1 (Spring 1975): 51–62.

————. "Hospital Output Indices," *Economic and Business Bulletin,* **24:**2 (Winter 1972): 21–27.

————. "Patterns of Hospital Use: An Analysis of Short-Run Variations," *Journal of Political Economy,* **79:**1 (January-February 1971): 154–165.

————, and Schweitzer, Stuart O. "Comparison of For-Profit and Nonprofit Hospitals: A Reevaluation," *Inquiry,* **11:**4 (December 1974): 304–309.

Ramsay, Thomas E., Jr., and Wright, Richard D. "Impacts of Health Maintenance Organizations' Growth on Community Health Care Costs," *Socio-Economic Planning Sciences,* **12** (1978): 241–249.

Raup, Ruth M., and Altenderfer, Marion E. *Medical Groups in the United States, 1959.* U.S. Public Health Service, July 1963, PHS Publication No. 1063.

Record, Jane Cassels, and Cohen, Harold R. "The Introduction of Midwifery in a Prepaid Group Practice," *American Journal of Public Health,* **62:**3 (March 1972): 354–360.

Record, Jane Cassels, and Greenlick, Merwyn. "New Health Professionals and the Physician Role: An Hypothesis from Kaiser Experience," *Public Health Reports,* **90:**3 (May-June 1975): 241–246.

Reimers, Wilbur L. "Experiences with Per Capita Payments for Outside Medical Services," in

Michael A. Newman (ed.), *The Medical Director in Prepaid Group Practice Health Maintenance Organizations.* Proceedings of a Conference, Denver, Colorado, April 1973, sponsored by U.S. Health Maintenance Organization Service.

Reinhardt, Uwe. "A Production Function for Physician Services," *Review of Economics and Statistics,* **54:**1 (February 1972): 55–66.

———. "Proposed Changes in the Organization of Health Care Delivery: An Overview and Critique," *Milbank Memorial Fund Quarterly,* **51:**2 (Spring 1973): 169–222.

———, and Yett, Donald E. *Physician Production Functions under Varying Practice Arrangements.* Community Profile Data Center, Community Health Service, HSMHA, Technical Paper 11, Revised, August 1972.

Reiser, Stanley Joel. "The Emergence of the Concept of Screening for Disease," *Milbank Memorial Fund Quarterly/Health and Society,* **56:**4 (Fall 1978): 403–426.

Reynolds, James A. "Group MD Fringe Benefits: Where Will They Stop?" *Medical Economics* (October 23, 1972): 211–218.

———. "A New Scheme to Force You to Compete for Patients," *Medical Economics* (March 21, 1977): 23–41.

Reynolds, Roger A. "Improving Access to Health Care Among the Poor—The Neighborhood Health Center Experience," *Milbank Memorial Fund Quarterly/Health and Society,* **54:**1 (Winter 1976): 47–82.

Rhee, Sang-O. "Factors Determining the Quality of Physician Performance in Patient Care," *Medical Care,* **14:**9 (September 1976): 733–750.

Richardson, Elliott. "Testimony Before the Subcommittee on Public Health and Environment," *Health Maintenance Organizations,* Hearings on HR 5615 and HR 11728, Committee on Interstate and Foreign Commerce, House of Representatives, Serial 92–88, April 11, 1972.

Richardson, William C. *Ambulatory Use of Physicians' Services in Response to Illness in a Low Income Neighborhood.* Chicago: Center for Health Administration Studies, Research Studies 29, 1971.

———. "*Group Payment Since the CCMC: Policy Implications of the Ignored and Unforeseen,*" presented at the Conference, "Health Care for the American People: Unfinished Agenda," held at Airlie House, Warrentown Virginia, May 18–20, 1977.

———, Shortell, S. M., and Diehr, P. K. "Access to Care and Patient Satisfaction," in William C. Richardson (ed.), *The Seattle Prepaid Health Care Project: Comparison of Health Services Delivery.* National Technical Information Service, PB 267488-SET, 1976.

Richardson, William C., et al. *The Seattle Prepaid Health Care Project: Comparison of Health Services Delivery.* "Chapter I: Introduction to the Project, the Study, and the Enrollees." National Technical Information Service, PB 267488-SET, 1976.

———. *The Seattle Prepaid Health Care Project: Comparison of Health Services Delivery.* Overview, Summary and References, Grant No. HS 01978, January 1977.

Riedel, Donald C., et al. *Federal Employees Health Benefits Program Utilization Study.* National Center for Health Services Research. Washington: USGPO, January 1975, U.S. Department of Health, Education and Welfare Publication No. (HRA) 75-3125.

Riessman, Catherine Kohler. "The Use of Health Services by the Poor," *Social Policy,* (May-June 1974): 41–49.

Rindfuss, Ronald R., and Ladinsky, Judith L. "Patterns of Birth: Implications for the Incidence of Elective Induction," *Medical Care,* **14:**8 (August 1976): 685–693.

Rivkin, Marian Osterweis, and Bush, Patricia J. "The Satisfaction Continuum in Health Care: Consumer and Provider Preferences," in Selma J. Mushkin (ed.), *Consumer Incentives for Health Care.* New York: Prodist, 1974.

Robert Wood Johnson Foundation. *Special Report,* 1 (1978), Princeton, N.J.

Robertson, Robert L. "Economic Effects of Personal Health Services: Work Loss in a Public School Teacher Population," *American Journal of Public Health,* **61:**1 (January 1971): 30–45.

———. "Comparative Medical Care Use under Prepaid Group Practice and Free Choice Plans: A Case Study," *Inquiry,* **9:**3 (September 1972): 70–76.

Roemer, Milton I. "Health Resources and Services in the Watts Area of Los Angeles," *California Health,* **23** (February-March 1966): 123–143.

———, and Gartside, Foline E. "Effect of Peer Review in Medical Foundations on Qualifications of Surgeons," *Health Services Reports,* **88:**9 (November 1973): 808–814.

Roemer, Milton I., and Shain, Max. *Hospital Utilization under Insurance.* Chicago: American Hospital Association, 1959.

Roemer, Milton I., and Shonick, William. "HMO Performance: The Recent Evidence," *Milbank Memorial Fund Quarterly/Health and Society,* **51:**3 (Summer 1973): 271–317.

Roemer, Milton I., et al. *Health Insurance Effects: Services, Expenditures, and Attitudes under Three Types of Plan.* Ann Arbor: University of Michigan, School of Public Health, 1972.

Roghmann, Klaus J., et al, "Who Chooses Prepaid Medical Care: Survey Results from Two Marketings of Three New Prepayment Plans," *Public Health Reports,* **90:**6 (November-December 1975): 516–527.

Roghmann, Klaus, Sorensen, Andrew, and Wells, Sandra. *A Summary and Discussion of: "A Cohort Analysis of the Impact of Three Health Maintenance Organizations on Inpatient Utilization."* Final Report for Contract No. HEW-100-88-0021, November 28, 1977.

Roman, S. A. "Health Maintenance Organizations: Are They for Inner Cities?" *Journal Community Health,* **1** (Winter 1975): 127–131.

Roney, James G., and Estes, Hilliard D. "Automated Health Testing in a Medical Group Practice," *Public Health Reports,* **90:**2 (March-April 1975): 126-132.

Roos, Noralou P., Roos, Leslie L., Jr., and Henteleff, Paul D. "Elective Surgical Rates—Do High Rates Mean Lower Standards?" *New England Journal of Medicine,* **297:**7 (August 18, 1977): 360–365.

Rosenberg, Charlotte L. "A Short-Stay Surgical Center for Your Patients," *Medical Economics,* **48:**23 (November 8, 1971): 114–135.

———. "Trouble in a Health Planners' Paradise," *Medical Economics,* **55:**16 (August 7, 1978): 177–182.

Ross, Austin, Jr. "A Report on Physician Terminations in Group Practice," *Medical Group Management,* **16:**5 (July 1969): 15–21.

Ross, Jancie. "Health Maintenance Organizations in the South," *Atlanta Economic Review,* **27:**6 (November-December 1977): 28–32.

Rothenberg, Robert E., Pickard, Karl, and Rothenberg, Joel E. *Group Medicine and Health Insurance in Action.* New York: Crown Publishers, 1949.

Ruchlin, Hirsch S., Pointer, Dennis D., and Cannedy, Lloyd L. "A Comparison of For-Profit Investor-Owned Chain and Non-Profit Hospitals," *Inquiry,* **10:**4 (December 1973): 13–23.

Sackett, David L. "Screening for Early Detection of Disease: To What Purpose?" *Bulletin of the New York Academy of Medicine,* **51:**1 (January 1975): 39–52.

Sagel, Stuart S., et al. "Efficacy of Routine Screening and Lateral Chest Radiographs in a Hospital Based Population," *New England Journal of Medicine,* **291:**19 (November 7, 1974); 1001–1004.

Salkever, David S. "Will Regulation Control Health-Care Costs?" *Bulletin of the New York Academy of Medicine*, **54**:1 (January 1978): 73–83.

⸺, et al. "Episodes of Illness and Access to Care in the Inner City: A Comparison of HMO and non-HMO Populations," *Health Services Research* (Fall 1976): 252–270.

Salmon, J. Warren. "The Health Maintenance Organization Strategy: A Corporate Takeover of Health Services Delivery," *International Journal of Health Services*, **5**:4 (1975): 609–624.

Sasuly, Richard, and Hopkins, Carl E. "A Medical Society-Sponsored Comprehensive Medical Care Plan: The Foundation for Medical Care of San Joaquin County, California," *Medical Care*, **5**:4 (July-August 1967): 234–248.

Saward, Ernest W. Personal communication, November 11, 1978.

⸺, and Greenlick, Merwyn R. "Health Policy and the HMO," *Milbank Memorial Fund Quarterly*, **50**:2 Part 1 (April 1972): 147–176.

Saward, Ernest W., Blank, Janet D., and Greenlick, Merwyn B. "Documentation of Twenty Years of Organizational Growth of a Prepaid Group Practice Plan," *Medical Care*, **6**:3 (May-June 1968): 231–244.

Saward, Ernest W., Blank, Janet, and Lamb, Henry. *Some Information Descriptive of a Successfully Operating HMO*. Health Maintenance Organization Service, U.S. Department of Health, Education and Welfare, 1973.

Saywell, Robert M., Jr., et al. "A Performance Comparison: USMG-FMG Attending Physicians," *American Journal of Public Health*, **69**:1 (January 1979): 57–62.

Scheffler, Richard M. "Further Considerations in the Economics of Group Practice in the Management Input," *Journal of Human Resources*, **10**:2 (Spring 1975): 258–263.

Schlenker, Robert E., et al. *HMO's in 1973: A National Survey*. Minneapolis: InterStudy, 1974.

Schroeder, Steven A., and Donaldson, Molla S. "The Feasibility of an Outcome Approach to Quality Assurance—A Report from One HMO," *Medical Care* **14**:1 (January 1976): 49–56.

Schroeder, Steven A., and O'Leary, Dennis S. "Differences in Lab Use and Length of Stay between University and Community Hospitals," *Journal of Medical Education*, **52** (1977): 418–420.

Schroeder, Steven A., and Showstack, J. A. *The Dynamics of Medical Technology Use: Analysis and Policy Options*. Paper presented at the Sun Valley Forum, August 1977.

⸺. "Financial Incentives to Perform Medical Procedures and Laboratory Tests: Illustrative Models of Office Practice" *Medical Care*, **16**:4 (April 1978): 289–298.

Schroeder, Steven A., Schliftman, Alan, and Piemme, Thomas E. "Variation among Physicians in Use of Laboratory Tests: Relation to Quality of Care," *Medical Care*, **12**:8 (August 1974): 709–713.

Schroeder, Steven A., et al. "Use of Laboratory Tests and Pharmaceuticals: Variation among Physicians and Effects of Cost Audit on Subsequent Use," *Journal of the American Medical Association*, **225**:8 (August 20, 1973): 969–973.

Schwartz, Harry. "Conflicts of Interest in Fee for Service and in HMOs," *New England Journal of Medicine*, **299**:19 (November 9, 1978).

⸺. "HIP's Troubles," *New York Times*, **121**:9e (April 30, 1972). Reprinted in *Medical Care Review*, **29**:5 (May 1972): 548–550.

Schwartz, Jerome L. "Consumer Sponsorship and Physician Sponsorship of Prepaid Group Practice Health Plans: Some Similarities and Differences," *Journal of the American Medical Association*, **55**:1 (January 1965), 94–102.

⸺. *Medical Plans and Health Care, Consumer Participation in Policy Making With a Special Section on Medicare*. Springfield, Illinois: Charles C. Thomas, 1968.

————. "Prepayment Medical Clinics of the Mesabi Iron Range: 1904-1964," *Journal of the History of Medicine and Allied Sciences,* **22** (April 1967): 139–151.

Scitovsky, Anne, Personal communication, Palo Alto, Ca., May 18, 1977.

————, and Snyder, Nelda M. "Effect of Coinsurance on Use of Physician Services," *Social Security Bulletin,* **35**:6 (June 1972): 3–19.

Scitovsky, Anne A., Benham, Lee, and McCall, Nelda. "Use of Physician Services under Two Prepaid Plans," *Medical Care,* **17**:5 (May 1979): 441–460.

Scitovsky, Anne A., and McCall, Nelda. "Use of Hospital Services Under Two Prepaid Plans," *Medical Care,* **18**:1 (January 1980): 30–41.

————, and Benham, Lee. "Factors Affecting the Choice between Two Prepaid Plans," *Medical Care,* **16**:8 (August 1978): 660–681.

Scitovsky, Anne, McCall, Nelda and Benham, Lee. "Use of Out-of-Plan Medical Services Under Two Prepaid Plans," in progress.

Seabrook, Charles. "Insurance Officials Considering New Kind of Health Care for Area," *Atlanta Journal* (March 22, 1979). Reprinted in *DHEW Green Sheet,* **26**:67 (April 6, 1979): R13.

Seldin, Donald W. "The Medical Model: Biomedical Science as the Basis of Medicine," in *Beyond Tomorrow: Trends and Prospects in Medical Science.* New York: Rockefeller University Press, 1977.

Shah, C. P., and Robinson, G. C. "Day-Care Surgery in British Columbia: A Seven-Year Experience (1968–1974)," *Canadian Medical Association Journal,* **116** (May 7, 1977): 1031–1032.

Shain, Max. "The Change to Experience Rating In The Michigan Blue Cross Plan," *American Journal of Public Health,* **56**:10 (October 1966): 1695–1698.

Shapiro, Sam. *Current Observations from a Test of the Efficacy of Breast Cancer Screening and Their Implications,* mimeo. Johns Hopkins University, Department of Health Services Administration, 1976.

————. "Evidence on Screening for Breast Cancer from a Randomized Trial," *Cancer,* **39** (1977): 2772–2782.

————, and Brindle, James. "Serving Medicaid Eligibles," *American Journal of Public Health,* **59**:4 (April 1969): 635–641.

Shapiro, Sam, Weiner, Louis, and Densen, Paul. "Comparison of Prematurity and Perinatal Mortality in a General Population and in the Population of a Prepaid Group Practice Medical Care Plan," *American Journal of Public Health,* **48**:2 (February 1958): 170–185.

Shapiro, Sam, et al. "Further Observations on Prematurity and Perinatal Mortality in a General Population and in the Population of a Prepaid Group Practice Medical Care Plan," *American Journal of Public Health,* **50**:9 (September 1960): 1304–1317.

————. "Patterns of Medical Use by the Indigent Aged under Two Systems of Medical Care," *American Journal of Public Health,* **57**:5 (May 1967): 784–790.

Shearn, Martin A. "Professional Education in a Service System," in Anne R. Somers (ed.), *The Kaiser-Permanente Medical Care Program: A Symposium.* New York: Commonwealth Fund, 1971, pp. 123–128.

Sheridan, Bart. "At Last—A Medicaid Program That Works!" *Medical Economics,* **55**:12 (June 12, 1978): 37–51.

Sherrick, John W. "Blue Cross Blues: Doctor's Use or Abuse of Voluntary Health Insurance Plans Determines Their Success," *Alameda-Contra Costa Medical Association Bulletin,* **7**:4 (April 1951): 8–11.

———. "A Further Report on Blue Cross," *Alameda-Contra Costa Medical Association Bulletin,* **8:**12 (December 1952): 11–14.

Shortell, Stephen M. "Continuity of Medical Care: Conceptualization and Measurement," *Medical Care,* **14:**5 (May 1976): 377–391.

———. "The Costs and Benefits of Closer Group Practice-Hospital Relationships," *Medical Group Management* (January-February, 1978): 16–22.

———, Becker, Selwyn W., and Neuhauser, Duncan. "The Effects of Management Practices on Hospital Efficiency and Quality of Care," in Stephen M. Shortell and Montague Brown (eds.), *Organizational Research in Hospitals.* Chicago: Blue Cross Association, 1976.

Shortell, Stephen M., et al. "The Relationship Among Dimensions of Health Services in Two Provider Systems: A Causal Model Approach," *Journal of Health and Social Behavior,* **18** (June 1977): 139–159.

Shortridge, Mary Helen. "Quality of Medical Care in an Outpatient Setting," *Medical Care,* **12:**4 (April 1974): 283–300.

Showstack, Jonathan A., et al. "Fee-For-Service Physician Payment: Analysis of Current Methods and Their Development," *Inquiry,* **16:**3 (Fall 1979): 230–246.

Shragg, Harry, et al. "Low Income Families in a Large Scale Prepaid Group Practice," *Inquiry,* **10:**2 (June 1973): 52–60.

Simler, Sheila L. "Orange's Hospital Center Sponsors the Struggling Central Essex Health Plan," *Modern Healthcare,* **7:**12 (December 1977): 32–35.

Simon, Herbert. *Models of Man.* New York: John Wiley and Sons, 1957.

Simon, Nathan, and Rubushka, Sanford. "Membership Attitudes in the Labor Health Institute of St. Louis," *American Journal of Public Health,* **46:**6 (June 1956): 716–722.

Skinner, Elizabeth A., et al. "Use of Ambulatory Health Services by the Near Poor," *American Journal of Public Health,* **68:**12 (December 1978): 1195–1201.

Skolnik, Alfred M. "Twenty-Five Years of Employee-Benefit Plans," *Social Security Bulletin,* **38:**9 (September 1976): 3–21.

Slayman, William O. "The Role of the Member in the Kaiser-Permanente Medical Care Program," in U.S. Health Maintenance Organization Service, *Selected Papers on Consumerism in the HMO Movement.* Washington, D.C.: USGPO, U.S. Department of Health, Education and Welfare Publication No. HSM 73-13012, July 1973.

Slee, Vergil, and Ament, R. P. "How Much Longer Do Patients Stay in Teaching Hospitals?" *PAS Reporter,* **6:**7 (1968).

Sleeth, James. "Section 1310 (Dual Option) Experience Noted by Qualified HMO," in U.S. Health Maintenance Organization Service, *HMO Update,* No. 4 (October 25, 1976).

Slesinger, Doris P., Tessler, Richard C., and Mechanic, David. "The Effects of Social Characteristics on the Utilization of Preventive Medical Services in Contrasting Health Care Programs," *Medical Care,* **14:**5 (May 1976): 392–404.

Sloan, Frank A. "Effects of Incentives on Physician Performance," in John Rafferty (ed.), *Health Manpower and Productivity.* Lexington, Mass.: D.C. Heath, 1974, pp. 53–84.

Sloan, Frank. "Real Returns to Medical Education: A Comment," *Journal of Human Resources,* **11:**1 (Winter 1976): 118–126.

———, Mitchell, J., and Cromwell, J. *Physician Participation in State Medicaid Programs.* Unpublished paper, January 1978.

Smillie, John G. "Recruitment of Physicians: Large Prepaid Group Practice," in Joseph L. Dorsey and Joseph Kane (eds.), *Physician Recruitment, Performance Evaluation, The Role of the Medical Director.* Washington, D.C.: Group Health Association of America, 1976.

———. "Testimony Before the U.S. House of Representatives, Subcommittee on Public Health and Environment of the Committee on Interstate and Foreign Commerce," *Health Maintenance Organizations,* Hearings, April 11–13, 1972, Serial 92–88.

Smith, Kenneth R., Miller, Marianne, and Golladay, Frederick L. "An Analysis of the Optimal Use of Inputs in the Production of Medical Services," *Journal of Human Resources,* 7:2 (Spring 1972): 208–225.

Somers, Anne R (ed.). *The Kaiser-Permanente Medical Care Program: A Symposium.* New York: The Commonwealth Fund, 1971.

Sorensen, Andrew, and Saward, Ernest. "An Alternative Approach to Hospital Cost Control: The Rochester Project," *Public Health Reports,* 93:4 (July-August 1978): 311–317.

Sorensen, Andrew A., et al. "A Note on the Comparison of the Hospital Cost Experience of Three Competing HMOs," *Inquiry,* 16:2 (Summer 1979): 167–171.

Sox, Harold, and Higgins, Michael. *Decision Rules, Decision Trees and the Evaluation of Chest Pain.* Stanford University, Health Services Research Seminar, May 22, 1978.

Sox, Harold C., Jr., Sox, Carol H., and Skeff, Kelley. *A Decision Rule for Estimating the Probability of Ischemic Heart Disease in Patients With Chest Pain,* mimeo. Palo Alto, Ca.: Veterans Administration Medical Center, 1979.

Sparer, Gerald, and Anderson, Arne. "Utilization and Cost Experience of Low Income Families in Four Prepaid Group Practice Plans," *New England Journal of Medicine,* 289:2 (July 12, 1973): 67–72.

Spitz, Bruce. "When a Solution Is Not a Solution: Medicaid and Health Maintenance Organizations," *Journal of Health Politics, Policy, and Law,* 3:4 (Winter 1979): 497–518.

Stacey, James. "The HMO That (Sort Of) Succeeded," *American Medical News* (January 9, 1978): 21–22.

Stamps, Paula L., et al. "Measurement of Work Satisfaction among Health Professionals," *Medical Care,* 16:4 (April 1978): 337–352.

Stanford Center for Health Care Research. "Comparison of Hospitals with Regard to Outcomes of Surgery," *Health Services Research,* 11:2 (Summer 1976): 112–127.

Stanford University Personnel Benefits Office. Personal communications, August-September 1979.

Starfield, Barbara, et al. "Coordination of Care and Its Relationship to Continuity and Medical Records," *Medical Care,* 15:11 (November 1977): 929–938.

———. "Continuity and Coordination in Primary Care: Their Achievement and Utility," *Medical Care,* 14:7 (July 1976): 625–636.

Starkweather, David. "The Laws Affecting Health Insurance in California," in Milton I. Roemer, Donald M. DuBois, and Shirley W. Rich (eds.), *Health Insurance Plans: Studies in Organizational Diversity.* Los Angeles: University of California, 1970.

Steinberg, Marcia K. *Consumer Participation in a Health Care Organization: The Case of the Health Insurance Plan of Greater New York.* Ph.D. dissertation, City University of New York, 1976.

Steinwachs, Donald M., and Yaffe, Richard. "Assessing the Timeliness of Ambulatory Care," *American Journal of Public Health,* 68:6 (June 1978): 547–556.

Steinwachs, Donald M., et al. "The Role of New Health Practitioners in a Prepaid Group Practice: Changes in the Distribution of Ambulatory Care Between Physician and Nonphysician Providers of Care," *Medical Care,* 14:2 (February 1976): 95–120.

Steinwald, Bruce, and Neuhauser, Duncan. "The Role of the Proprietary Hospital," *Law and Contemporary Problems,* 35 (Autumn 1970): 817–838.

Steinwald, Carolynn. "Foundations for Medical Care," *Blue Cross Reports, Research Studies,* 7 (August 1971).

Stevens, Carl M. *HMOs: What Makes Them Tick?* Boston: Harvard Center for Community Health and Medical Care, Health Care Policy Discussion Paper 8, June 1973.

Stevens, Rosemary. *American Medicine and the Public Interest.* New Haven: Yale University Press, 1971.

Strumpf, George B., and Garramone, Marie A. "Why Some HMOs Develop Slowly," *Public Health Reports,* **91**:6 (November-December 1976): 496–503.

Strumpf, George B., et al. "Health Maintenance Organizations, 1971–1977: Issues and Answers," *Journal of Community Health,* **4**:1 (Fall 1978): 33–54.

Studney, Donald, et al. "A Computerized Prenatal Record," *Obstetrics and Gynecology,* **50**:1 (July 1977): 82–87.

Sullivan, Judith A., et al. "Overcoming Barriers to the Employment and Utilization of the Nurse Practitioner," *American Journal of Public Health,* **68**:11 (November 1978): 1097–1103.

Sullivan, Ronald. "Highly Rated Health-Care System in Jersey Is Believed in Jeopardy," *New York Times,* **126**: (July 25, 1977): 25c. Reprinted in *Medical Care Review* (1977): 934–935.

Tessler, Richard C., and Mechanic, David. "Consumer Satisfaction with Prepaid Group Practice: A Comparative Study," *Journal of Health and Social Behavior,* **16**:1 (March 1975): 95–113.

———. "Factors Affecting the Choice Between Prepaid Group Practice and Alternative Insurance Programs," *Milbank Memorial Fund Quarterly/Health and Society,* **53**:2 (Spring 1975): 149–172.

Thomas, Robert L. Letter to the Editor, *San Francisco Medical Society Bulletin,* **24**:10 (October 1951): 4, 42.

Thompson, Hugh C., and Osborne, Charles E. "Office Records in the Evaluation of Quality Care," *Medical Care,* **14**:4 (April 1976): 294–314.

Thompson, Robert S. "Approaches to Prevention in an HMO Setting," *Journal of Family Practice,* **9**:1 (1979): 71–82.

Thurlow, Ralph M. "Short-Stay Surgery at Half the Hospital Cost," *Medical Economics,* **47**:8 (April 27, 1970): 152.

Tilson, Hugh H. "Stability of Physician Employment in OEO Neighborhood Health Centers," *Medical Care,* **11**:5 (September-October 1973): 384–400.

———. "The Physician in Neighborhood Health Centers," *Inquiry,* **10**:2 (June 1973): 27–38.

Ting, Harold Montford. *The Economics of Health Maintenance Organizations.* Unpublished Ph.D. Dissertation, Stanford University, June 1975.

Ullman, Ralph. *Geographic Mobility and Location of Prepaid Group Practice: A Matrix Accounting Approach.* Presented at the National Center for Health Statistics, Data Use Conference, November 1978.

U.S. Bureau of the Census. "Population Estimates," *Current Population Reports,* Series P-25. Washington, D.C.: USGPO.

———. *Money Income and Poverty Status in 1975 of Families and Persons in the United States and the West Region, by Divisions and States.* Series P. 60, No. 113. Washington, D.C.: USGPO, July 1978.

U.S. Bureau of Labor Statistics. *Autumn 1974 Urban Family Budgets and Comparative Indexes for Selected Urban Areas.* San Francisco: U.S. Department of Labor, Bureau of Labor Statistics, (circa 1975).

U.S. Civil Service Commission. *Annual Report of Federal Civilian Employment in the United States by Geographical Area,* Yearly, circa December 31, 1964–76.

———, *Blue Cross/Blue Shield Utilization Reports.* Washington, D.C.: U.S. Civil Service Commission, Annual.

————, Bureau of Retirement, Insurance, and Occupational Health. *Annual Reports.* Washington, D.C.: USGPO.

————, Annual Unpublished Data, 1961–76.

U.S. Congress. *Health Maintenance Organization Act of 1973,* Public Law 93-222, 93rd Congress, S. 14 (December 29, 1973).

U.S. Congressional Budget Office. *Profile of Health Care Coverage: The Haves and Have-Nots.* Washington, D.C.: USGPO, 1979.

U.S. Department of Health, Education and Welfare. "Certificate-of-Need: Press Release" (April 2, 1979). Reprinted in *Medical Care Review,* **36:**5 (May 1979): 472–473.

————. "Health Maintenance Organizations," *Federal Register,* **39:**203 (October 18, 1974): 37,308–37,323.

U.S. Federal Trade Commission. *In the Matter of Medical Service Corporation of Spokane County, A Corporation, and Medical Service Bureau of Spokane County, an Association,* Docket No. C-2853, December 1976.

U.S. General Accounting Office. *Better Controls Needed for Health Maintenance Organizations under Medicaid in California.* Washington, D.C.: GAO, September 10, 1974.

————. *Civil Service Should Audit Kaiser Plans' Premium Rates under the Federal Employees Health Benefits Program to Protect the Government.* Washington, D.C.: USGPO, 1978.

————. *Effectiveness of Grant Programs Aimed at Developing Health Maintenance Organizations and Community Health Networks.* Washington, D.C., November 1975, MWD-75-98.

————. *Relationship Between Nonprofit Prepaid Health Plans with California Medicaid Contracts and For Profit Entities Affiliated With Them.* November 1, 1976, HRD-77-4.

U.S. Health Care Financing Administration. *Alternative Models for Pre-paid Capitation of Health Care Services for Medicare/Medicaid Recipients.* Washington, D.C.: Health Care Financing Administration, September 1978. RFP No. HCFA-78-OPPR-22/PHG.

U.S. Health Maintenance Organization Service. *1976 Census of HMOs.* Washington, D.C.: Health Maintenance Organization Service, 1977.

————. *1977 Census of HMOs.* Washington, D.C.: Health Maintenance Organization Service, 1978.

U.S. House, Committee on Interstate and Foreign Commerce. *Health Maintenance Organization Amendments of 1975.* Report together with Dissenting and Supplemental Views. September 26, 1975, 94th Congress, First Session. Washington, D.C.: USGPO, 1975.

U.S. House, Committee on Interstate and Foreign Commerce, Subcommittee on Oversight and Investigations. *Cost and Quality of Health Care: Unnecessary Surgery.* Washington, D.C.: USGPO, January 1976.

U.S. House, Committee on Interstate and Foreign Commerce, Subcommittee on Oversight and Investigations. *Getting Ready for National Health Insurance: Unnecessary Surgery: Hearings.* July 15, 17, 18, and September 3, 1975. Washington, D.C.: USGPO, 1975.

U.S. National Center for Health Statistics. "Advance Report, Final Mortality Statistics, 1975," *Monthly Vital Statistics Report,* **25:**11 (Supplement) (February 11, 1977).

————. Balamuth, Eve. "Health Interview Responses Compared with Medical Records." *Vital and Health Statistics,* Series 2, No. 7, Washington, D.C.: USGPO, July 1965, Publication No. 1000.

————. Blanken, Gary E. "Surgical Operations in Short-Stay Hospital, U.S., 1971," *Vital and Health Statistics,* Series 13, No. 18. Washington, D.C.: USGPO, November 1974.

————. "Comparison of Hospitalization Reporting in Three Survey Procedures," *Vital and Health Statistics,* Series 2, No. 8. Washington, D.C.: USGPO, July 1965, Publication No. 1000.

————. "Current Estimates From the Health Interview Survey: United States, 1977," *Vital and Health Statistics,* Series 10, No. 126. Washington, D.C.: USGPO, September 1978, Department of Health, Education and Welfare Publication No. (PHS) 78-1554.

————. Danchik, Kathleen M. "Physician Visits: Volume and Interval Since Last Visit, U.S.-1971," *Vital and Health Statistics,* Series 10, No. 97. Washington, D.C.: USGPO, March 1975, (HRA) 75-1524.

————. DeLozier, James. "The National Ambulatory Medical Care Survey: 1973 Summary, U.S., May 1973-April 1974," *Vital and Health Statistics,* Series 13, No. 21. Washington, D.C.: USGPO, October 1975.

————. *Health, United States, 1975.* Department of Health, Education and Welfare Publication No. (HRA) 76-1232. Washington, D.C.: USGPO, 1976.

————. "Hospital and Surgical Insurance Coverage: United States, 1974," *Vital and Health Statistics,* Series 10, No. 117. Washington, D.C. USGPO, August 1977, Department of Health, Education and Welfare Publication No. (HRA) 77-1545.

————. Laurent, Andre, Cannell, Charles, and Marquis, Kent. "Reporting Health Events in Household Interviews: Effects of an Extensive Questionnaire and a Diary Procedure," *Vital and Health Statistics,* Series 2, No. 49. Washington, D.C.: USGPO, April 1972, (HSM) 72-1049.

————. Marquis, Kent, and Cannell, Charles. "Effect of Some Experimental Interviewing Techniques on Reporting in the Health Interview Survey," *Vital and Health Statistics,* Series 2, No. 41. Washington, D.C.: USGPO, May 1971, Publication No. 1000.

————. Marquis, Kent, Cannell, Charles, and Laurent, Andre. "Reporting Health Events in Household Interviews: Effects of Reinforcement, Question Length and Reinterviews," *Vital and Health Statistics,* Series 2, No. 45. Washington, D.C.: USGPO, March 1972, (HSM) 72-1028.

————. "Personal Out-of-Pocket Health Expenses: United States, 1975," *Vital and Health Statistics,* Series 10, Number 122. Washington, D.C.: USGPO, November 1978, Department of Health, Education and Welfare Publication No. (PHS) 79-1550.

————. "Persons Hospitalized by Number Episodes and Days Hospitalized in a Year, U.S.-1972," *Vital and Health Statistics,* Series 10, No. 116. Washington, D.C., USGPO., August 1977.

————. "Physician Visits, Volume and Interval Since Last Visit: United States, 1975," *Vital and Health Statistics,* Series 10, Number 128, Washington, D.C.: USGPO, April 1979, Department of Health, Education and Welfare Publication No. (PHS) 79-1556.

————. Ranofsky, Abraham. "Inpatient Utilization of Short-Stay Hospitals by Diagnosis, U.S.-1971," *Vital and Health Statistics,* Series 13, No. 16. Washington, D.C., USGPO, July 1974.

————. "Reporting of Hospitalization in the Health Interview Survey," *Vital and Health Statistics,* Series 2, No. 6. Washington, D.C.: USGPO, July 1965, Publication No. 1000.

————. Ries, Peter W. "Current Estimates from the Health Interview Survey, U.S.-1974," *Vital and Health Statistics,* Series 10, No. 100. Washington, D.C.: USGPO, September 1975.

————. *State Estimates of Disability and Utilization of Medical Services: United States, 1969-71.* Washington, D.C.: USGPO, Department of Health, Education and Welfare Publication No. (HRA) 77-1241, January 1977.

————. "A Summary of Studies of Interviewing Methodology," *Vital and Health Statistics,* Series 2, No. 69. Washington, D.C.: USGPO, March 1977, Department of Health, Education and Welfare Publication No. (HRA) 77-1343.

————. Wilder, Charles. "Hospital Discharges and Length of Stay: Short-Stay Hospitals, U.S., July 1963-June 1964," *Vital and Health Statistics,* Series 10, No. 30. Washington, D.C.: USGPO, June 1966.

———. Wilder, Charles. "Physician Visits: Volume and Interval Since Last Visit, U.S.-1969," *Vital and Health Statistics*, Series 10, No. 75. Washington, D.C.: USGPO, July 1972, (HSM) 72-1064.

U.S. Office of Health Maintenance Organizations. *1977 Census of HMOs*. Washington, D.C.: USGPO, 1978.

U.S. Office of the White House Press Secretary. *Major Features of the Comprehensive Health Policy for the 70's*, for release February 18, 1971.

U.S. Public Health Service, Division of Public Health Methods. "Hospitalization: Patients Discharged From Short-Stay Hospitals, United States, July 1951-June 1958," *Reports From the U.S. National Health Survey*, Series B-7. Washington, D.C.: USGPO, 1958, Publication No. (PHS) 584-B7.

U.S. Senate, Committee on Governmental Affairs, Permanent Subcommittee on Investigations. *Prepaid Health Plans and Health Maintenance Organizations*, 95th Congress, 2nd Session, Report 95-749. Washington, D.C.: USGPO, 1978.

———. *Prepaid Health Plans*, Hearings, March 13 and 14, 1975, 94th Congress, First Session. Washington, D.C.: USGPO, 1975.

U.S. Senate, Special Committee on Aging. *Kickbacks Among Medicaid Providers: Committee Reports*, 95th Congress, First Session. Washington, D.C.: USGPO, 1977.

———. Subcommittee on Long-Term Care. *Fraud and Abuse among Practitioners Participating in the Medicaid Program*. A Staff Report, 94th Congress, 2nd Session. Washington, D.C.: USGPO, August 1976.

Vahovich, Stephen G. "Physicians' Supply Decisions by Specialty: 2SLS Model," *Industrial Relations*, **16**:1 (February 1977): 51–60.

Varady, Paul D., and Maxwell, Morton H. "Assessment of Statistically Significant Changes in Diastolic Blood Pressures," *Journal of the American Medical Association*, **221**:4 (July 24, 1972): 365–368.

Vayda, Eugene. "The Community Health Foundation of Cleveland," *Bulletin of New York Academy of Medicine*, **44**:11 (November 1968): 1307–1311.

———. "Stability of the Medical Group in a New Prepaid Medical Care Program," *Medical Care*, **8**:2 (March-April 1970): 161–168.

———. "A Comparison of Surgical Rates in Canada and in England and Wales," *New England Journal of Medicine*, **289**:23 (December 6, 1973): 1224–1229.

Vial, Don. "Negotiated Health Programs: The California Experience," *Monthly Labor Review*, **98**:4 (April 1975): 37–42.

Vignola, Margo L. *Curbing Health Expenditures: An Evaluation of State Prepaid Medicaid Contracts*. Presented at the Annual Meeting of the American Public Welfare Association, June 21, 1977.

Von Berg, William G. "Experiments in the Development of Prepaid Group Practice." Remarks to the Group Health Institute. Sponsored by the Group Health Association of America, Detroit, May 16, 1972.

Vuori, Hannu, et al. "Doctor-Patient Relationship in the Light of Patients' Experiences," *Social Science and Medicine*, **6** (1972): 723–730.

Waitzkin, Howard, and Stoeckle, John D. "Information Control and the Micropolitics of Health Care: Summary of an Ongoing Research Project," *Social Science and Medicine*, **10** (1976): 263–276.

Wall Street Journal. "Fringe Benefits Average Nearly $4,000," *Wall Street Journal* (June 13, 1978): 1.

Wall Street Journal Staff Reporter. "Breast Cancer Screening Project Finds Some Women Had Unnecessary Surgery," *Wall Street Journal* (September 19, 1977).

Walsh, Diana Chapman, and Egdahl, Richard H. *Payer, Provider, Consumer: Industry Confronts Health Care Costs.* New York: Springer-Verlag, 1977.

Ware, John E., Jr. "Effects of Acquiescent Response Set on Patient Satisfaction Ratings," *Medical Care,* **16**:4 (April 1978): 327–336.

————, and Snyder, Mary K. "Dimensions of Patient Attitudes Regarding Doctors and Medical Care Services," *Medical Care,* **13**:8 (August 1975): 669–682.

————, and Wright, W. Russell. *Development and Validation of Scales to Measure Patient Satisfaction with Health Care Services,* 2 volumes of a final report. Carbondale, Ill.: Southern Illinois University School of Medicine, 1976.

Ware, J. E., Jr., Wright, W. R. and Snyder, M. K. "Consumer Perceptions of Health Care Services: Implications for Academic Medicine," *Journal of Medical Education,* **50**:9 (September 1975): 839–848.

Wasserman, Fred William. *Health Maintenance Organizations: Determinants of Failure or Success.* Ph.D. dissertation, University of California, Los Angeles, 1976.

Watkins, Richard N., and Howell, Linda. *A Population Based Quality Assessment of the Treatment of Appendicitis.* Seattle, Wash. Group Health Cooperative of Puget Sound, 1977.

Watkins, Richard N., Hughes, Edward F. X., and Lewit, Eugene M. "Time Utilization of a Population of General Surgeons in a Prepaid Group Practice," *Medical Care,* **14**:10 (October 1976): 824–838.

Weil, Peter A. "Comparative Costs to the Medicare Program of Seven Prepaid Group Practices and Controls," *Milbank Memorial Fund Quarterly/Health and Society,* **54**:3 (Summer 1976): 339–365.

Weinerman, E. Richard. "An Appraisal of Medical Care in Group Health Centers," *American Journal of Public Health,* **46**:3 (March 1956): 300–309.

————. "Patients' Perceptions of Group Medical Care," *American Journal of Public Health,* **54**:6 (June 1964): 880–889.

————. "Problems and Perspectives of Group Practice," 1968 Health Conference of the New York Academy of Medicine, *Bulletin of the New York Academy of Medicine,* **44**:11 (November 1968).

Weisbrod, Burton A. "Collective-Consumption Services of Individual-Consumption Goods," *Quarterly Journal of Economics* (1964).

Weiss, Carol H. *Evaluation Research: Methods for Assessing Program Effectiveness.* Englewood Cliffs, N.J.: Prentice-Hall, 1972.

Weiss, James E., and Greenlick, Merwyn R. "Determinants of Medical Care Utilization: The Effects of Social Class and Distance on Contacts with the Medical Care System," *Medical Care,* **8**:6 (November-December 1970): 456–462.

Weissman, Arthur, Presentation of Director of Medical Economics, Kaiser Foundation Health Plan, Oakland, before Committee on Medical Economics, Commission on the Cost of Medical Care, January 19, 1962.

Wennberg, John E. and Gittelsohn, Alan. "Health Care Delivery in Maine I: Patterns of Use of Common Surgical Procedures," *Journal of Maine Medical Association,* **66**:5 (May 1975): 123–130, 149.

————. "Small Area Variations in Health Care Delivery," *Science,* **182**:4117 (December 14, 1973): 1102–1108.

————, and Soule, David. "Health Care Delivery in Maine II: Conditions Explaining Hospital Admission," *Journal of Maine Medical Association*, **66**:10 (October 1975): 255–261, 269.

Wersinger, Richard P. *The Analysis of Three Prepaid Health Care Plans in Monroe County, New York; Part III: Inpatient Utilization Statistics, January 1, 1974-December 31, 1974*. Rochester, N.Y.: University of Rochester School of Medicine and Dentistry, Department of Preventive Medicine and Community Health, October 1975.

————. Personal communication, May 1, 1979.

————, and Roberts, J. *A Comparative Analysis of the Enrollment and Utilization Experience of a Federally Qualified Prepaid Group Practice: HMO, The First Three Years Experience*. Presented at the 1977 Group Health Institute, Long Beach, Ca., June 19–22, 1977.

Wersinger, Richard, et al. "Inpatient Hospital Utilization in Three Prepaid Comprehensive Health Care Plans Compared with a Regular Blue Cross Plan," *Medical Care*, **14**:9 (September 1976): 721–732.

Wescott, Lloyd B. "Columbia-Hunterdon: Similar But Different," *New England Journal of Medicine*, **295**:22 (November 25, 1976): 1250–1252.

————. "Discussion Of the Role Of The Community in Developing Improved Health Care," *Bulletin of the New York Academy of Medicine*, **46**:12 (December 1970): 1042–1047.

West, Sheila K., et al. "Drug Utilization Review in an HMO: I. Introduction and Examples of Methodology," *Medical Care*, **15**:6 (June 1977): 505–514.

West Bay Health Systems Agency. *Staff Analysis: Kaiser Permanente Medical Center, San Francisco, Certificate of Need Application 78-036, Open Heart Surgery Unit*. San Francisco: West Bay Health Systems Agency, August 25, 1978.

Wetherille, Rhona L., and Quale, Jean N. *A Census of HMOs*. Minneapolis: InterStudy, August 1973 and quarterly thereafter.

Whipple, David. *Capitation/Incentive Project: Working Papers and Supporting Documents*. Final Report, Monterey Ca., Naval Postgraduate School, January 1977.

Williams, Greer. *Kaiser-Permanente Health Plan: Why It Works*. Oakland, Ca.: Henry J. Kaiser Foundation, February 1971.

Williams, Ronald L. "Measuring the Effectiveness of Perinatal Medical Care," *Medical Care*, **17**:2 (February 1979): 95–110.

Williams, Stephen J., et al. "A Causal Model of Health Services for Diabetic Patients," *Medical Care*, **16**:4 (April 1978): 313–326.

Williamson, John W., Alexander, Marshall, and Miller, George E. "Continuing Education and Patient Care Research: Physicians Response to Screening Test Results," *Journal of American Medical Association*, **201**:12 (September 18, 1967): 938–942.

————, et al. "Health Accounting: An Outcome Based System of Quality Assurance: Illustrative Application to Hypertension," *Bulletin of New York Academy of Medicine*, **51**:6 (June 1975): 727–738.

Wilson, Glenn, and Begun, James W. "Trends in Physicians' Patient Volume," *Inquiry*, **14**:2 (June 1977): 171–175.

Winickoff, Richard N., et al. *Quality Assurance in a Prepaid Group Practice*. Presented at the American Public Health Association, November 1, 1977.

Wisconsin Physicians Service Insurance Corporation. *An Overview of Wisconsin Physicians' Services Health Maintenance Program*. Madison: Wisconsin Physicians Service, March 1977.

Wolfman, Burton. "Medical Expenses and Choice of Plans: A Case Study," *Monthly Labor Review*, **84** (November 1961): 1186–1190.

Wollstadt, Lloyd J., Shapiro, Sam, and Bice, Thomas W. "Disenrollment from a Prepaid Group Practice: An Actuarial and Demographic Description," *Inquiry,* **15:**2 (June 1978): 142–150.

Worth, Robert M. "Comparison of Fee-For-Service and Capitation Medicine in Low Income Group in Honolulu," *Hawaii Medical Journal,* **33:**3 (March 1974): 91–96.

Worthington, Nancy L. "Expenditures for Hospital Care and Physicians' Services: Factors Affecting Annual Changes," *Social Security Bulletin,* **38:**11 (November 1975): 3–15.

Yale Law Journal Editors. "The American Medical Association: Power, Purpose and Politics in Organized Medicine," *Yale Law Journal,* **63:**7 (May 1954): 938–1022.

Yankauer, Alfred, Connelly, John P., and Feldman, Jacob J. "Physician Productivity and the Delivery of Ambulatory Care: Some Findings from a Survey of Pediatricians," *Medical Care,* **8:**1 (January-February 1970): 35–46.

Yedidia, Avram. "Dual Choice Programs," *American Journal of Public Health,* **49:**11 (November 1959): 1475–1480.

————. *Planning and Implementation of the Community Health Foundation of Cleveland, Ohio.* Division of Medical Care Administration, U.S. Public Health Service, 1968.

Yett, Donald E. "An Evaluation of Alternative Methods of Estimating Physicians' Expenses Relative to Output," *Inquiry,* **4:**1 (March 1967): 3–27.

Zako, Louis. "My Year with an HMO Was One Year Too Many," *Medical Economics,* **53:**8 (April 19, 1976): 79–85.

Zeckhauser, Richard, and Eliastam, Michael. "The Productivity Potential of the Physician Assistant," *Journal of Human Resources,* **9:**1 (Winter 1974): 95–116.

Zelten, Robert A. *The Study of Enrollment in Prepaid Group Practice Plans; Final Report to the Robert Wood Johnson Foundation.* University of Pennsylvania, Leonard Davis Institute of Health Economics, August 1, 1977.

Zwick, Daniel I. "Some Accomplishments and Findings of Neighborhood Health Centers," *Milbank Memorial Fund Quarterly,* **50:**4 (October 1972), Part I: 387–420.

Zyzanski, S. J., Hulka, B. S., and Cassel, J. C. "Scale for the Measurement of Satisfaction with Medical Care: Modifications in Content, Format and Scoring," *Medical Care,* **12:**7 (July 1974): 611–620.

Index